RD 93 .T79 1991
21670584
Wounds and lacerations

D1272602

THE RICHARD STOCKTON COLLEGE
OF NEW JERSEY LIBRARY
POMONA, NEW JERSEY 08240-0195

WOUNDS AND LACERATIONS

EMERGENCY CARE AND CLOSURE

WOUNDS AND LACERATIONS

EMERGENCY CARE AND CLOSURE

Alexander Trott, M.D.

Associate Professor of Emergency Medicine
Department of Emergency Medicine
University of Cincinnati College of Medicine
Cincinnati, Ohio

with 294 illustrations

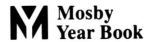 **Mosby**
Year Book

St. Louis   Baltimore   Boston   Chicago   London   Philadelphia   Sydney   Toronto

THE RICHARD STOCKTON COLLEGE
OF NEW JERSEY LIBRARY
POMONA, NEW JERSEY 08240-0195

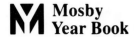
Mosby Year Book

Dedicated to Publishing Excellence

Editor Richard A. Weimer
Assistant Editor Adrianne H. Cochran
Production Editor Cynthia A. Miller
Manuscript Editor Radhika Rao Gupta
Design Candace F. Conner
Illustrators Joe Chovan
            Tony Poole
            Carl Jones

Copyright © 1991 by Mosby–Year Book, Inc.
A Mosby imprint of Mosby–Year Book, Inc.

All rights reserved. No part of this publication may be reproduced, stored in a retrieval system, or transmitted, in any form or by any means, electronic, mechanical, photocopying, recording, or otherwise, without prior written permission from the publisher.

Printed in the United States of America

Mosby–Year Book, Inc.
11830 Westline Industrial Drive
St. Louis, Missouri 63146

Library of Congress Cataloging-in-Publication Data
Trott, Alexander.
    Wounds and lacerations : emergency care and closure / Alexander
Trott.
       p.   cm.
    Includes index.
    ISBN 0-8016-5154-9
    1. Wounds and injuries--Surgery.   2. Surgical emergencies.
 I. Title.
    [DNLM: 1. Emergencies. 2. Wound Healing. 3. Wounds and Injuries-
-therapy.   WO   700   T858w]
    RD93.T79   1991
    617.1'026--dc20
    DNLM/DLC
    for Library of Congress
                                      90-6468
                                      CIP

C/D/D 9 8 7 6 5

To Jennifer, my wife,
who is always my source of vision and strength.

To Buffy, Hays, and Alexandra, my daughters,
who make it all worthwhile.

Preface

With the growth and maturation of the specialty of emergency medicine there has come a new and strong interest in wound care. Traditional methods for caring for wounds and lacerations have undergone intense scientific scrutiny. Old ideas and concepts have been challenged and new materials and procedures have been developed. The net result is that practitioners of wound care have been able to achieve much higher levels of knowledge and expertise. The purpose of this book is to provide the reader with an up-to-date source of the principles and techniques of emergency wound care. The goal was to create a work written and structured in the context of knowledge gained by recent scientific investigations, but that retained valid, time-honored concepts and procedures.

Wounds and Lacerations: Emergency Care and Closure was written for all medical personnel actively caring for emergency wounds or in training to do so. This book is directed to emergency physicians, family practitioners, pediatricians, house officers, medical students, wound-care technicians, military medics, and other individuals directly involved in wound care. The wound-care problems that can be encountered by these groups are commonly seen in emergency departments, clinics, private offices, dispensaries, and first-aid stations. In addition to basic wound-care techniques, this book presents strategies to manage more complicated wounds and lacerations.

Emergency wound care is not simply a technical exercise. A thorough comprehension of skin anatomy, wound healing, and the causes of wound infection is necessary to minimize complications and yield the best functional and cosmetic result. With an understanding of general wound-care fundamentals, basic and advanced techniques can be applied. Wound-care problems covered in this text include simple and complex lacerations, specific anatomic site problems, bite wounds, rabies exposure, abrasions, soft-tissue foreign bodies, burns, and disorders of the fingertip (trauma and infection). Wound preparation, anesthetic techniques, dressing principles, and tetanus prophylaxis are described as well. Finally, the various issues surrounding patient discharge and follow up are discussed.

Alexander Trott

Acknowledgments

Several people deserve recognition for their contributions to the production of this manuscript. LaVerne Young diligently and patiently typed the entire manuscript and put up with my need to have it done "today." I also wish to thank Edward Otten, M.D., Kenneth Gardner, M.D., and Lawrence Kurtzman, M.D. for their review of portions of the manuscript and their comments and suggestions for the text. Finally, I owe a special thanks to Joe Chovan, Tony Poole, and Carl Jones for their creative and professional production of the illustrations.

Contents

1 *Patient Arrival—the First Ten Minutes, 1*

Initial Steps, 1
Basic History, 3
Screening General Physical Exam, 3
Preparation for Specific Care, 3

2 *The Anatomy of Wound Repair, 5*

Anatomy of the Skin and Fascia, 5
Skin Tension Lines, 8
Alterations of Skin Anatomy, 11

3 *Surface Injury and Wound Healing, 12*

Mechanism of Injury, 12
Normal Wound Healing, 15
Categories of Wound Healing, 19
Alterations of Wound Healing, 19
Abnormal Scar Formation, 21

4 *The Potential for Wound Infection, 24*

Epidemiology, 24
Microbiology of Wound Infection, 25
Factors that Increase Risk of Infection, 25

5 *Infiltration and Nerve Block Anesthesia, 29*

    Pharmacology of Local Anesthetics, 30
    Toxicity of Local Anesthetics, 30
    Allergy to Local Anesthetics, 32
    Alternative Anesthetic Strategies for the Allergic Patient, 32
    Anesthetic Solutions, 33
    Topical Anesthesia, 34
    Buffering Anesthetics to Reduce Pain of Injection, 34
    Patient Sedation, 35
    Choice of Needles and Syringes, 36
    Anesthesia Techniques, 36

6 *Wound Cleansing and Irrigation, 55*

    Wound Cleansing Solutions, 55
    Preparation for Cleansing, 58
    Techniques for Wound Cleansing, 61

7 *Instruments and Suture Materials, 66*

    Basic Instruments, 66
    Suture Materials, 76
    Needle Types, 79

8 *Decisions Before Closure—Timing, Debridement, and Consultation, 80*

    Timing of Closure, 81
    Wound and Laceration Exploration, 84
    Hemostasis, 85
    Tissue Debridement and Techniques, 88
    Surgical Drains, 92
    Indications for Intravenous Antibiotic Therapy, 92
    General Guidelines for Consultation, 93

9 *Basic Laceration Repair—Principles and Techniques, 96*

Definition of Terms, 96
Basic Knot-Tying Techniques, 97
Principles of Wound Closure, 110

10 *Complicated Lacerations and Wounds: Problems and Solutions, 122*

Long, Straight Lacerations, 123
Beveled Edges, 128
Medium-Deep Lacerations, 129
Pull-Out Dermal Closure, 130
Corners and Uncomplicated Flaps, 131
Complicated Flap (Partial Avulsion) Lacerations, 132
Geographic Lacerations, 135
Wounds with Tissue Loss, 139
"Dog-Ear" Deformities, 142
Parallel Lacerations, 142
Thin-Edge, Thick-Edge Wound, 142
Laceration in an Abrasion, 146
Aged Skin, 146

11 *Special Anatomic Sites, 148*

Scalp, 149
Forehead, 154
Eyebrow and Eyelid, 156
Cheek or Zygomatic Area, 159
Nasal Structures, 162
Ear, 163
Lips, 168
Oral Cavity, 171
Perineum, 173
Knee, 174
Lower Leg, 174
Foot, 176

12 *The Hand, 177*

Initial Treatment, 177
Patient History, 178
Terminology, 180
Examination of the Hand, 182
Circulation, 193
Radiography, 194
Wound Exploration, 194
Selected Hand Injuries and Problems, 195

13 *Wound Taping and Stapling, 214*

Wound Taping, 214
Wound Stapling, 220

14 *Bite Wounds, 227*

Animal and Human Bites, 227
Microbiology of Bite Wounds, 228
Animal Bite Risk Factors, 230
Animal Bite Wound Management, 232
Specific Injuries, 233
Wound After-Care and Follow-Up, 236
Rabies Exposure and Prophylaxis, 236
Post-Exposure Prophylaxis, 242

15 *Foreign Bodies, Puncture Wounds, and Abrasions, 247*

Foreign Bodies, 247
Puncture Wounds, 252
Fishhooks, 254
Abrasions, 256

16 *Minor Burns, 260*

Initial Management and General Patient Assessment, 260
Burn Assessment, 261
Guidelines for Hospital Vs. Non-Hospital Management of Burn Victims, 266
Treatment of Minor Burns, 267

17 *Wound Dressing and Bandaging Techniques, 275*

Wound Dressing Principles, 275
Basic Wound Dressing, 278
Home Care and Dressing Change Intervals, 281
Body Area Dressings, 281

18 *Patient Discharge and Follow-up Care, 309*

Tetanus Prophylaxis, 309
Suture Removal, 311
Prophylactic Antibiotics for Emergency Wounds, 314
Analgesia, 315
Instructions to the Patient, 315
Advising Patients about Wound Healing, 317

WOUNDS AND LACERATIONS
EMERGENCY CARE AND CLOSURE

1 *Patient Arrival—the First Ten Minutes*

Initial Steps
    Patient Comfort and Safety
    Initial Hemostasis
    Jewelry Removal
    Pain Relief
    Wound Care Delay

Children with Lacerations
Basic History
Screening General Physical Exam
Preparation for Specific Care
References

Before repair of wounds or lacerations is initiated, a thorough evaluation of the patient must be done. The combination of wound characteristics, anatomic site, and underlying host conditions affects the management of every wound. Each patient is unique and requires individualized treatment. The basic history, general physical exam survey, and wound area exam will help define the repair strategy and will identify more serious injuries or problems that may necessitate more specialized or intensive care. It is important to keep in mind that all wounds can be potentially life-threatening, so initial attention should be directed to the patency of the airway and the stability of the vital signs.

INITIAL STEPS

Patient Comfort and Safety

If there is the slightest question about a patient's ability to cope with his or her injury, the patient is placed in a supine position on a stretcher. Loss of blood, deformity, and pain are sufficient to provoke vasovagal syncope (fainting), which can cause further injury from an unexpected fall during evaluation or treatment. Be aware that accompanying relatives or friends can also respond in a similar manner.

Initial Hemostasis

Any bleeding can be stopped with simple pressure and compression dressings. There is no need for dramatic clamping of bleeders. Clamping, if necessary at all, is reserved for the actual exploration and repair of the wound under controlled, well-lighted conditions. Blind application of hemostats in an actively bleeding wound can lead to the crushing of normal nerves, tendons, or other important structures.

1

Jewelry Removal

Rings and other jewelry must be removed as quickly as possible from injured hands or fingers. Swelling progresses rapidly after wounding, causing rings to act as constricting bands. A finger can become ischemic and the outcome can be disastrous. Most items of jewelry can be removed with soap or lubricating jelly. Occasionally, ring cutters have to be used. Never let the sentimental value of a wedding ring impede good medical judgment. A jeweler can always restore a ring that has been cut or damaged during removal. Another technique for ring removal that does not require cutting is described in Chapter 12.

Pain Relief

Pain relief usually is achieved by gentle, emphathetic, and professional handling of the patient. Occasionally it is necessary to give parenteral sedative medications to patients being treated in the emergency wound care setting. Sedation and specific pain relief measures are discussed more completely in Chapter 5.

Wound Care Delay

If there is likely to be a delay from initial wound evaluation to repair, the wound is covered with a saline-moistened dressing to prevent drying. The dressing need not be soaked and dripping wet. Delays that extend beyond an hour or more will require that the wound be thoroughly cleansed and irrigated before the saline dressing is applied. If extended delays are inevitable, antibiotics are occasionally considered in order to suppress bacterial growth. If antibiotics are administered, they must be given early to provide the maximum protective benefit.[3] One experimental study has demonstrated that the benefit decreases significantly if the time between wounding and administration exceeds 3 hours.[2] See Chapter 8 for further discussion and recommendations.

Children with Lacerations

Particular care has to be taken with children who have wounds and lacerations. The pain and fear generated by the experience can be significantly reduced by a few simple measures. Allow the child to remain in the parent's lap for as long as possible. Most of the physical exam can be carried out at that time. If hemostasis is required and if the parent is willing to cooperate, allow him or her to tamponade small, bleeding wounds. Parents can also apply topical anesthesics. Finally, careful judgment has to be used when handling children and their parents. It is not uncommon for some parents to be unable to tolerate the situation, and they often do better in the waiting room while care is being delivered.

BASIC HISTORY

The patient's current and past medical history, present medications, allergies, and tetanus immunization status can have a significant impact on emergency wound care. Diseases like diabetes and peripheral vascular disease can increase the risk of wound infection and cause delayed or poor wound healing.[1,4] It is well known that corticosteroids adversely affect the normal healing process.[5] Finally, a careful detailing of allergies is necessary to prevent an untoward reaction to local anesthetics or antibiotics that might be administered to the patient.

SCREENING GENERAL PHYSICAL EXAM

The examination of every patient with a minor laceration or injury includes measuring the basic vital signs. Each vital sign can provide information pertinent to the management of the patient. Hypotension and tachycardia are the classic signs of hypovolemia. Innocuous-looking scalp wounds can bleed profusely, causing clinically significant blood loss with concomitant hypotension. A patient with hypertension who sustains a laceration will often have brisk bleeding that can be difficult to control during repair. An elevated temperature in a patient with a wound that is several hours or days old is an indicator of early wound infection, particularly if the wound is associated with heavy contamination.

A rapid general survey of the patient can reveal other injuries not reported by the patient. Because of the nature of a traumatic episode, patients often cannot accurately report all that has happened to them. A man who falls and strikes his head may only be aware of a bleeding laceration of the forehead. Only when the examiner reveals the presence of other injuries does the patient understand the extent of the injuries.

Wounds and lacerations are often the result of or the cause of systemic problems and illnesses. Patients who fall and sustain minor injuries may need to be questioned and examined for causes of syncope. Any patient with a scalp laceration caused by blunt trauma has to be suspected to have a more serious intracranial injury. In addition to wound repair, a trauma-oriented neurologic exam is often necessary.

PREPARATION FOR SPECIFIC CARE

The patient is now ready for the next level of care. Chapter 8 details the steps taken to examine and explore the wound itself. Specific types of wounds, different anatomic sites, and other special problems are approached through specialized exams that are discussed in later chapters and sections in this text.

References

1. Altemeier W: Principles in the management of traumatic wounds and in infection control, Bull NY Acad Med 55:123-138, 1979.
2. Burke J: The effective period of preventive antibiotic action in experimental incisions and dermal lesions, Surgery 50:161-168, 1961.
3. Edlich RF et al: Principles of wound management, Ann Emerg Med 17:1284-1302, 1988.
4. Hunt T: Disorders of wound healing, World J Surg 4:271-277, 1980.
5. Pollack S: Systemic medications and wound healing, Int J Dermatol 21:489-496, 1982.

2 The Anatomy of Wound Repair

Anatomy of the Skin and Fascia
   Epidermis and Dermis (Skin or
      Cutaneous Layer)
   Superficial Fascia (Subcutaneous Layer)

Deep Fascia
Skin Tension Lines
Alterations of Skin Anatomy
References

The primary anatomic focus in surface wound care is the skin. Underlying the skin are two equally important structures, the superficial (subcutaneous) fascia and the deep fascia. The skin is a complex organ that provides basic protection against mechanical trauma, heat injury, and bacterial invasion. The skin serves to regulate heat loss and gain through its rich vascular network and sweat glands. It contains the sensory organs that register stimuli from the environment. The fascias act not only as a supportive base to the skin, but also carry nerves and vessels that eventually branch into it.

All the layers of the skin and fascia are present in every body site, but they vary considerably in thickness. Most skin is 1 to 2 mm thick, but can increase to 4 mm over the back. This variability often dictates the choice of suture needles. Larger, stronger needles are required to penetrate the skin on the palms of the hand and soles of the feet. Very small and delicate needles should be used on the thin skin of the eyelids. Knowledge of these and other properties of the skin, which are discussed below, helps in the choice of the correct wound-care materials and appropriate closure techniques.

ANATOMY OF THE SKIN AND FASCIA

Although the skin and fascia comprise a complex system of organs and anatomic features, it is the layer arrangement that is most important for wound closure (Fig. 2-1). These layers include the epidermis, dermis, superficial fascia (commonly referred to as the subcutaneous or subcuticular layer), and deep fascia. These layers should be thought of as planes that need to be carefully and accurately reapproximated when disrupted by trauma. Each one has its own set of characteristics that are important to proper wound closure and healing.

5

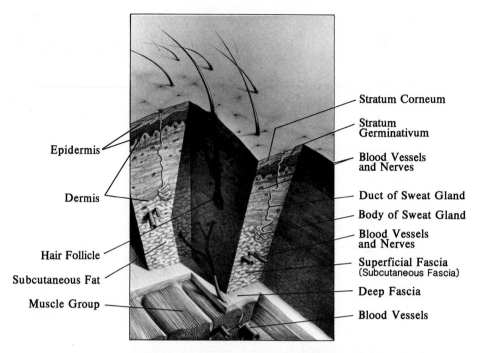

Epidermis

Dermis

Hair Follicle

Subcutaneous Fat

Muscle Group

Stratum Corneum

Stratum Germinativum

Blood Vessels and Nerves

Duct of Sweat Gland

Body of Sweat Gland

Blood Vessels and Nerves

Superficial Fascia (Subcutaneous Fascia)

Deep Fascia

Blood Vessels

FIG. 2-1 Anatomy of the skin illustrating structures pertinent to wound repair.

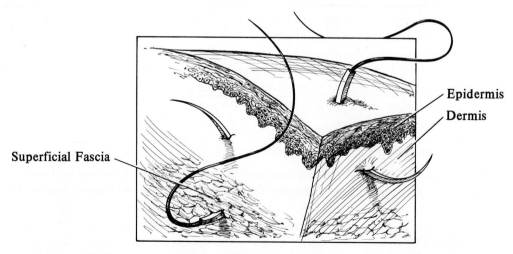

Superficial Fascia

Epidermis

Dermis

FIG. 2-2 Demonstration of either percutaneous or deep suture closure. Note that the needle is anchored in the dermis for each suture placement.

Epidermis and Dermis (Skin or Cutaneous Layer)

The epidermis is the outermost layer of the skin or cutaneous layer. It is also called the cutaneous layer. The epidermis consists totally of squamous epithelial cells and contains no organs, nerve endings, or vessels. Its primary function is to provide protection against the ingress of bacteria and toxic chemicals and the inappropriate egress of water and electrolytes.

There are four microscopic layers of the epidermis, of which two are important in emergency wound care. The stratum germinativum, or basal layer, is the parent layer for new cells. This layer provides the cells for new epidermis formation during wound healing after injury. The stratum corneum is the keratinized or horny layer that is derived from migrating and maturing basal cells. This layer is the most superficial and gives skin its final cosmetic appearance.

Although the epidermis is an anatomically separate layer, it is only a few cell layers thick. During wound repair, it cannot be seen by the naked eye as being separate from the dermis. Therefore, correct approximation of the epidermis will naturally result from careful apposition of the lacerated edges of the dermis.

The dermis lies immediately beneath the epidermis. It is much thicker than the epidermis and is primarily composed of connective tissue. The main cell type in the dermis is the fibroblast, which elaborates collagen, the basic structural component of skin. Other cells found in the dermis are macrophages, mast cells, and lymphocytes. Along with fibroblasts, these components are all active during wound healing.

The dermis is composed of two layers, the papillary dermis and the reticular dermis. The richly vascular papillary dermis interdigitates with the epidermis and provides nutrients to that layer. The deeper reticular dermis contains the bulk of adnexal structures of the skin. These include the hair follicles and vascular plexi. Nerve fibers branch and differentiate into specialized nerve endings that invest both layers of the dermis.

The dermis is the key layer for achieving proper wound repair. It is easily identifiable and provides the anchoring site for both superficial or percutaneous and deep sutures (Fig. 2-2). Every effort is made to cleanse, judiciously debride, and accurately approximate the dermal edges to allow for optimal wound healing with minimal scar formation.

Superficial Fascia (Subcutaneous Layer)

Deep to the dermis is a layer of very loose connective tissue that encloses a varying amount of fat. Fat makes the superficial fascia easily recognizable in a laceration. Fascia provides insulation against heat loss as well as some measure of protection against trauma.

There are several consequences of injury to this layer. Devitalized fat can promote bacterial growth and infection.[3] Every effort is made not to place sutures in fatty tissue because of its propensity for ischemia and infection. Fortunately, it can be liberally debrided so that any devitalized portion can be completely excised. Injuries to the superficial fascia also have the potential for creating dead space. Failure to evacuate this space properly can lead to an increased risk of infection.

The sensory nerve branches to the skin travel in the superficial fascia just deep to the dermis. When injecting a local anesthetic, the needle is directed along the plane between the dermis and superficial fascia. Anesthetic spreads easily in this area and will quickly abolish sensation from the skin.

Deep Fascia

Deep fascia is a relatively thick, dense, and discrete fibrous tissue layer. It acts as a base for the superficial fascia and as an enclosure for muscle groups. The main function of the deep fascia is to support and protect muscles and other soft tissue structures. It also provides a barrier against the spread of infection from the skin and superficial fascia into muscle compartments. Lacerations of the deep fascia are easily recognized and require closure to re-establish the protective and supportive functions of this layer.

SKIN TENSION LINES

There are two anatomic forces inherent in skin that have an important impact on the final scar morphology of healed lacerations. One is a static force and the other is dynamic. As it naturally lies over the body framework, the skin is under constant static tension.[5] The arrangement, orientation, and distensibility of collagen fibers allows skin to act as a relatively taut covering, which, when interrupted by trauma, causes a wound to retract open. The degree to which the retraction or "gaping" takes place is an indicator of how wide the resulting scar may eventually be. Lacerations of the lower extremity, particularly over the anterior tibia, tend to retract under great tension, and they scar conspicuously. A healed horizontal laceration of the skin of the eyelid, on the other hand, becomes virtually unnoticeable with time.

Static skin tension plays an important role in wound edge debridement and revision. It is tempting to want to excise jagged wound edges to convert an irregular laceration into a straight one. If the wound is already gaping because of static tension, then debridement of tissue might increase the tension necessary to pull the straight edges together. An irregular laceration will often heal with a less noticeable scar than a straight wound. As a rule, a ragged wound with viable tissue edges is repaired by putting the "puzzle pieces" back together and preserving as much tissue as possible. If the wound needs later revision, the preserved tissue will be welcomed by the plastic surgeon.

Different from static forces but equally important are the dynamic forces on the skin. These are created by the underlying muscles in any given body area and correspond to wrinkles created by compression of skin during muscle contraction.[1,4] These forces are most dramatically visible in the face during the various changes in facial expression. Lacerations that are perpendicular to these lines tend to heal with wider scars than do those that are parallel. In choosing elective incisions of the face, surgeons will apply the scalpel to correspond with these lines (Figs. 2-3 and 2-4). Dynamic tension forces are important in emergency wound care for several reasons. The final appearance of the scar will be affected by the direction of the wound, and the patient should be counseled accordingly. If foreign bodies are excised, the incision must be parallel to the lines created by dynamic tension forces.

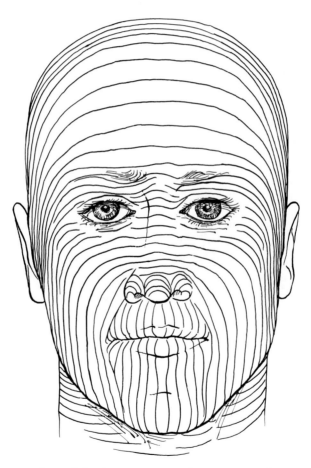

FIG. 2-3 Skin tension lines of the face. Incisions or lacerations parallel to these lines are less likely to create widened scars than those that are perpendicular to these lines. (Adapted from Simon R and Brenner B: Procedures and techniques in emergency medicine, Baltimore, 1982, Williams & Wilkins.)

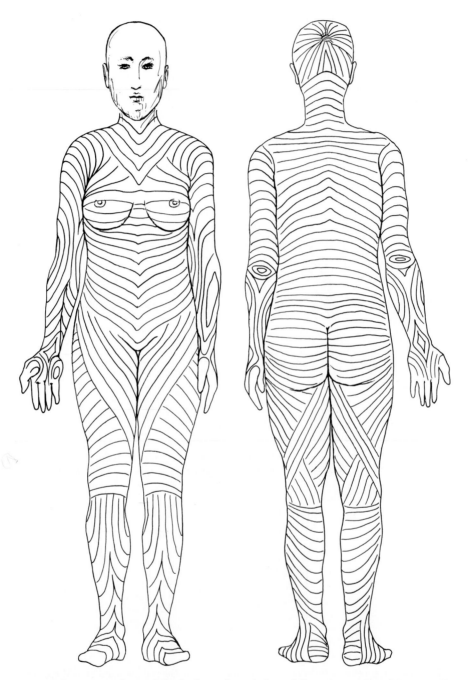

FIG. 2-4 Skin tension lines of the body surface. (Adapted from Simon R and Brenner B: Procedures and techniques in emergency medicine, Baltimore, 1982, Williams & Wilkins.)

ALTERATIONS OF SKIN ANATOMY

Often, there are clinical situations in which the anatomic structure of the skin is altered so much that it requires special wound care. The most common skin changes in this setting are those caused by aging and chronic corticosteroid administration.[2,6]

In aging, there is a flattening of the dermo-epidermal junction with an accompanying decrease in the prominence of the dermal papilli. This effacement appears to result in a reduction of vascularity and nutrient supply to the epidermis. The dermis itself loses its thickness and becomes increasingly acellular and avascular. The net result is that the tensile strength of the dermis decreases significantly, which makes it less resistant to injury. More important to wound care is that the dermis does not support sutures well: they tend to "tear" the skin or cause ischemia because the dermis has a low resistance to suture tension. Although sutures can be effective in younger patients, wound tapes are more appropriate in many lacerations that occur in older people.

Corticosteroids have a profound effect on collagen deposition through inhibition of collagen fiber synthesis and accelerated collagen degradation. The dermis becomes atrophic, thin, and poorly resistant to trauma. Small vessels appear to become increasingly fragile and readily cause ecchymoses in response to even the most trivial trauma. As in aging, the poor quality of the skin makes it less able to support sutures. Skin tapes or simple bandages are often preferable for managing these wounds.

References

1. Borges A and Alexander J: Relaxed skin tension lines, Z-plasties on scars and fusiform excision of lesions, Br J Plast Surg 15:242-254, 1962.
2. Gilchrest B: Age-related changes in skin. In Cape R, Coe R, and Rossman I, editors: Fundamentals of geriatric medicine, New York, 1983, Raven Press.
3. Haury B et al: Debridement: an essential component of traumatic wound care, Am J Surg 135:238-242, 1978.
4. Kraissl C: The selection of lines for elective surgical incisions, Plast Reconstr Surg 8:1-28, 1951.
5. Thacker J et al: Practical applications of skin biomechanics, Clin Plast Surg 4:167-171, 1977.
6. Warrenfeltz A and Graham W: Avulsion injuries in patients receiving corticosteroids, Am Fam Prac 11:74-81, 1975.

3 *Surface Injury and Wound Healing*

Mechanism of Injury
  Shearing
  Tension
  Compression
Normal Wound Healing
  Immediate Response to Injury
  Inflammatory Phase
  Epithelialization
  Neovascularization
  Collagen Synthesis

Wound Contraction
Categories of Wound Healing
Alterations of Wound Healing
  Technical Factors
  Anatomic Factors
  Associated Conditions and Diseases
  Drugs
Abnormal Scar Formation
References

One of the realities of wound care is that many of the elements of scar formation are beyond the control of the person repairing a traumatic wound. Unlike surgical incisions, wounds and lacerations are not planned with regard to location, length, depth, or cosmetic concerns. Wounds caused at random present a variety of biologic and technical problems that need to be solved in order to produce the best repair result. It is incumbent on the operator to have a thorough understanding of the mechanisms of injury and wound healing to increase the chances of achieving a cosmetically acceptable scar. Age, race, body region, skin tension lines, associated conditions and diseases, drugs, type of wound, and technical considerations all affect scar formation. The choice of repair strategy depends on these and other factors. Finally, knowledge of the spectrum of wound healing will ensure that patients with traumatically induced wounds receive the proper advice and counseling.

MECHANISM OF INJURY

The mechanism of injury is important because it is a significant determinant in the choice of management technique as well as in predicting the possibility of the wound becoming infected. The injury mechanism also plays a role in scar formation and in the eventual cosmetic outcome. The mechanism involved in causing surface wounds, and in particular, lacerations, can be divided into three forces that are applied to the skin under injury conditions: shearing, tension, and compression forces.[7,19]

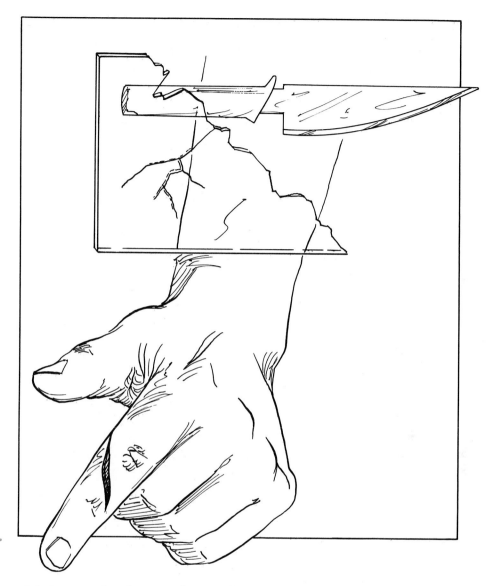

FIG. 3-1 Examples of injuring objects and a resulting laceration caused by shearing forces.

Shearing

Shearing injuries, which result in a simple dividing of tissues, are those caused by sharp objects such as knives or glass (Fig. 3-1). The skin is divided traumatically, but little energy is imparted to the tissues and minimal cell destruction occurs outside the confines of the laceration. Such lacerations can be repaired primarily (primary intention) and they have a low incidence of wound infection. The resulting scar is usually thin and cosmetically acceptable.

Tension

Tension injuries occur as a result of a blunt or semi-blunt object striking the skin at an angle of less than 90 degrees (Fig. 3-2). Under these conditions a triangular flap of skin is often created. Because the blood supply is interrupted on two sides of the flap, ischemia can occur, leading to devitalization and necrosis. The remaining blood vessels entering the flap from the base have to be preserved by careful handling and special suturing techniques, which are described later. The energy necessary to create this type of wound is greater than that caused by the shearing force. The combination of greater cell destruction and potential ischemia, therefore, can increase the risk of wound infection. These wounds also tend to lead to greater scar formation.

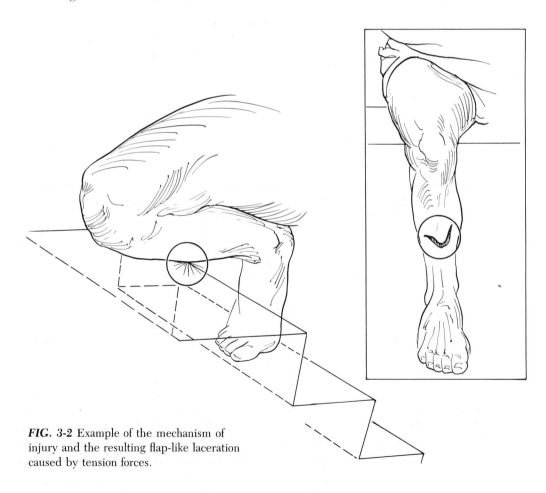

FIG. 3-2 Example of the mechanism of injury and the resulting flap-like laceration caused by tension forces.

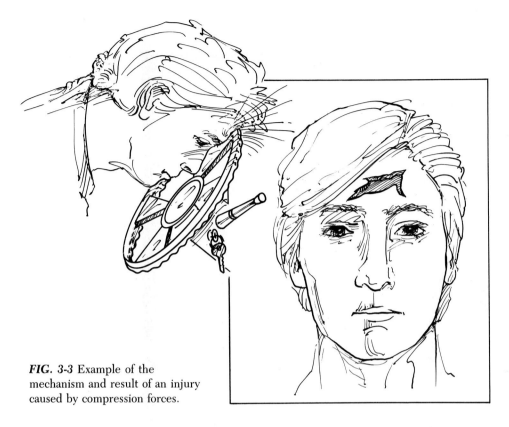

***FIG.** 3-3* Example of the mechanism and result of an injury caused by compression forces.

Compression

Crushing or compression injuries occur when a relatively blunt object strikes the skin at right angles (Fig. 3-3). These lacerations often have ragged edges and are accompanied by a significant amount of devitalization of skin and superficial fascia (subcutaneous tissue). Such wounds require extensive cleansing, irrigation, and debridement to decrease the already significant chance of developing infection.[2] In spite of meticulous repair, the resulting scars can be cosmetically unacceptable to patients and, consequently, are subject to consideration for later plastic surgery.

NORMAL WOUND HEALING

Once injury has occurred by whatever mechanism, normal wound healing is a process that proceeds unimpeded unless there is undue interference from infection, excessive tissue devitalization, poor wound repair technique, underlying patient conditions and diseases, and inhibitory drugs. Although wound healing is commonly described as occurring in phases, it is actually a continuum of overlapping events. These are described individually for the sake of clarity and their interrelationships are depicted graphically in Fig. 3-4.

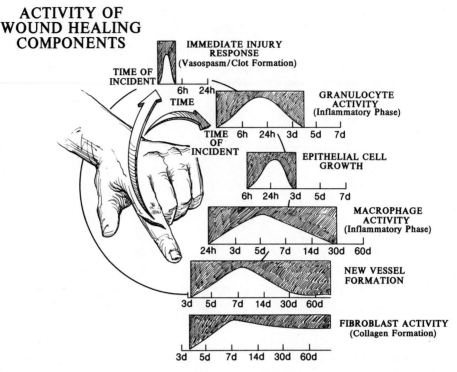

FIG. 3-4 Graphic illustration of the various components of wound healing and their time frames.

Immediate Response to Injury

At the moment of injury, several events take place that culminate in rapid hemostasis. The traumatic insult causes changes in skin architecture that result in tissue retraction and contraction, which leads to the compression of small venules and arterioles. Vessels undergo intense reflex vasoconstriction for up to 10 minutes. Platelets begin to aggregate in the lumens of severed vessels as well as on the exposed wound surfaces. The clotting cascade is activated by tissue clotting factors, and, within minutes, the wound begins to fill with a hemostatic coagulum. As hemostasis is secured, vasoactive amines are released into the wound region, leading to the dilatation of uninjured capillaries and the initiation of wound exudation.

Inflammatory Phase

Once hemostasis has been achieved and exudation begins, the inflammatory response rapidly follows. The complement system is activated, and chemotactic factors, which attract granulocytes to the wound area, are released. These cells are followed shortly by lymphocytes. Peak granulocyte numbers can be found between 12 to 24 hours after the injury has been sustained. The chief function of granulocytes and lymphocytes appears to be the control of bacterial growth and, therefore, the suppression of infection. These cells are aided by immunoglobulins that are included in the wound exudate. In most simple wounds granulocyte counts markedly diminish after 3 days.

After 24 to 48 hours, macrophages can be detected in large numbers, and by day 5, they are the predominant inflammatory cells in the wound area. These cells play a major role in the inflammatory responses and in the early fibroblast and collagen formation responses. Their first responsibility appears to be phagocytosis and ingestion of wound debris. As part of this process, these cells return usable substrates (amino acids and simple sugars) back to the wound exudate. Macrophages also appear to be important in stimulating fibroblast reproduction and neovascularization. Finally, these remarkable cells produce and release a chemotactic factor that attracts more of its kind to the wound region.

Epithelialization

While the inflammatory response proceeds, epithelial cells at the stratum germinativum or basal layer of the epidermis undergo morphologic and functional changes. Within 12 hours intact cells at the wound edge begin to form pseudopod-like structures that facilitate cell migration. Replication takes place and the cells begin to move over the wound surface. An advancing layer can be seen to travel over the damaged dermis and under the hemostatic coagulum. Once these cells reach the inner wound area, they begin to meet other advancing epithelial extensions. The original cuboidal shape of the epithelial cells is regained and desmosomal attachments to other cells are made. Continued replication eventually re-establishes the normal layers of epidermis. For lacerations caused by shearing forces, initial epithelialization can take place within 24 hours, but the architecture and thickness of this layer continually changes over the months of the wound maturation process.

Neovascularization

Crucial to wound repair is the phenomenon of new vessel formation. These vessels replace the old injured network and bring oxygen and nutrients to the healing wound. Neovascularization is evident by day 3 and is most active by day 7. The marked erythematous appearance of the wound at the time of suture removal can thus be explained. Vascularity decreases rapidly by day 21, with continued regression as the wound matures. New vessels form loops of capillaries that are surrounded by actively growing fibroblasts. These two components on the wound surface give it the classic appearance referred to as granulation. Granulation tissue is most often seen in open wounds that are allowed to heal by secondary intention.

Collagen Synthesis

With the establishment of a vascular supply and stimulation by macrophages, fibroblasts rapidly undergo mitosis. They begin to produce new collagen fibrils by the

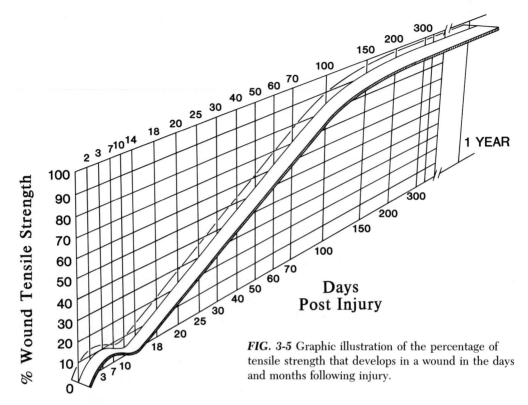

FIG. *3-5* Graphic illustration of the percentage of tensile strength that develops in a wound in the days and months following injury.

second day. Peak synthesis occurs between days 5 to 7, and the wound has its greatest collagen mass by 3 weeks. By then, the wound is devoid of inflammatory infiltrate and edema.

New collagen is laid down in a random, amorphous pattern. It is basically a gel with little tensile strength. Over the months, however, this gel continually remodels itself, creating an organized basket-weave pattern that is achieved by the cross-linking of collagen fibers. In order for this process to proceed without excess collagen formation, collagen lysis takes place. Hydrolysis and collagenase activity break down old and damaged collagen, permitting ingestion by macrophages. New collagen takes its place. The balance between synthesis and lysis creates a vulnerable period approximately 7 to 10 days after injury, when the wound is most prone to unwanted opening or dehiscence. Explaining this possibility to the patient may prevent the development of this unwanted complication. The wound will have only 5% of its original tensile strength at 2 weeks and 35% at 1 month (Fig. 3-5). Final tensile strength is not achieved for several months.

Wound Contraction

Every wound undergoes some degree of wound contraction. It is most pronounced, however, in full-thickness skin losses. The scar that forms gradually contracts centripetally over the wound defect through the action of specialized fibroblasts called myofibroblasts. Contraction pulls normal surrounding skin over the defect. Practically speaking, a properly everted suture line will contract to a flat, cosmetically acceptable scar, whereas a wound closed with the edges already inverted will form an unsightly depression in the epidermis that will stand out because of shadow formation from incident light (see Chapter 9 for further details).

CATEGORIES OF WOUND HEALING

For clinical purposes, wound healing is often categorized into three types or intentions: primary, secondary, and tertiary. These divisions provide general guidelines that help determine proper wound management based on time from injury, level of contamination, and degree of tissue devitalization. Chapter 8 further describes the categories of wound healing and choices of management for each.

ALTERATIONS OF WOUND HEALING

Several factors can alter the process and final outcome of wound healing. These factors are summarized and discussed in the box below.

Alterations of Wound Healing

TECHNICAL FACTORS

Inadequate wound preparation
Excessive suture tension
Reactive suture materials
Local anesthetics

ANATOMIC FACTORS

Static skin tension
Dynamic skin tension
Pigmented skin
Oily skin
Body region

ASSOCIATED CONDITIONS AND DISEASES

Advanced age
Severe alcoholism
Acute uremia
Diabetes
Ehlers-Danlos syndrome
Hypoxia
Severe anemia
Peripheral vascular disease
Malnutrition

DRUGS

Corticosteroids
Nonsteroidal anti-inflammatories
Penicillamine
Colchicine
Anticoagulants
Antineoplastic agents

Technical Factors

Any wound that becomes infected will heal with a larger, more noticeable, and cosmetically less acceptable scar. Inadequate cleansing, irrigation, or debridement of contaminated and devitalized tissues will increase the chance of infection.[10]

Excessive tension created by improper suture technique can cause unnecessary wound ischemia.[16] Ischemia promotes cellular necrosis with greater inflammatory and scarring responses. Deep sutures, undermining, and increasing the number of sutures per laceration are methods that can reduce the danger of excessive tension.

Because tissue reactivity and inflammation vary with different suture materials, these materials can have differing effects on the healing process.[18] Although silk has excellent mechanical properties, it has a propensity for causing marked tissue reactivity. Nylon and polypropylene, however, are the least reactive of the nonabsorbable materials. Absorbable sutures still act as foreign material, and excessive numbers can increase the risk of infection and may provoke a greater scarring response.[6,14]

Experiments have shown that local anesthetics can cause retardation of wound healing.[3] This negative effect is enhanced by increasing concentrations of local anesthetics as well as the use of adrenalin in anesthetic solutions.[13] There is no question, however, that local anesthetics need to be used in wound care. Judicious amounts at the lowest concentrations possible are recommended.

Anatomic Factors

Body region and skin tension lines have a significant effect on wound healing, specifically on final scar morphology (see Chapter 11). Wounds over the anterior thorax or the extremities heal with the most evident scars, while wounds of the eyelid heal with the least obvious scars. Pigmented and oily skin also tends to heal with greater scar formation than fairer, less oily skin.

Associated Conditions and Diseases

Several conditions and diseases cause an alteration in wound healing. Advanced age has been implicated in slower healing of wounds.[9] However, if the patient is basically healthy, normal healing and scar formation will ultimately take place.[8] Wound healing can be retarded in the chronic alcoholic who has advanced liver disease and impaired protein synthesis.[1] Acute uremia has long been thought to impede healing.[5] In uremics, there is an inhibition of fibroblast growth and a decrease in tensile strength during wound healing. Diabetics have numerous problems with wound healing.[12] Not only do they have an increased chance of wound infection, but there is also retardation of neovascularization and collagen synthesis. A rare disease that causes problems with collagen formation and wound healing is Ehlers-Danlos syndrome.[4]

Any condition that leads to failure of oxygen and nutrient delivery to the wound will profoundly affect wound healing.[11] Shock, severe anemia, peripheral vascular disease, and malnutrition all fall into this category. Patients with severe underlying diseases such as advanced cancer, hepatic failure, and severe cardiovascular disease will exhibit one or more of these clinical states and be subject to poor wound healing. Victims of major trauma, particularly those who have undergone prolonged shock and complicated resuscitations, are also at risk for poor wound healing.

Drugs

Numerous drugs and pharmacologic preparations alter wound healing.[15] Drugs that appear to have negative effects include corticosteroids, nonsteroidal anti-inflammatory agents (aspirin, phenylbutazone), pencillamine, colchicine, anticoagulants, and antineoplastic agents. Of these drugs, corticosteroids have the most profound effect on healing and interfere with the process at many points. They adversely alter the inflammatory response, fibroblast activity, neovascularization, and epithelialization. Nonsteroidal anti-inflammatory compounds depress the normal inflammatory response and can decrease overall wound tensile strength. Anticoagulants and aspirin increase the possibility of wound hematoma formation with subsequent delays in healing time. Although in theory antineoplastic agents have a good reason to inhibit wound healing, in actual practice it is not clear that they do so in a clinically significant manner.

Vitamins C and A, zinc sulfate, and anabolic steroids have a generally positive effect on wound repair.[15] Vitamin C deficiency profoundly impairs collagen formation, but normal synthesis can be restored with administration of ascorbic acid. Vitamin A and anabolic steroids are able to reverse corticosteroid-induced suppression of the inflammatory response. Zinc deficiency appears to play a role in slowing the healing process. Correction of the deficiency will reverse that effect. Use of zinc ointments in nonzinc-deficient patients can cause a cross-linking failure during collagen maturation.[15] Experimental evidence that zinc sulfate can retard wound contraction is supportive of this observation.[17]

ABNORMAL SCAR FORMATION

A keloid is an inappropriate accumulation of scar tissue that originates from a wound and extends beyond its original boundaries (Fig. 3-6). Keloids are more common in blacks, but can occur in darkly pigmented skin areas of people of different races. These scars tend to be more commonly located on the ears, upper extremities, lower abdomen, and sternum. Treatments for keloids have included corticosteroid injection, compressive dressings, and surgical excision followed by radiation therapy. Eventual outcome and treatment depends on early recognition of keloid formation and prompt therapy.

Hypertrophic scars also have excessive bulk, but unlike keloids, they are confined to the original borders of the wound (Fig. 3-7). They tend to occur in areas of

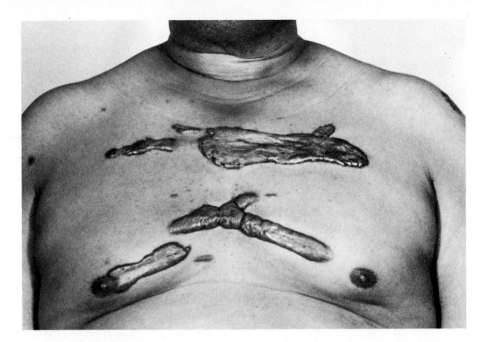

FIG. 3-6 An example of a keloid scar. Note that the scar extends beyond the margins of the original wound.

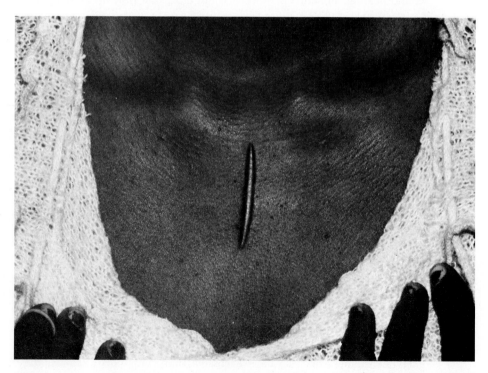

FIG. 3-7 An example of a hypertrophic scar. Note that the scar remains confined to the original borders of the wound.

tissue stress such as flexion creases across joints. The cause of this excessive scar response is not known. Physical therapy and splinting can be used during healing in patients who have a history of hypertrophic scarring. Corticosteroids and radiation therapy are other therapeutic alternatives.

References

1. Benveniste K and Thut P: The effect of chronic alcoholism on wound healing, Proc Soc Exp Biol Med 166:568-575, 1981.
2. Cardany R et al: The crush injury: a high risk wound, J Am Coll Emerg Phys 5:965-970, 1976.
3. Chvapil M et al: Local anesthetics and wound healing, J Surg Res 27:367-371, 1979.
4. Cohen I, McCoy B, and Biegelmann, R: An update on wound healing, Ann Plast Surg 3:264-272, 1979.
5. Colin J, Elliot P, and Ellis H: The effect of uraemia upon wound healing: an experimental study, Br J Surg 60:793-797, 1979.
6. Edlich R et al: Technique of closure: contaminated wound, J Am Coll Emerg Phys 3:375-381, 1974.
7. Edlich R, Rodeheaver G, and Thacker J: Technical factors in the prevention of disease. Simmons RL, Howard RJ, and Henriksen AI, editors: Surgical infectious diseases, New York, 1982, Appleton-Century-Crofts.
8. Goodson W and Hunt T: Wound healing and aging, J Invest Dermatol 73:88-912, 1979.
9. Grove G: Age-related differences in healing of superficial skin wounds in humans, Arch Dermatol Res 272-381-385, 1982.
10. Haury B et al: Debridement: an essential component of traumatic wound care, Am J Surg 135:238-242, 1978.
11. Hotter A: Physiologic aspects and clinical implications of wound healing, Heart Lung 11:522-530, 1982.
12. Hunt T: Disorders of wound healing, World J Surg 4:271-277, 1980.
13. Morris T and Appleby R: Retardation of wound healing by procaine, Br J Surg 67:391-392, 1980.
14. Paterson-Brown S et al: Suture materials in contaminated wounds: a detailed comparison of a new suture with those currently in use, Br J Surg 74:734-735, 1987.
15. Pollack S: Systemic medications and wound healing, Int J Dermatol 21:491-496, 1982.
16. Price P: Stress, strain, and sutures, Ann Surg 128:408-421, 1948.
17. Soderberg T and Hallmans G: Wound contractions and zinc absorption during treatment with zinc tape, Scand J Reconstr Surg 16:255-259, 1982.
18. Swanson N and Tromovitch T: Suture materials: properties, uses and abuses, Int J Dermatol 21:373-378, 1982.
19. Trott AT: Mechanisms of surface soft tissue trauma, Ann Emerg Med 17:1279-1283, 1988.

4 *The Potential for Wound Infection*

Epidemiology

Microbiology of Wound Infection

Factors that Increase Risk of Infection

    Wound Characteristics

Technical Elements

    Patient Condition

References

The most common and serious complication of wound and laceration repair is infection. Because virtually all accidentally induced wounds occur in unsterile conditions, they have to be considered contaminated with micro-organisms. The stratum corneum of the epidermis normally acts as an effective barrier against the penetration of bacteria into the deeper layers of the skin and superficial fascia. Any violation of the stratum corneum provides a pathway for bacterial invasion. Not only do environmental micro-organisms find their way into wounds, but the skin, which is richly populated with a variety of endogenous microflora, can harbor a potentially infective inoculum of pathogenic bacteria.[16]

EPIDEMIOLOGY

In spite of the ubiquity of pathogenic micro-organisms and the traumatic, unsterile conditions under which wounds occur, there is a low incidence of infection in simple, uncomplicated wounds and lacerations. Several clinical studies performed on patients treated in emergency departments place the rate of infection for simple lacerations between 4.5% and 6.3%.[10,22,12,28]

Wounds caused by animal and human bites often have a greater potential for and a higher incidence of infection. Depending on the anatomic site involved, the reported rate of infection following human bites has been reported to range from 1% (human lip) to 40% (hand), with an average for all sites of 17.7%.[14,13,15] Animal bites vary considerably in rate of infection, ranging from 4.3% in dog bites to 50% in cat bites.[2,7] Animal bites also require consideration of special factors such as exposure to rabies. Bite injuries, the spectrum of infecting organisms, and treatment considerations are discussed at length in Chapter 14.

MICROBIOLOGY OF WOUND INFECTION

The actual development of wound infection depends on a multitude of factors. The mere presence of bacteria alone does not inevitably lead to this complication. The type of injury, time from injury, size of inoculum, presence of foreign material, condition of the host, and a variety of other factors can lead to circumstances favorable for reaching an infective bacterial count level. The prime goal of proper wound preparation is to prevent the establishment of wound infection.

In non-animal bite wounds, if infection does occur, it is most likely to be caused by *Staphylococcus aureus*. In one study of lacerations, 44% of the wounds that became infected after repair grew pure *S. aureus* in culture.[10] Of the infected wounds 39% yielded *S. aureus* mixed with a variety of other gram-positive and gram-negative bacteria. Of all the lacerations reported to have become infected in another emergency department study, 80% revealed *S. aureus* as the primary pathogen.[12]

An investigation of patients with somewhat larger and more extensive surface wounds and lacerations than those usually managed in emergency departments alone revealed that 60% of all recovered organisms were identified as gram-positive cocci.[23] Slightly less than one-half of these cocci were *S. aureus*, with a variety of streptococci and *Staphylococcus epidermidis* making up the rest of the gram-positive group. The remaining 40% of the culturable bacteria were gram-negative rods (*Escherichia coli*, *Proteus* species, *Enterobacter* species, and *Klebsiella pneumoniae.*)

FACTORS THAT INCREASE RISK OF INFECTION

Below are listed numerous factors that potentially can increase the rate of minor wound infection after closure. For the most part, these variables can be altered to decrease the risk of developing infection. Knowledge of their importance, along with appropriate wound management, can lessen their infection potentiating effect. These factors can be divided into three categories: wound characteristics, technical elements, and underlying patient condition.

Wound Characteristics

An important determinant of wound infection is the time from injury to cleansing and repair. By using quantitative bacterial screening of wounds in patients treated for lacerations, it has been observed that wounds repaired after 5 hours consistently grow greater than 100,000 (10^5) organisms, which is a potentially infective inoculum.[19] It is well known, however, that many lacerations can be primarily repaired safely after 5 hours. Clean wounds that are not visibly soiled or devitalized and are in highly vascular areas like the face, for example, can be safely repaired up to 12 to 24 hours after injury. Careful clinical judgment is required to select the timing of wound repair. A more detailed discussion of the timing of repair can be found in Chapter 8.

The mechanism of injury and extent of tissue damage have profound effects on the potential for infection. Experimental studies support the clinical observation that crushing injuries produce extensive devitalized tissue that makes wounds more susceptible to bacterial invasion.[3,11] Leukocyte phagocytic and bactericidal activity, crucial to infection control, is adversely affected by an anaerobic environment, a condition that can exist with crushing wounds.[3] Soiling of the wound with dirt and foreign material is commonly believed to produce an increased chance of wound infection. Investigators have studied the infection potential of various soils.[20] They were able to demonstrate in an experimental model that soil, and, in particular, clay, reduced an infection-producing inoculum of S. aureus from 1,000,000 (10^7) to 100 (10^2) organisms.

Several clinical studies have shown that lacerations in different body regions have a variable propensity for infection.[12,22,28] Wounds and lacerations occurring below the knee resulted in the highest infection rate, up to 17.5%.[12] The next highest incidence occurred in the upper extremity, including the hand, with an infection rate varying between 3.8% and 9%.[12,22] Facial lacerations accounted for 2.6% to 4.3% of wound infections, and scalp lacerations, 1.5% to 2.6%.[12,28]

Technical Elements

Although wound cleansing is a key step in wound management, the improper use of certain cleansing solutions can increase the chance of wound infection. Agents like povidone-iodine scrub and hexachlorophene surgical scrub contain ionic detergents. In an experimental study performed on animals, these detergents were found to have an adverse effect on the ability of a wound to resist infection.[4] Povidone-iodine solution, (1%) without detergent retains the same antibacterial activity as the detergent-containing scrub solution but appears to be nontoxic to tissues.[8,9]

Local anesthetics with the vasoconstrictor epinephrine are commonly used to achieve hemostasis during wound repair. There is experimental evidence that vasoconstrictors used under these circumstances reduce infection-fighting capabilities of wounds.[25] This adverse effect varies directly with the concentration of epinephrine.

Proper tissue handling and suture technique can reduce the incidence of wound infection. Poor hemostasis and the accumulation of unwanted hematoma provide a good medium for bacterial growth. Excessive suture tension creates unnecessary compression of tissue at the wound edges. The ischemia that develops creates further damage to the tissues and can increase the probability of wound infection. Ischemia also causes a greater inflammatory response that can lead to a cosmetically less acceptable scar.

The choice of suture material can play a role in the extent of inflammation and the potential for wound infection. Experimental studies tend to confirm the clinical observations that of the absorbable sutures, polyglycolic acid sutures elicit the least inflammatory response and are associated with a lower rate of infection than chromic or gut sutures.[5,27] Monofilament suture material, nylon and polypropylene, is the least reactive of the nonabsorbable suture materials.[5,27] The least reactive of all wound closure methods, however, appears to be wound taping. In a contaminated wound guinea pig model, wound tapes were able to resist infection far better than nylon.[6] In recent animal comparison trials of staples versus standard suture techniques, resistance to infection was greater for staples than for sutures.[21,26]

Wound dressings are considered a necessary part of wound care. Under experimental conditions early after injury, wounds appear to be susceptible to surface contamination with *S. aureus* or *E. coli*.[24] By 72 hours, however, wounds do not develop infection after attempted surface contamination with these agents. A frequently used dressing adjunct, tincture of benzoin, impairs the ability of precontaminated experimental wounds to resist infection.[17] Tincture of benzoin deliberately spilled into wounds increases the rate of infection. In actual clinical settings, this risk has not been documented, but when applying wound tapes, there is the potential to spill this substance into a laceration because it is commonly painted close to the laceration edge.

Patient Condition

It has been well demonstrated that certain conditions and diseases increase the rate of post-surgical wound infection. There is virtually no research documenting the wound infection rate in patients (who have associated diseases) with emergency department wounds. Nonetheless, the potential remains for an increased infection rate under certain circumstances. In a large multicenter study of surgical patients, wound infections were increased in patients over the age of 50, patients who had diabetes, patients receiving corticosteroids, and those suffering from malnutrition.[18] Other diseases that have been associated with increased wound infection are cirrhosis of the liver and uremia.[1]

References

1. Altemeier W: Principles in the management of traumatic wounds and in infection control, Bull NY Acad Med 55:123-138, 1979.
2. Aghababian R and Conte J: Mammalian bite wounds, Ann Emerg Med 9:79-83, 1980.
3. Cardany C et al: The crush injury: a high risk wound, J Am Coll Emerg Phys 5:965-970, 1976.
4. Custer J et al: Studies in the management of the contaminated wound, Am J Surg 121:5672-575, 1971.
5. Edlich R et al: Physical and chemical configurations of sutures in the development of surgical infection, Ann Surg 177:679-687, 1973.
6. Edlich R et al: Technique of closure: contaminated wounds, J Am Coll Emerg Phys 3:375-381, 1974.

7. Elenbaas R, McNabney W, and Robinson W: Prophylactic oxacillin in dog bite wounds, Ann Emerg Med 11:248-251, 1982.

8. Faddis D, Daniel D, and Boyer J: Tissue toxicity of antiseptic solutions, J Trauma 17:895-897, 1977.

9. Gravett A et al: A trial of povidone-iodine in the prevention of infection in sutured lacerations, Ann Emerg Med 16:167-171, 1987.

10. Gosnold J: Infection rate of sutured wounds, Practitioner 2218:584-585, 1977.

11. Haury B et al: Debridement: an essential component of traumatic wound care, Am J Surg 135:238-242, 1978.

12. Hutton P, Jones B, and Lasw D: Depot penicillin as prophylaxis in accidental wounds, Br J Surg 65:549-550, 1978.

13. Lindsey D et al: Natural course of the human bite wound: incidence of infection and complications in 434 bites and 803 lacerations in the same group of patients, J Trauma 27:45-48, 1987.

14. Losken HW and Auchincloss JA: Human bites of the lip, Clin Plast Surg 1984, 11:773-775.

15. Malinowski R et al: The management of human bites of the hand, J Trauma 19:655-658, 1979.

16. Marples M: Life on the human skin, Sci Am 220:108-1115, 1969.

17. Panek P, et al: Potentiation of wound infection by adhesive adjuncts, Am Surg 38:343-345, 1972.

18. Postoperative wound infections. Report of an Ad Hoc Committee on Trauma, Division of Medical Sciences, National Academy of Sciences, Ann Surg 160(suppl):32-58, 1964.

19. Robson M, Duke W, and Krizek T: Rapid bacterial screening in treatment of civilian wounds, J Surg Res 14:426-480, 1973.

20. Rodeheaver G et al: Identification of the wound infection-potentiating factors in soil, Am J Surg 138:8-14, 1974.

21. Roth JH and Windle BH: Staple versus skin incisions closure in pig model, Can J Surg 31:19-20, 1988.

22. Rutherford W and Spence R: Infection in wounds sutured in the accident and emergency department, Ann Emerg Med 9:350-352, 1980.

23. Sanford J: Microbiology of open wounds. In Rund D and Wolcott B, editors: Emergency medicine annual, East Norwalk, Conn, 1983, Appleton-Century-Crofts.

24. Schauerhamer R, Edlich R, and Panek P: Studies in the management of the contaminated wound, Am J Surg 122:74-77, 1971.

25. Stevenson T et al: Damage to tissue defenses by vasoconstrictors, J Am Coll Emerg Phys 4:532-535, 1975.

26. Stillman RM, Marino CA, and Seligman SJ: Skin staples in potentially contaminated wounds, Arch Surg 119:821-822, 1984.

27. Swanson N and Tromovitch T: Suture material, 1980s: properties, uses, and abuses, Int J Dermatol 21:373-378, 1982.

28. Thirlby R and Blair A: The value of prophylactic antibiotics for simple lacerations, Surg Gynecol Obstet 156:212-216, 1983.

5 Infiltration and Nerve Block Anesthesia

Pharmacology of Local Anesthetics
Toxicity of Local Anesthetics
 Management of the Toxic Reaction
Allergy to Local Anesthetics
 Management of Allergic Responses
Alternative Anesthetic Strategies for the
 Allergic Patient
Anesthetic Solutions
 Lidocaine
 Mepivacaine (Carbocaine)
 Bupivacaine (Marcaine)
Topical Anesthesia
 Technique for Topical Anesthesia
Buffering Anesthetics to Reduce Pain of
 Injection
 Technique for Buffering Anesthetics
Patient Sedation
 Intramuscular Sedation
 Technique for Intravenous Fentanyl
  Sedation
Choice of Needles and Syringes
Anesthesia Techniques
 Direct Wound Infiltration
 Indications
 Anatomy
 Technique for direct infiltration
 Parallel Margin Infiltration (Field Block)
 Indications
 Anatomy
 Technique for parallel margin
  infiltration
 Supraorbital and Supratrochlear Nerve
  Blocks (Forehead Block)
 Indications
 Anatomy
 Technique for forehead block
Infraorbital Nerve Block

 Indications
 Anatomy
 Technique for infraorbital nerve block
Mental Nerve Block
 Indications
 Anatomy
 Technique for mental nerve block
Auricular Block
 Indications
 Anatomy
 Technique for auricular block
Digital Nerve Blocks (Finger and Toe
 Blocks)
 Indications
 Anatomy
Techniques
 Technique for digital block
 Alternative toe block technique
Median Nerve Block
 Indications
 Anatomy
 Technique for median nerve block
Ulnar Nerve Block
 Indications
 Anatomy
 Technique for ulnar nerve block
Radial Nerve Block
 Indications
 Anatomy
 Technique for radial nerve block
Sural and Tibial Nerve Block (Sole of
 Foot Blocks)
 Indications
 Anatomy
 Technique for sural nerve block
 Technique for posterior tibial nerve
  block
References

Anesthesia for wounds and lacerations is not difficult to accomplish. As for any procedure, a thorough understanding of the properties of anesthetic solutions and injection techniques is required. The choice of anesthetics and techniques must be individualized for every patient. The type, location, and extent of the wound, level of contamination, and estimated length of time for repair are variables that make each patient unique. Besides technical considerations, patients have differing emotional characteristics and responses. They often fear that injections and needles will cause excessive pain. Therefore, gentle handling and proper counseling of the patient during the procedure are required to achieve proper analgesia.

PHARMACOLOGY OF LOCAL ANESTHETICS

Upon injection, local anesthetics infiltrate tissues and diffuse across neural sheaths and membranes. They act by interfering with neural depolarization and transmission of impulses along axons.[9] The myelin sheath coverings of nerve fibers within the axon vary in diameter and thickness. Fibers that carry stimuli from pain receptors in the skin have no myelin sheath and have the smallest diameter. The sensations of pressure and touch are transmitted by larger, myelinated fibers. The thin pain fibers are more rapidly and easily blocked by local anesthetic solutions. The significance of this fact in wound care is that a solution of 1% lidocaine can block pain stimuli but often leaves the sensation of touch and pressure intact.[12] Therefore, an overly anxious patient may react to touch and pressure as if it were pain and ask why the wound is not completely numb. A higher concentration of lidocaine (2%) will in all likelihood abolish all awareness of stimuli, including touch and pressure, from the wound area.

There are three main pharmacologic properties that are important to consider in delivering local anesthetics: onset of action, duration, and toxicity of anesthesia. These properties are discussed with each anesthetic solution and are summarized in Table 5-1. They vary widely according to local vascularity of a given body area, type and amount of anesthetic, concentration, technique, accuracy of injection, and adjunctive use of epinephrine. Although epinephrine in low concentrations (1:100,000 or 1:200,000) is mixed in anesthetic solutions to prolong duration as well as to decrease bleeding, it has potential complications. Under experimental conditions, this adjunct has been shown to potentiate wound infection.[10,17] Anesthetics with vasoconstrictors also cannot be used in anatomic areas that have terminal vasculature, like the fingers, toes, ears, penis, and the tip of the nose because these vasoconstricting effects can lead to local skin necrosis.

TOXICITY OF LOCAL ANESTHETICS

There are three toxic reactions that can occur with the injection of local anesthetics. These are cardiovascular reactions, excitatory central nervous system effects, and vasovagal syncope secondary to pain and anxiety. Cardiovascular reactions include

Table 5-1 *Summary of Local Anesthetics for Minor Wound Care*

AGENT	CONCEN-TRATION	Onset of Action INFILTRA-TION	BLOCK	DURATION OF ACTION	MAXIMUM ALLOWABLE DOSE ONE TIME
Lidocaine (Xylocaine)	1.0%	Immediate	4-10 min.	60-120 min. (for block)	4.5 mg/kg of 1% (30 cc per average adult)
Mepivicaine (Carbocaine)	1.0%	Immediate	6-10 min.	90-180 min. (for block)	5 mg/kg of 1% (30 cc per average adult)
Bupivicaine (Marcaine)	0.25%	Slower	8-12 min.	240-480 min. (for blocks)	3 mg/kg of 0.25% (50 cc per average adult)
TAC	See text	5-10 min.	—	Approx 20 min.	2-5 cc of mixture

hypotension and bradycardia and are caused by a myocardial inhibitory effect of the anesthetic.[6] Local anesthetic solutions can cause excitatory phenomena in the central nervous system that ultimately can culminate in seizure activity. Both the cardiovascular and nervous system effects are commonly caused by an inadvertent injection of a solution directly into a vessel, causing a bolus effect on the heart or brain. Therefore, a key principle in the use of local anesthetics is always to aspirate the syringe before injection to check for blood return. If blood is aspirated, the needle has to be moved in order to avoid injecting the solution into a vein or artery.

The most common reaction to local anesthetics is vasovagal syncope (fainting). The anxiety and pain of injection can cause dizziness, pallor, bradycardia, and hypotension. This reaction can largely be avoided by gentle handling of the patient, proper counseling, and slow, careful injection technique. No anesthetic infiltration is ever carried out on a patient who is not in the supine position. Preferably, the patient should also be placed so that he or she cannot see the injection being administered.

Local complications to anesthetic infiltration are unusual but can include infection, hematoma formation, and, potentially, permanent nerve damage to peripheral nerves anesthetized during block procedures.

Management of the Toxic Reaction

Treatment of toxic reactions is largely supportive. The airway is appropriately protected and ventilations are maintained. Hypotension and bradycardia are usually self-limited and can be reversed by placing the patient in the Trendelenburg position. An intravenous line is started with normal saline, and a bolus of 250 to 500 mL is infused to counteract hypotension in any patient who does not respond to that maneuver. Cardiac monitoring with frequent vital signs is instituted. Seizures are also self-limited but may need to be controlled by intravenous diazepam (Valium®).

ALLERGY TO LOCAL ANESTHETICS

Allergic reactions are uncommon with the newer amide local anesthetics such as lidocaine, mepivacaine, and bupivicaine. Reactions were more frequent with the older ester solutions, procaine and tetracaine.[12] Multiple-dose vials still contain the preservative methylparaben, which has been implicated as a possible mediator of allergic responses.[12] Allergic reactions are characterized by either delayed appearances of skin rashes or the acute onset of localized or general urticaria. Rarely, outright anaphylactic shock can occur. True allergic responses occur in less than 1% of patients receiving local anesthetics.[13] This observation has recently been confirmed in a study of 59 patients who reported prior reactions to local anesthetic agents. None responded adversely to skin testing and provocative drug challenge.[3]

Management of Allergic Responses

Allergic responses are managed in the standard manner with airway control, establishment of intravenous access, and by administering epinephrine, diphenhydramine, and steroids as needed.

ALTERNATIVE ANESTHETIC STRATEGIES FOR THE ALLERGIC PATIENT

Because patients cannot always accurately describe a prior adverse reaction to a local anesthetic and it is usually impossible to perform skin testing in an emergency department setting, the clinician may be faced with a patient who is truly allergic to local anesthetics. The following strategies are suggested:

Use no anesthetic at all for calm patients who have very small lacerations. Often the pain of injection exceeds the pain of placing two or three sutures.

Use normal saline alone as the injecting agent. This alternative often provides for just enough anesthesia to suture small wounds.

Ice placed directly over the wound can provide a short period of decreased pain sensation.

Because the preservative methylparaben has been implicated in allergic reactions, use local anesthetic preparations prepared for spinal, epidural, and intravenous anesthesia. They are preservative free.

If the allergy-causing drug can be identified as an ester (tetracaine, benzocaine, chloroprocaine, cocaine, procaine), then it can be substituted with an amide (lidocaine, mepivacaine, bupivacaine, Benadryl).

Diphenhydramine (Benadryl) has similar anesthetic properties to standard local anesthetics. A 50 mg (1 cc) vial is dilated in a syringe with 4 cc of normal saline to produce a 1% solution. Local infiltration is carried out in the usual manner.

ANESTHETIC SOLUTIONS

There are three anesthetic solutions commonly in use for local infiltration and simple nerve block. These are lidocaine (Xylocaine® 1% and 2%, with and without epinephrine), mepivacaine (Carbocaine® 1% and 2%), and bupivacaine (Marcaine® 0.25% and 0.5%). The amide derivatives have largely replaced the older ester compounds like procaine (Novocain®).

Lidocaine (Xylocaine®)

Lidocaine is the most commonly used anesthetic solution. The drug has a rapid onset of action that is almost immediate in local infiltration. Lidocaine's tissue-spreading properties are good and it readily penetrates nerve sheaths. Duration of action for nerve blocks is approximately 75 minutes with a range of 60 to 120 minutes. Although there is no clear information in the literature concerning the duration of action for direct wound infiltration, the anesthetic effect appears to wear off much sooner, in approximately 20 to 30 minutes. A small group of patients appear to metabolize lidocaine very rapidly and require repeated local injections. With the addition of epinephrine, the duration of action is increased and local hemostasis is better achieved.[10] The maximum allowable doses of lidocaine and the other local anesthetics are summarized in Table 5-1.

Mepivacaine (Carbocaine®)

Mepivacaine is widely used as an emergency wound anesthetic but has some properties that are different than lidocaine. The drug has a slightly slower onset of action: 6 to 10 minutes for a simple block. The duration of action is 30 to 60 minutes longer than lidocaine, and this drug is preferred for longer procedures. Mepivacaine has less of a vasodilatory effect than lidocaine and usually does not require the use of epinephrine for local wound area hemostasis.

Bupivacaine (Marcaine®)

Bupivacaine is a newer amide that is not widely used in emergency wound care. Although it is a very effective anesthetic, its chief drawback is that it has slow onset of action, approximately 8 to 12 minutes for simple blocks of small nerves. The main advantage of bupivacaine is its duration of action, which is considerably longer than lidocaine and mepivacaine. In a recent study comparing lidocaine with bupivacaine, no significant difference was noted in the pain of local infiltration, onset of action, and level of satisfactory anesthesia.[8] Because the anesthesic effects of bupivacane lasted four times longer than lidocaine and significantly extended the period of pain relief, bupivacaine was recommended by the authors to be considered for anesthesia of lacerations sutured in the emergency department.

TOPICAL ANESTHESIA

Topical anesthesia is a promising method to anesthetize very simple lacerations and wounds, especially in pediatric patients. A mixture of equal parts of tetracaine (0.5%), epinephrine (1:2000 concentration), and cocaine (11.8%) can be applied directly to the wound to achieve local anesthesia. This mixture is often referred to by the acronyms TAC or TEC. A more recent investigation has found that the deletion of cocaine with a concomitant increase (to 1.87%) in the concentration of tetracaine and a decrease in the concentration of adrenaline (to 1:15,000) achieves statistically equivalent levels of anesthesia.[16] The deletion of the cocaine eliminates the concern that is usually generated in the emergency department over handling that controlled substance.

Experimentally, TAC has been associated with a higher potential for wound infection.[1] However, in a study of 158 primarily pediatric patients this potential for increased infection was not observed when TAC was compared to local needle infiltration.[15] In the study comparing TA and TAC, the rate of wound infection was 1% to 2% for each group.[16]

Technique for Topical Anesthesia

A 2 × 2 inch sponge is saturated, but should not be left dripping with the solution. The sponge is placed around and in the laceration and left for approximately 5 to 15 minutes. The parent can apply the sponge to further ease a child's fear. The maximum dose of the solution is 2 to 5 mL. Even though local infiltration analgesia has been shown to have similar efficacy when compared to TAC, occasionally supplemental infiltration is required to achieve complete anesthesia.[16,15] The chief advantage of TAC or TA, especially for children, is that no needle-stick is required. This anesthesic cannot be used on the ear, tip of the nose, or penis. A recent report of the death of a 7½-month-old infant whose nasal mucous membranes and lips were inadvertently exposed to 10 mL of the solution underscores the need to be cautious when using this method of anesthesia, especially near these highly permeable tissues.[5]

BUFFERING ANESTHETICS TO REDUCE PAIN OF INJECTION

A promising new approach to reducing the pain of local anesthetic infiltration is to add sodium bicarbonate buffer to lidocaine. The rationale is that the relatively acidic pH of lidocaine is one of the causes of pain. A recent study showed a significant reduction in the pain of injection when the pH of lidocaine, which 6.49, was corrected to 7.38.[11] Mepivacaine can be buffered in a similar manner as can lidocaine plus epinephrine.[4]

Technique for Buffering Anesthetics

Buffering of lidocaine or mepivacaine can be achieved by adding 1 mL of sodium bicarbonate (1 meq/mL solution) to 10 cc of a 1% concentration of these anesthetics.

Once buffering has been carried out, the shelf life of the lidocaine and mepivacaine is markedly reduced, and the buffered solution should be discarded and replaced after 24 hours.

PATIENT SEDATION

Several methods have been used over the years to control pediatric patients with wounds and lacerations that require emergency care and repair. These methods have ranged from "mummifying" patients with sheets and tape, to using pre-designed "papoose" boards, to "cardiac" sedative cocktails consisting of an opiate and a tranquilizer. Recently, the short-acting synthetic narcotic fentanyl (Sublimaze®) has gained favor for difficult wound repairs in children. In a series of 2000 pediatric cases with facial trauma, fentanyl sedation was used successfully to aid the emergency department repair process.[2] Of the 2000 cases, three episodes of apnea occurred that were easily reversed with airway control and the administration of naloxone. The average dose of anesthesic lasted 30 to 40 minutes, long enough in the vast majority of cases to carry out the closure. *Caution:* No parenteral sedation should ever be given without the ready availability of airway support equipment and narcotic antagonists.

Intramuscular Sedation

In a single, mixed, intramuscular injection, the following drugs can be delivered for the sedation of an uncooperative or excessively fearful pediatric patient:

Meperidine (Demerol®) 1 mg/kg
Promethazine (Phenergan®) 0.5 mg/kg

Maximum sedative benefit is achieved in 30 to 60 minutes. Although uncommon, the patient has to be carefully observed for respiratory depression. Occasionally, a patient will exhibit paradoxical excitation.

Technique for Intravenous Fentanyl Sedation

In every case where fentanyl sedation is used, the proper airway support equipment (appropriate airway cannulas, Ambu-masks, intubation blades, and endotracheal tube sizes) and narcotic reversal drugs have to be available, tested, and operational. Candidates for sedation need to have been screened for other serious medical problems, such as blood loss and head injury, in order not to increase the possibility of an untoward reaction or complication.

Either a free-running intravenous line or a heparin "well" arrangement can be used to gain venous access. The dose of fentanyl is calculated on the patient's weight at 2 to 3 µg per kg, delivered over 3 to 5 minutes. This amounts to 1 cc of fentanyl per 50 lbs. While injecting, the respirations and speech pattern of the patient are closely monitored. Most problems, particularly respiratory depression, occur as a direct result of excessive rates of administration. Another potential pitfall is being unaware of the amount of fentanyl left in the surgical tubing. A careful, slow flush of the IV line or immediate termination of infusion will eliminate unwanted, excessive infusion of the substance. Patients 18 to 36 months of age usually require the full dose. Older patients may reach adequate sedation with a smaller dose.

CHOICE OF NEEDLES AND SYRINGES

There is a large variety of needles and syringes available to deliver local anesthetics. For emergency wound care, the choices can be limited to three or four needle gauges and one or two syringe volumes.

For local, direct, and parallel wound infiltration, a 25, 27, or 30 gauge needle can be used. The least amount of pain during injection is achieved by the 30 gauge needle (the smallest in diameter of the group), which is recommended for children.[7] Depending on the amount of anesthetic required, a 6 or 10 cc syringe will usually suffice. For nerve blocks, the larger 25 gauge needle attached to a 10 cc syringe is recommended.

ANESTHESIA TECHNIQUES

Most minor lacerations and wounds can be managed by administering a local anesthetic directly into or around (parallel to) the wound area. Other wounds are best served by the application of a nerve block. The following are descriptions of the techniques of administering local anesthesics most useful for emergency wound and laceration repair.

Direct Wound Infiltration
Indications

Direct infiltration is indicated for most minimally contaminated lacerations in anatomically uncomplicated areas.

Anatomy

The proper plane of injection is immediately beneath the dermis at the junction of the superficial fascia (subcutaneous tissue; Fig. 5-1). Direct injection into the der-

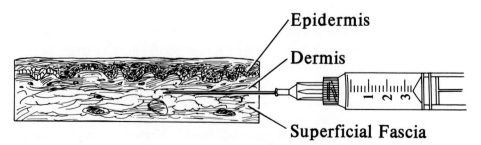

Epidermis

Dermis

Superficial Fascia

FIG. 5-1 The plane of anesthesia for local skin infiltration is just below the dermis at the junction of the superficial fascia (subcutaneous tissue).

mis has been shown to be considerably more painful as compared to injection into the superficial fascia.[14] Tissue resistance is less in this plane, and sensory nerves are easily reached by the spreading solution. Direct infiltration is less painful than other techniques because the needle does not pass through intact, sensory-active skin.

Technique for Direct Infiltration

Insert the needle through the open wound into the superficial fascia (subcutaneous fat) parallel to and just deep to the dermis (Fig. 5-2). Inject a small bolus of anesthetic solution. Remove the needle and inject another bolus at an adjacent site, but just inside the margin of anesthesia of the previous injection. This ensures greater patient comfort. Repeat this process until all edges and corners of the wound are anesthetized. A simple laceration approximately 3 to 4 cm in length will require 3 to 4 mL of an anesthetic solution.

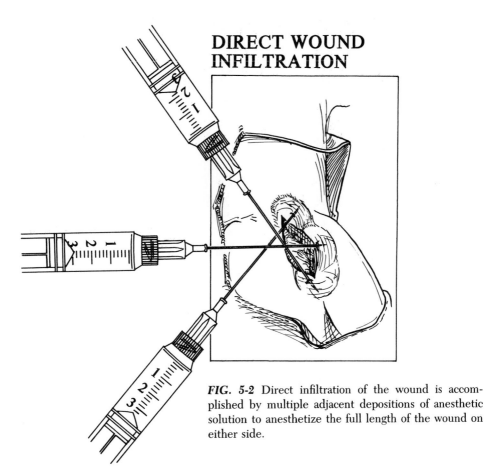

DIRECT WOUND INFILTRATION

FIG. 5-2 Direct infiltration of the wound is accomplished by multiple adjacent depositions of anesthetic solution to anesthetize the full length of the wound on either side.

Parallel Margin Infiltration (Field Block)

Indications

This technique is an alternative to direct wound infiltration and has the advantage of requiring fewer needle sticks. It is preferred in wounds that are grossly contaminated so that the needle does not inadvertently carry debris or bacteria into uncontaminated tissues.

Anatomy

The same plane as described above for direct wound infiltration is used but it is approached through intact skin.

Technique for Parallel Margin Infiltration

The needle is inserted into the skin at one end of the laceration. The needle is advanced to the hub parallel to the derma-superficial fascia plane (Fig. 5-3). Aspiration is followed by slow injection of a "track" of anesthetic as the needle is with-

PARALLEL MARGIN INFILTRATION
(Field Block)

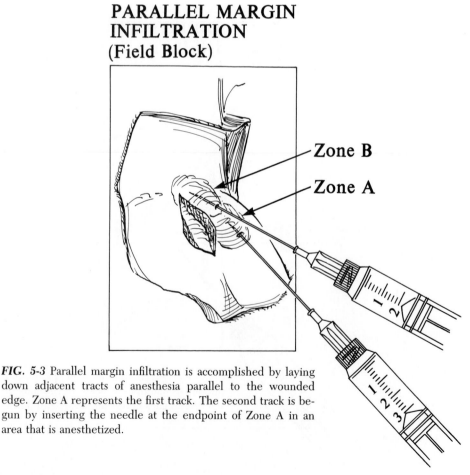

FIG. 5-3 Parallel margin infiltration is accomplished by laying down adjacent tracts of anesthesia parallel to the wounded edge. Zone A represents the first track. The second track is begun by inserting the needle at the endpoint of Zone A in an area that is anesthetized.

drawn down the tissue plane to the insertion site. The needle is then reinserted at the end of the first track where the skin is beginning to become anesthetized. The second insertion (if needed) will be less painful. Reinsertion and injection is repeated on all sides of the wound until complete infiltration has been achieved.

Supraorbital and Supratrochlear Nerve Blocks (Forehead Block)
Indications

For extensive lacerations and wounds of the forehead and anterior scalp.

Anatomy

The supraorbital and supratrochlear nerves supply sensation to the forehead and anterior scalp and exit from foramina located along the supraorbital ridge (Fig. 5-4, *A*).

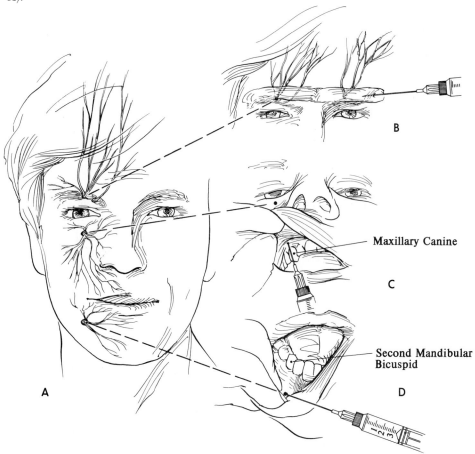

Maxillary Canine

Second Mandibular
Bicuspid

FIG. 5-4 A, Position and course of the supraorbital, supratrochlear, infraorbital, and mental nerves. **B,** Technique for deposition of anesthesia to accomplish a supratrochlear and supraorbital (forehead) nerve block. **C,** Intraoral technique to anesthetize the infraorbital nerve. **D,** Intraoral technique to anesthetize the mental nerve.

Technique for Forehead Block

The easiest manner to block the nerves as well as their many branches is to lay a continuous subcutaneous track at brow level as shown in Fig. 5-4, *B*. The actual injection technique is similar to that discussed above in the section on parallel margin infiltration.

Infraorbital Nerve Block
Indications

Lacerations of the upper lip are very common. Local anesthetic infiltration can cause anatomic distortion leading to difficulty with exact wound edge approximation and repair. An infraorbital nerve block can circumvent this problem. This block can also be used to repair lacerations of the lateral-inferior portion of the nose and lower eyelid.

Anatomy

The location and distribution of the infraorbital nerve is illustrated in Fig. 5-4, *A*. The infraorbital foramen is located approximately 1.5 cm below the inferior rim of the orbit and 2 cm from the lateral edge of the nose. This foramen can often be palpated. If not, its location can be found along an imaginary line illustrated in Fig. 5-4, *A*. This line extends from the supraorbital foramen, the nasal portion of the pupil, across the infraorbital foramen, to the corner of the mouth and over the mental foramen.

Technique for Infraorbital Nerve Block

The infraorbital nerve can be approached both intraorally and extraorally. By the intraoral route the upper lip is retracted, revealing the maxillary canine tooth. Before actual injection, the site of needle entry into the buccal mucosa can be pretreated with a topical anesthetic like viscous lidocaine (Xylocaine® viscous). A cotton-tipped applicator soaked in this solution is applied to the gingival-buccal margin for 1 to 2 minutes before the insertion of the needle. The needle is introduced at the gingival-buccal margin at the anterior margin of that tooth (Fig. 5-4, *C*). It is advanced parallel to the maxillary bone until the area of the infraorbital foramen is reached. If paresthesia results, pull the needle back slightly before injection in order to avoid injecting into the foramen and causing unwanted pressure on the nerve. One to two cc of anesthetic are deposited and anesthesia results within 4 to 6 minutes.

The extraoral route to the infraorbital nerve is less commonly used. The foramen is approached by introducing the needle directly into the skin approximately 1.5 cm below the infraorbital foramen and directing it toward the nerve. The same amount of anesthetic is injected.

Mental Nerve Block
Indications

To repair lower lip lacerations without distorting the anatomy by local infiltration.

Anatomy

The mental nerve foramen lies just inferior to the second mandibular biscuspid, midway between the upper and lower edges of the mandible, and 2.5 cm from the midline of the jaw. This nerve provides sensation to the lower half of the lip but only a portion of the chin.

Technique for Mental Nerve Block

As in the infraorbital technique, the mucosal injection site can be pre-treated with viscous lidocaine as described above for the infraorbital nerve block. The lower lip is retracted and the needle is introduced at the gingival-buccal margin inferior to the second bicuspid (Fig. 5-4, *D*). Once the foramen is approximated, 1 to 2 cc of anesthetic is injected after careful aspiration. Full anesthesia is achieved reached within 4 to 6 minutes.

Auricular Block
Indications

Lacerations of the auricle of the ear are not uncommon. The skin is tightly adherent to the cartilaginous skeleton and the deposition of an anesthesic for large or complicated wounds can be difficult or may excessively distort the local tissue relationships. The auricular block is indicated for more extensive repairs of the ear.

Anatomy

Sensory innervation of the auricle arises from branches of the auriculotemporal, greater auricular, and lesser occipital nerves. Sensory supply to the meatus derives additionally from the branch of the vagus. For this reason, an auricular block does not always completely block the meatal opening.

Technique for Auricular Block

The technical goal of the auricular block is to achieve circumferential anesthesia around the ear. Beginning just below the lobule, fully insert a 2.5 inch needle attached to a pre-loaded syringe with 10 cc of anesthetic (without adrenalin) into the sulcus behind the ear, parallel to the bone (see Fig. 5-5). Leave approximately 3 to 5 cc of anesthetic in a track back to the insertion site. Without leaving the insertion site, redirect the needle anterior to the lobule and tragus. Leave a similar track in that area. Reload the syringe if necessary. Starting at a point just behind the superior portion of the helix, leave a similar track behind the superior portion of the ear.

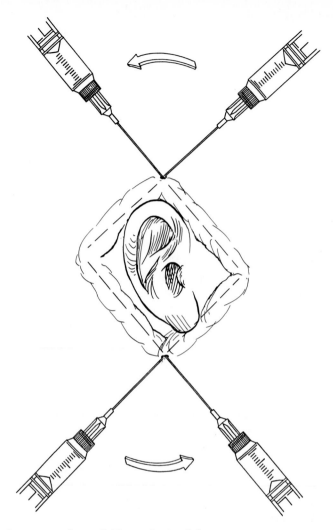

FIG. 5-5 Technique to achieve field anesthesia of the ear.

Again, without leaving the injection site, deposit a bolus of anesthetic backwards from the tragus. Anesthesia should be accomplished in 10 to 15 minutes.

Digital Nerve Blocks (Finger and Toe Blocks)
Indications

The most common nerve block in minor wound care is the digital block. The block is the anesthetic method recommended for lacerations distal to the level of the mid-proximal phalanx of the finger or toe. It is the procedure preferred for nail removal, paronychia drainage, as well as repair of lacerations of the digits.

Anatomy

There are four digital nerves for each finger or toe, including the thumb and great toe (Fig. 5-6). The palmar digital nerves have the most extensive sensory distribu-

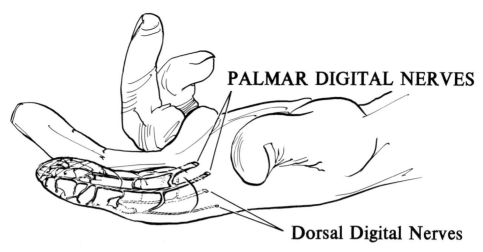

PALMAR DIGITAL NERVES

Dorsal Digital Nerves

FIG. 5-6 Illustration of the four digital nerves of the digit. Note that the two palmar digital nerves are dominant and provide sensation to the volar surface of the finger as well as the entirety of the volar pad and nail bed area.

tion and are responsible for distal finger and fingertip sensation, including the dorsum. Although the dorsal nerves have a lesser distribution, there is sufficient overlap with the palmar nerves that all four branches on each finger have to be blocked for wounds on the dorsum of the finger at and proximal to the proximal interphalangeal joint. The digital nerves are immediately adjacent to the phalanges and these structures act as landmarks for locating the nerves.

Techniques
Techniques for Digital Block

No more than a total of 4 mL of 1% lidocaine without epinephrine or 1% mepivacaine are recommended. The needle is introduced into the dorsal-lateral aspect of the proximal phalanx in the portion of the web space just distal to the metacarpal-phalangeal joint (Fig. 5-7). This precaution prevents the build up of excessive pressure on the nerves and digital blood vessels. The needle is advanced until it touches bone. Approximately .5 cc of anesthetic is delivered to the dorsal digital nerve (Fig. 5-8). The needle is then passed closely adjacent to the bone of the phalanx to the volar surface of the digit and 1 cc of solution is deposited at the site of the volar or palmar nerve. The procedure is repeated on the opposite side of the digit to achieve full finger or toe anesthesia. A complete block is usually achieved within 4 to 5 minutes.

If anesthesia is necessary only for the fingertip, then just the volar digital nerves need to be blocked. This block can be accomplished by inserting the needle into the web space, just adjacent and parallel to the affected finger. The needle is advanced proximally to the palmar aspect of the head of the metacarpal (palpable as a bony prominence in the palm, just proximal to the finger). One to two ccs of anesthetic are deposited. This process is repeated on the opposite side to complete the block of both palmar nerves.

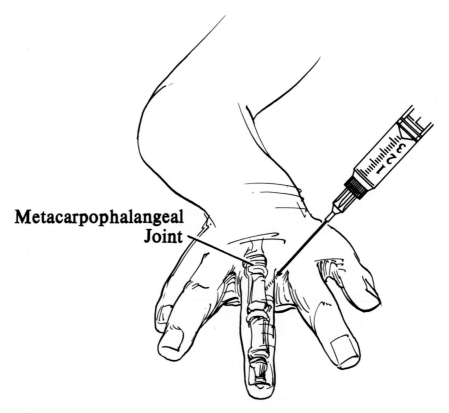

Metacarpophalangeal
Joint

FIG. 5-7 The digital nerve block is initiated by introducing the needle into the dorsal aspect of the digit just distal to the metacarpal phalangeal joint in the web space.

Alternative Toe Block Technique

Because the second to fifth toes are relatively thin at the proximal phalanx, a single midline dorsal needlestick can be used to anesthetize both sides of the toe. After depositing the anesthesic on one side, the needle is withdrawn and passed down

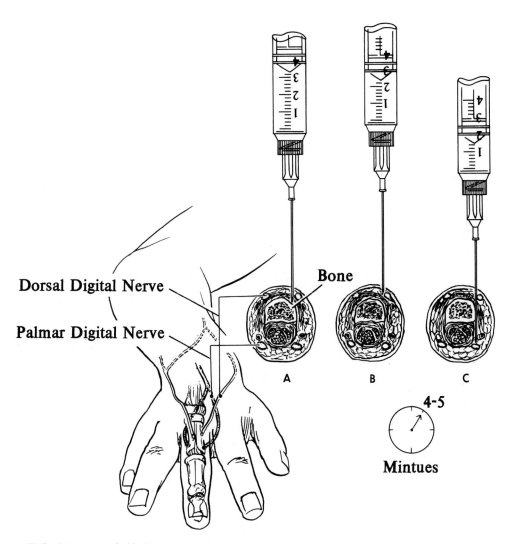

Dorsal Digital Nerve

Palmar Digital Nerve

Bone

A   B   C

4-5

Mintues

FIG. 5-8 A, One half of a cc of an anesthetic is deposited at the dorsal digital nerve after introduction of the needle as illustrated in Fig. 5-7. Note that the bone is used as a landmark to find the proper plane of the dorsal digital nerve. **B,** The needle is slightly withdrawn from the bone after injection of the dorsal digital nerve. **C,** The needle is advanced along the bone to the level of the palmar digital nerve and 1 cc of the anesthetic is deposited at that point. The process is repeated on the opposite side of the digit.

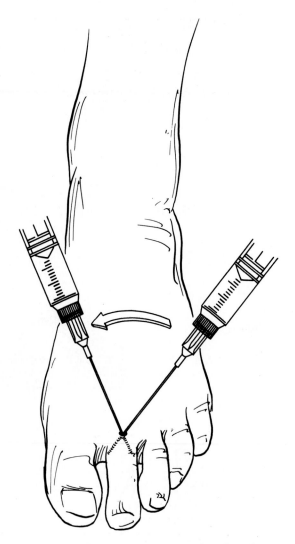

FIG. 5-9 Technique to provide anesthetic to toes other than the great toe (see text).

the opposite side without leaving the original puncture site (Fig. 5-9). Standard digital technique described above is best for the great toe.

Median Nerve Block
Indications

For lacerations and wounds of the palmar aspect of the thumb, index, and middle
fingers and the radial half of the palm.

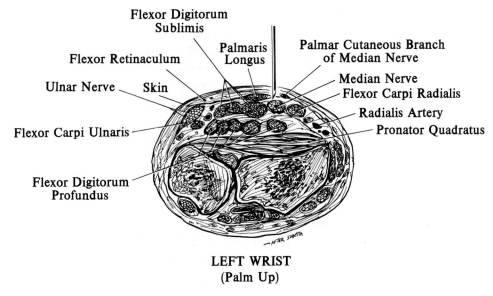

LEFT WRIST
(Palm Up)

FIG. 5-10 Cross sectional anatomy of the wrist. Note the positions of the palmaris longus, flexor digitorum sublimus, and median nerve.

Anatomy

The median nerve can be found at the proximal flexor crease of the wrist between the palmaris longus and the flexor carpi radialis tendon, closer to the latter (Fig. 5-10). The two tendons can be identified by having the patient voluntarily close his fingers into a fist and slightly flexing the wrist. Some patients do not have a palmaris longus tendon, in which case the nerve is just radial to the flexor sublimis tendons of the fingers, which usually lie below the palmaris longus tendon.

Technique for Median Nerve Block

Upon identifying the palmaris longus tendon, or in its absence, the flexor digitorum sublimis tendon at the proximal flexor crease of the wrist, the needle is introduced immediately radial to it (Fig. 5-11). The needle is passed just deep to the flexor retinaculum. An attempt is made to elicit paresthesias by passing the needle slowly deeper into the wrist. If paresthesias are elicited, 2 cc of solution is deposited adjacent to but not into the nerve. If none are elicited, 5 cc of solution is injected. Anesthesia might not be complete for at least 20 minutes.

Ulnar Nerve Block
Indications

Repair of wounds to the dorsal and palmar aspects of the hand, fifth finger, and ulnar side of the fourth finger.

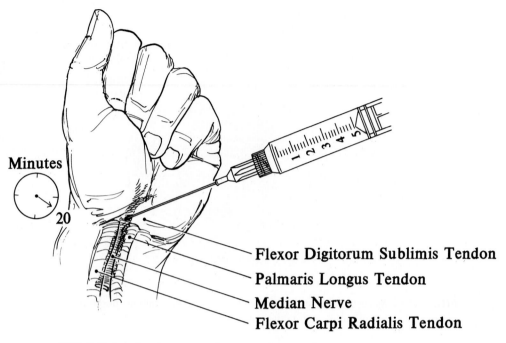

Minutes

20

Flexor Digitorum Sublimis Tendon
Palmaris Longus Tendon
Median Nerve
Flexor Carpi Radialis Tendon

FIG. 5-11 Level and position of injection for a median nerve block (see text).

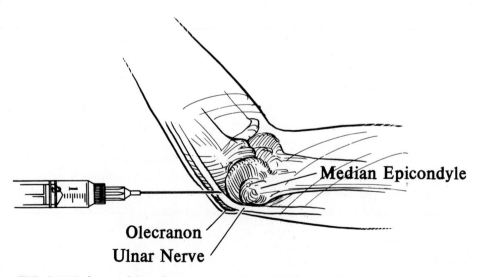

Median Epicondyle

Olecranon
Ulnar Nerve

FIG. 5-12 Technique for performing an anesthetic block of the ulnar nerve at the elbow (see text).

Anatomy

The ulnar nerve has two branches that provide sensory innervation to the ulnar side of the hand. The palmar branch of the ulnar nerve is found immediately radial to the flexor carpi ulnaris tendon at the proximal wrist crease. The dorsal branch of the ulnar nerve divides from the palmar branch approximately 4 to 5 cm proximal from the wrist and courses under the flexor carpi ulnaris tendon to the dorsal-ulnar side of the hand. Because of this division, attempts to block the nerve at the wrist are not always successful and often require blocking both branches. The easiest way to block the ulnar nerve is at the elbow where the nerve courses .5 cm below the skin between the medial epicondyle and the olecranon (Fig. 5-12).

Technique for Ulnar Nerve Block

The ulnar nerve can be palpated between the medial epicondyle and the olecranon. Inject 2 to 3 cc of anesthetic on either side of the nerve but not directly into it. Paresthesias indicate proximity; therefore, the needle has to be moved slightly away from the nerve before injection.

Radial Nerve Block
Indications

For wounds located on the dorsum of the thumb, index and middle fingers, and radial portion of the dorsum of the hand.

Anatomy

Approximately 7 cm proximal to the wrist a superficial cutaneous branch leaves the main radial nerve. At the level of the wrist, this branch begins to fan out in several rami and provides sensory innervation to the dorsal-radial aspect of the hand. The rami lie in the superficial fascia just deep to the skin.

Technique for Radial Nerve Block

Starting at the dorso-radial aspect of the wrist, a continuous subcutaneous track of anesthesic is laid down in order to block all the sensory branches (Fig. 5-13). Approximately 10 cc of anesthetic is required. Up to 5 to 10 minutes are necessary for this block to abolish sensation.

Sural and Tibial Nerve Block (Sole of Foot Blocks)
Indications

One of the most painful areas in which to inject local anesthetic is the sole of the foot. This area is commonly injured and subject to puncture wounds, lacerations, and the embedding of foreign bodies. Sural and tibial nerve blocks are recommended. These blocks are much less painful to the patient than direct infiltration.

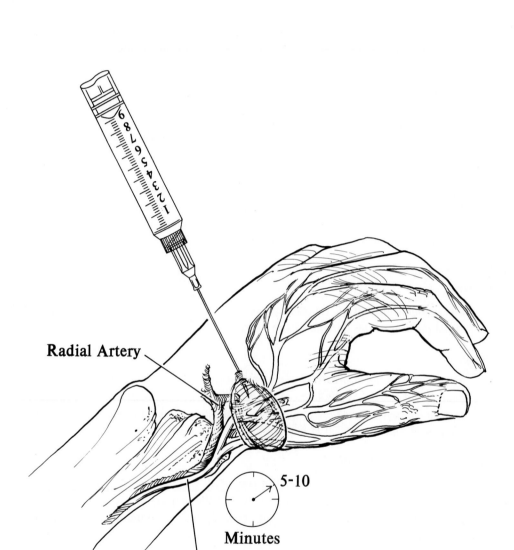

Radial Artery

5-10

Minutes

Radial Nerve

FIG. 5-13 Technique for performing a radial nerve block (see text).

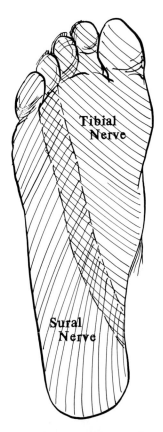

FIG. 5-14 Plantar surface of the foot. Distribution of sural and tibial nerve sensory component. Note that there is overlap between the two distributions.

Anatomy

The sural nerve courses behind the fibula and lateral malleolus to supply the heel and lateral aspect of the foot. The tibial nerve can be found between the Achilles tendon and the medial malleolus. It can be easily located because it accompanies the posterior tibial artery at that level. This nerve supplies a large portion of the sole and medial side of the foot. As denoted in Fig. 5-14, there is some overlap of distribution of these nerves as well as some overlap of sensation with the anteriorly located saphenous and superficial peroneal nerves. Complete anesthesia is not always achieved by a single block. It can be supplemented by local infiltration with minimal discomfort to the patient because of the pre-existing partial anesthesia from the block.

Technique for Sural Nerve Block

The needle is introduced just lateral to the Achilles tendon approximately 1 to 2 cm proximal to the level of the distal tip of the lateral malleolus (Fig. 5-15). The needle

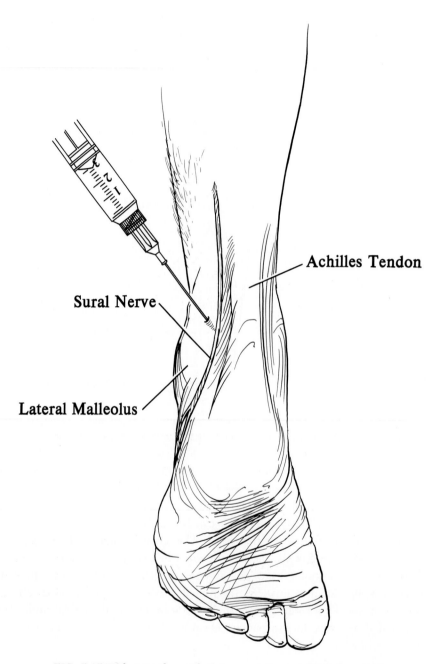

FIG. 5-15 Technique for performing a sural nerve block (see text).

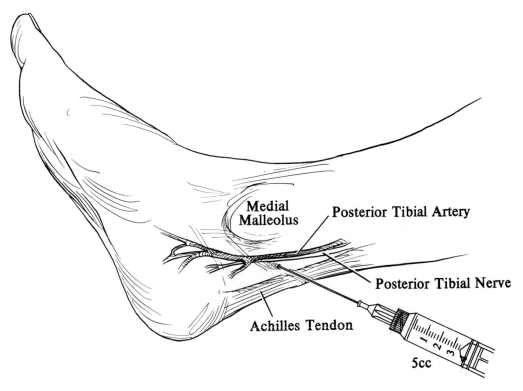

FIG. 5-16 Technique for performing a posterior tibial nerve block (see text).

is directed to the posterior medial aspect of the fibula and 5 cc of anesthetic is deposited after aspiration of the syringe. To make sure all the boundaries of the sural nerve are properly infiltrated, a fan-shaped motion is made with the needle and multiple small boluses are delivered.

Technique for Posterior Tibial Nerve Block

The posterior tibial artery is palpated as a landmark. The needle is passed adjacent to the Achilles tendon toward the posterior tibial artery behind the medial malleolus (Fig. 5-16). Once the area of the artery is approximated, careful aspiration of the syringe is carried out. If there is no blood return, 5 cc of anesthetic is injected. Blocks of the posterior tibial and sural nerve take approximately 5 to 10 minutes to achieve appropriate anesthetic levels.

References

1. Barker W et al: Damage to tissue defenses by a topical anesthetic agent, Ann Emerg Med 11:307-310, 1982.
2. Billmire DA, Neale HW, and Gregory RO: The use of intravenous fentanyl in the outpatient treatment of pediatric facial trauma, J Trauma 25:1079-1080, 1985.
3. Chandler MJ, Grammer LC, and Patterson R: Provocative challenge with local anesthetics in patients with a prior history of reaction, J Allergy Clin Immunol 79:883-886, 1987.
4. Christoph RA et al: Pain reduction in local anesthetic administration through pH buffering, Ann Emerg Med 17:117-120, 1988.
5. Dailey RH: Fatality secondary to misuse of TAC solution, Ann Emerg Med 17:159-160, 1988.
6. deJong R: Toxic effects of local anesthetics, JAMA 239:1166-1168, 1978.
7. Edlich RF, Smith JF, Mayer NE: Performance of disposable needle syringe systems for local anesthesia, J Emerg Med 5:83-90, 1987.
8. Fariss BL et al: Anesthetic properties of bupivacaine and lidocaine for infiltration anesthesia, J Emerg Med 5:275-282, 1987.
9. Goth A: Pharmacology of local anesthesia. In Medical pharmacology: principles and concepts, St Louis, 1981, The CV Mosby Co.
10. Larrabee WF, Lanier BJ, and Miekle D: Effect of epinephrine on local cutaneous blood flow, Head and Neck Surg 9:287-289, 1987.
11. MacKay W, Morris R, and Mushlin P: Sodium bicarbonate attenuates the pain on skin infiltration with lidocaine, with or without epinephrine, Anesth Analg 66:572-574, 1987.
12. Mather M and Cousins M: Local anesthetics and their current clinical use, Drugs 18:185-205, 1979.
13. Moore DC: Systemic toxic reactions to high blood levels of local anesthetic drugs. In Regional block: a handbook for use in the clinical practice of medicine and surgery, Springfield, Ill, 1976, Charles C Thomas, Publisher.
14. Morris R et al: Comparison of pain associated with intradermal and subcutaneous infiltration with various local anesthetic solutions, Anesth Analg 66:1180-1182, 1988.
15. Pryor G, Kilpatrick W, and Opp D: Local anesthesia in minor lacerations: topical TAC versus lidocaine infiltration, Ann Emerg Med 9:568-571, 1980.
16. Ross D: Personal communication, 1989.
17. Stevenson T et al: Damage to tissue defenses by vasoconstrictors, J Am Coll Emerg Phys 4:532-535, 1975.

6 Wound Cleansing and Irrigation

Wound Cleansing Solutions
  Povidone-Iodine
  Chlorhexidine
  Polaxamer 188
  Hexachlorophene
  Hydrogen Peroxide
Preparation for Cleansing
  Hand Washing for Wound Care
    Personnel
  Personnel Precautions
  Wound Area Hair Removal
  Anesthesia

Foreign Material
Wound Immersion and Soaking
Techniques for Wound Cleansing
  Materials
  Periphery Cleansing Techniques
    Technique for scrubbing the wound
      periphery
  Irrigation
    Technique for wound irrigation
  Topical Infection Control
  Debridement
References

Wound cleansing and preparation is the most important step for reducing the risk of wound infection. In wound management it is often this step that is most time consuming and tedious. It is essential, however, that all contaminants and devitalized tissue are removed prior to wound closure. If not, the risk of infection and of a cosmetically poor scar are greatly increased. Neither good suturing technique nor the use of prophylactic antibiotics can replace meticulous cleansing and irrigation, and judicious debridement.

WOUND CLEANSING SOLUTIONS

There are several commercially available skin-cleansing preparations (Table 6-1). Most of the clinical data that compare the efficacy of these agents come from studies of elective surgery patients or experiments on laboratory animals.[25,1,4,11] There is very little actual clinical information detailing the use of skin-cleansing preparations in traumatic wound settings. Nonetheless, based on the various characteristics and properties of these solutions, some guidelines for proper use can be made.

Povidone-Iodine

Povidone-iodine is a complex of the potent bactericidal agent iodine with a carrier molecule, povidone. Upon contact with tissues, the carrier complex slowly releases

Table 6-1 *Summary of Wound Cleansing Agents*

Skin Cleanser	Antibacterial Activity	Tissue Toxicity	Systemic Toxicity	Potential Uses
Povidone-iodine surgical scrub	Strongly bactericidal against gram (+) and gram (−) bacteria	Detergent can be toxic to wound tissues	Painful to open wounds Other reactions extremely rare	Hand cleanser
Povidone-iodine solution	Same as povidone-iodine scrub	Minimally toxic to wound tissues	Extremely rare	Wound-periphery cleanser
Chlorhexidine	Strongly bactericidal against gram (+) organisms, less strong against gram (−) bacteria	Detergent can be toxic to wound tissues	Extremely rare	Hand cleanser Alternative wound periphery cleanser
Polaxamer 188	No antibacterial activity	None known	None known	Wound cleanser (particularly useful on face)
Hexachlorophene	Bacteriostatic against gram (+), poor activity against gram (−) bacteria	Detergent can be toxic to wound tissues	Teratogenic with repeated use	Alternative hand cleanser
Hydrogen peroxide	Very weak antibacterial agent	Toxic to red cells	Extremely rare	Wound cleanser adjunct

free iodine. The gradual release decreases tissue irritation and reduces potential toxicity while preserving germicidal activity. Povidone-iodine is very effective against gram-positive and gram-negative bacteria, fungi, and viruses. The solution is currently in widespread use for hand washing, pre-operative skin preparation, and skin cleansing around traumatic wounds. When compared to other agents such as chlorhexidine and hexachlorophene, povidone-iodine appears to have a greater bactericidal effect against gram-negative bacteria.[1,5,11,23] However, unlike chlorhexidine and hexachlorophene, it has a shorter protective effect against bacterial buildup on the skin after hand washing and appears to be less effective than these agents for that purpose.[11,18]

Povidone-iodine is manufactured as a solution by itself (povidone-iodine solution) or in conjunction with an ionic detergent (povidone-iodine scrub preparation). The detergent in the scrub preparation appears to be toxic to several normal tissues as well as to components of an open wound.[4,8] The solution without detergent has little inherent tissue toxicity.[8] Excessive exposure of open wounds to scrub solutions, as a result of thorough scrubbing or soaking is not recommended.

A study that demonstrates the inherent lack of clinical toxicity of povidone-iodine without detergent was carried out on 225 patients undergoing ophthalmologic surgery.[2] Povidone-iodine solution, diluted to half strength with saline, was used to prepare the eye and its surrounding structures for surgery. The authors reported no corneal, conjunctival, or other tissue toxicity. In the emergency wound care setting, povidone-iodine solution, without the scrub detergent component, can be safely recommended for basic wound cleansing.

Povidone-iodine is available in several preparations. The concentration of povidone-iodine varies between 7.5% and 10% with 0.75% to 1% free iodine liberated during use. Adverse and allergic reactions are extremely rare, even when the solution is used in known iodine-allergic patients.[20]

Chlorhexidine

Chlorhexidine is an anti-bacterial biguanide that is very effective against gram-positive bacteria. This agent is also effective against gram-negative bacteria, but slightly less so than povidone-iodine.[5] Its action against viruses is uncertain.[10] Chlorhexidine is currently most often used for hand washing. Repeated use can lead to buildup on the skin and prolonged suppression of hand bacterial count.[18] Chlorhexidine is less often used for skin preparation around wounds. Under normal conditions of use, it has an exceedingly low toxicity. The skin cleanser does, however, contain an ionic detergent like the povidone-iodine scrub preparation, and direct contact with an open wound is discouraged.[2]

Polaxamer 188

A new and potentially useful wound cleanser is the non-ionic detergent, polaxamer 188 (Shur Clens®).[6] It is a surface-active agent with the cleansing properties of soap but virtually no tissue toxicity, including to the eye and cornea. Unlike povidone-iodine and chlorhexidine, it has no demonstrable adverse effects if used directly on a wound. It has been used successfully in a large trial of over 3000 patients without serious side effects.[6] The major drawback of polaxamer 188 is that it has no antibacterial activity. For this reason, alternative cleansing agents might be preferable for heavily contaminated wounds. Conversely, polaxamer 188 is very well suited for use on the face because that area is naturally resistant to infection.

Hexachlorophene

Hexachlorophene is a bacteriostatic agent with good activity against gram-positive bacteria, but it is not very effective against gram-negative organisms. Although this skin cleanser once enjoyed widespread popularity as a cleansing agent, it has been replaced by povidone-iodine and chlorhexidine. In recent years, new discoveries of its potential toxicity and teratogenicity have led to a further decline in its use.[11] Because hexachlorophene has a cumulative and protective buildup in the skin, it remains an alternative for hand washing before minor wound procedures.

Hydrogen Peroxide

Hydrogen peroxide is commonly used along with other cleansing solutions and wound preparations. Because of its inherent instability in tissue, it rapidly breaks down to water and oxygen. This reaction creates a foaming process and is thought to dislodge bacteria, debris, and other contaminants from small crevices in tissues. Hydrogen peroxide also aids in removing coagulated blood from wounds. The germicidal action of hydrogen peroxide is weak and brief at best.[10] In a controlled study of appendectomy wound incisions, hydrogen peroxide topically applied to the incision before suture closure did not reduce the infection rate when compared to the control.[12]

PREPARATION FOR CLEANSING

Before actually cleansing and irrigating a laceration or wound, several issues have to be considered. These include hand washing, personnel precautions, hair removal, anesthesia, foreign material, and wound soaking.

Hand Washing for Wound Care Personnel

Because of the unsterile nature of traumatic wounds, fixed-time hand washing with pre-operative scrubbing techniques is not necessary. Although a simple, brief hand washing will suffice before each procedure, it is necessary to make sure that the fingernails have been well cleaned because they harbor more bacteria than other parts of the hand.[7,15] Chlorhexidine appears to be a good choice for hand washing. As a skin cleaner it is well tolerated by users, it has a propensity to build up in the skin, with an accompanying prolonged antibacterial effect, and it does not stain clothing like povidone-iodine does.

Personnel Precautions

Because the process of preparing and cleansing a wound brings wound care personnel into contact with blood and other secretions, it is recommended that appropriate protective gloves and eyewear be worn at all times. Gowns are also recommended but not always practical. The main infective agents that are of concern in these settings are hepatitis B and the human immunodeficiency virus (HIV).

Wound Area Hair Removal

The practice of shaving hair around a traumatic wound remains controversial. Two studies have shown an increase in wound infection rates in shaved versus non-shaved patients, but the patients investigated had been pre-operatively shaved for surgery.[3,19] There are no data concerning shaving and traumatic wounds. Although hair shafts harbor bacteria, the deeper structures such as roots, glands, and follicles do not appear to contain high levels of organisms under normal conditions.[15] Hair can be easily and successfully cleansed using standard techniques for applying antiseptic solutions.

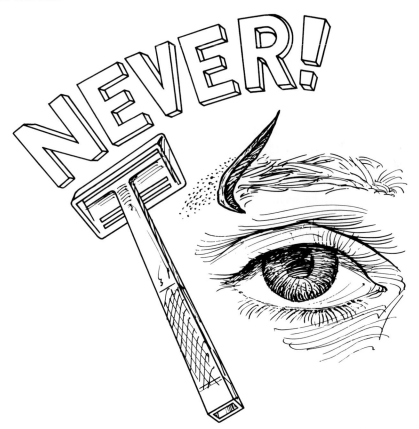

FIG 6-1 Because hair grows inconsistently on the eyebrow, this structure is never shaved.

A case for some hair removal can be made on technical grounds. In areas like the scalp it is much easier to close lacerations without having the suture material become entangled with hair. There is experimental evidence that if hair becomes inadvertently buried in wounds, infection can result.[14] Clipping hair about the wound with scissors or shaving with a razor with a recessed blade, is recommended if either of these problems should arise because these techniques reduce the chance of epidermal or dermal injuries, which can act as portals of entry for bacterial invasion and possible infection.[7]

The only site from which hair is absolutely not removed is the eyebrow (Fig. 6-1). The unpredictability of hair growth in that area makes it cosmetically important not to remove that hair. Furthermore, the eyebrow hairs provide excellent landmarks to aid in proper alignment during wound closure.

Anesthesia

Because wound cleansing can be uncomfortable if not outright painful, most wounds should be anesthetized before cleaning. Not only will the patient be more comfortable, but the cleansing can be more vigorous and possibly more effective. Techniques for administering anesthesics are discussed fully in Chapter 5.

An issue that often arises concerning the administration of anesthesics prior to wound cleansing is whether bacteria can be embedded further into a wound if a needle is passed through a contaminated surface. In clean, sharp wounds this issue is of no concern and direct wound infiltration can be safely carried out. For wounds that are visibly and heavily contaminated, the parallel injection technique or an appropriate nerve block can be used.

Foreign Material

As part of wound preparation it is very important to determine the presence or absence of foreign bodies in the wound. An alert patient can usually give an accurate history of the nature of the injury and can report the "sensation" of a foreign body still in the wound. Foreign materials of all types should be considered harmful and as having the potential for becoming infected if left in the tissues. Although irrigation will remove most debris, direct visualization and removal by instruments are often required. Radiographs are particularly useful to find tooth fragments, metallic objects, and glass. Contrary to popular opinion, glass, even as small as 0.5 mm in size, can be seen without difficulty.[24] More detail on the removal of foreign bodies is contained in Chapter 15.

Wound Immersion and Soaking

Wound soaking is a common practice in minor wound care. Soaking is believed to loosen debris, break up blood coagulum, and help sterilize the wound. However, in an experimental animal study povidone-iodine solution was unable to penetrate beyond 1.5 mm of tissue to effectively kill bacteria in spite of 20 minutes of wound soaking.[17] It was also observed that the overall bacterial count of contaminated wounds would not be sufficiently reduced by this practice. Wound soaking has some value in loosening, softening, and removing gross contaminants from the skin surrounding the wound, but it is not a substitute for thorough mechanical skin cleansing and wound irrigation.

TECHNIQUES FOR WOUND CLEANSING

As in any procedure, proper preparation is essential. The patient is placed in a comfortable position, usually supine. It is impossible to predict how he or she will react to the discomfort of wound cleansing, the sight of blood, or the appearance of a wound. Vasovagal reactions (fainting) can occur if the patient is upright. Harmful injuries can be sustained if he or she falls to the floor during the procedure. It is also prudent to ask relatives to leave the area, or, at least to watch their response to blood and the procedures that are being performed. They can have vasovagal syncope as well.

Materials

The materials necessary for wound cleansing include several 4 × 4 fine-pore sponges (90 pores per inch, as opposed to the traditional coarse gauze 45 pores per inch) an appropriate wound-cleansing solution such as povidone-iodine solution, sterile saline for irrigation, a 35-cc syringe with an attached 18-gauge needle or catheter, and two all-purpose bowls. The cleansing solution is placed in one bowl and diluted by one half with saline. Dilution decreases the overall viscosity of the wound-cleansing solution and allows for easier cleaning. Normal saline is placed in the second bowl for irrigation.

Periphery Cleansing Techniques

The main purpose of scrubbing with the wound cleanser is to clean the skin surrounding the wound. If solutions that do not have a detergent component are used, then any accidental spills into the wound are unimportant. In fact, the detergent soaked sponge can be useful in the mechanical dislodging of adherent, gross contaminants from within the wound itself. Whether periphery cleansing of the wound or irrigation of the wound should be done first has never been scientifically investigated.

Technique for Scrubbing the Wound Periphery

The actual technique for scrubbing the wound periphery is illustrated in Fig. 6-2. It is essential to be gentle and to start at the wound itself. Exposed dermis and other wound tissues should not be further damaged by overly vigorous scrubbing. The motion should be circular, with gradually larger circles away from the wound. The sponge is then discarded. At no time should the sponge be brought from the periphery back toward the wound because this maneuver will carry unwanted organ-

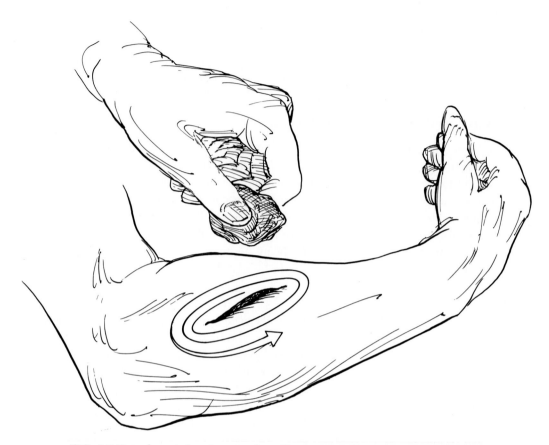

FIG. 6-2 Note the spiral technique of scrubbing a wound periphery by beginning at the center and moving away to the periphery without crossing back over the actual wound area.

isms from unsterile skin areas back to the area of the cleansed wound site. Scrubbing continues until the skin is visibly free from contaminants and dried blood. There is no specified amount of time for scrubbing, but it should last for at least 2 to 3 minutes.

Irrigation

"The solution to pollution is dilution" is an old maxim of wound care that still rings true today. Wound irrigation is probably the most effective way to remove debris and contaminants. Irrigation is also the single most effective method of reducing bacterial counts on wound surfaces.[16] In comparing methods of irrigation for highly contaminated wounds, high-pressure streams of saline are clearly superior to low-pressure streams such as those that might be obtained with a bulb-type syringe.[16,22] For "clean" wounds with low levels of contamination, some authorities recommend

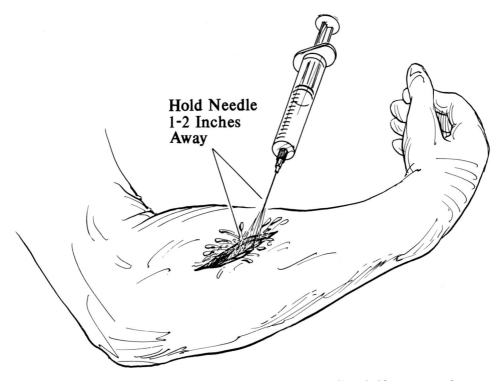

**Hold Needle
1-2 Inches
Away**

FIG. 6-3 Technique for wound irrigation. Note that the needle is held approximately 1 to 2 inches from the wound.

reducing the force of the stream to minimize any potential for unnecessary tissue trauma from the irrigation itself.[6]

Technique for Wound Irrigation

A practical and effective method of irrigation of minor wounds is through an 18-gauge needle or plastic catheter attached to a 35-cc syringe.[22] The amount of irrigation fluid can vary from 100 cc to 250 cc or more, depending on the level of contamination of the wound. Irrigation is carried out by creating a stream of saline solution (Fig. 6-3). The needle or catheter is held approximately 1 to 2 inches from the wound so that the force of the stream is not dissipated by distance. The syringe is refilled as often as is necessary to achieve maximum reduction of wound contaminants. Care is taken not to inject the needle or catheter into the wound directly and dissect irrigation solution into tissue. The goal of irrigation is to achieve a wound that has no visible gross dirt, debris, or hematoma.

Topical Infection Control

In a controlled study of 500 emergency department patients with traumatic lacerations, irrigation was followed by instillation for 60 seconds of 1% povidone-iodine solution with a sponge. The povidone-iodine was not removed through further irrigation.[9] The authors report a significantly decreased infection rate in the povidone-iodine group: 5.4% versus 15.4% for the control group. Povidone-iodine has also been delivered into surgical wounds through irrigation, and similarly reduced infection rates have been reported.[21] In another study of patients with lacerations repaired in the emergency department, the instillation of a 5% solution of penicillin directly into the wound before repair was shown to be effective in decreasing the subsequent rate of infection.[13]

Closer analysis of the emergency department studies reveals that the reported infection rates in the control groups (15.4% and 31%) are much higher than those rates (4.5% and 6.3%) found by other investigators reporting on the incidence of infection for lacerations repaired in emergency departments. Although these studies are promising, topical infection control has to be viewed with caution until further investigations are carried out. Topical application of antiinfectives cannot be clearly recommended for routine emergency wound care.

Debridement

In spite of efforts to cleanse and irrigate the wound, gross contaminants can still remain adhered to the injured tissues. If this occurs, sharp debridement should be carried out prior to closure. Removal of imbedded or adherent debris can be accomplished with tissue scissors or by scalpel excision. This procedure is more fully discussed in Chapter 8.

References

1. Berry A et al: A comparison of the use of povidone-iodine and chlorhexidine in the prophylaxis of postoperative wound infection, J Hosp Infect 3:55-63, 1982.
2. Caldwell DR et al: Povidone-iodine: its efficacy as a pre-operative conjunctival and periocular preparation, Ann Ophthalmol 16:577-588, 1984.
3. Cruse P and Foord R: A five-year prospective study of 23,649 surgical wounds, Arch Surg 107:206-209, 1973.
4. Custer J et al: Studies in the management of the contaminated wound, Am J Surg 121:572-575, 1971.
5. Dineen P: Hand washing degerming: a comparison of povidone-iodine and chlorhexidine, Clin Pharmacol Ther 23:63-67, 1978.
6. Edlich RF et al: Principles of emergency wound management, Ann Emerg Med 17:1284-1302, 1988.
7. Edlich R, Rodeheaver G, and Thacker J: Technical factors in the prevention of wound infection. In Simmons R and Howard R, eds: Surgical infectious diseases, New York, 1980, Appleton-Century-Crofts.
8. Faddis D, Daniel D, and Boyer J: Tissue toxicity of antiseptic solutions, J Trauma 17:895-897, 1977.
9. Gravett A et al: A trial of povidone-iodine in the prevention of infection in sutured lacerations, Ann Emerg Med 16:167-171, 1987.

10. Harvey S: Antiseptics and disinfectants; fungicides; ectoparasticides. In Goodman A, Goodman L, and Gilman A, eds: The pharmacologic basis of therapeutics, Macmillan Publishing Co, New York, 1980.

11. Kaul A and Jewett J: Agents and techniques for disinfection of the skin, Surg Gynecol Obstet 152:677-685, 1981.

12. Lau HY and Wong SH: Randomized, prospective trial of topical hydrogen peroxide in appendectomy wound infection, Am J Surg 142:393-397, 1981.

13. Lindsey D, Nava C, and Marti M: Effectiveness of penicillin irrigation in control of infection in sutured lacerations, J Trauma 22:186-188, 1982.

14. Mahlor D, Rosenberg L, and Goldstein J: The fate of buried hair, Ann Plast Surg 5:131-138, 1980.

15. Pecora D, Landis R, and Martin E: Location of cutaneous microorganisms, Surgery 64:1114-1117, 1968.

16. Peterson L: Prophylaxis of wound infections, Arch Surg 50:177-183, 1945.

17. Rodeheaver G et al: Bactericidal activity and toxicity of iodine-containing solutions in wounds, Arch Surg 117:181-185, 1982.

18. Rotter M, Koller W, and Wewalka G: Povidone-iodine and chlorhexidine gluconate containing detergents for disinfection of wounds, J Hosp Infect 1:149-158, 1980.

19. Seropian R and Reyolds B: Wound infections after preoperative depilatory versus razor preparation, Am J Surg 121:251-254, 1971.

20. Shelanski H and Shelanski M: PVP-iodine: history, toxicity, and therapeutic uses, J Int Coll Surg 25:727-734, 1956.

21. Sindelar WF and Mason GR: Efficacy of povidone-iodine in prevention of surgical wound infections, Surg Forum 28:48-52, 1977.

22. Stevenson T et al: Cleansing the traumatic wound by high-pressure syringe irrigation, J Am Coll Emerg Phys 5:17-21, 1976.

23. Synder I and Finch R: Antiseptics, disinfectants, and sterilization. In Craig C and Stitzel R, eds: Modern pharmacology, Boston, 1982, Little, Brown & Co.

24. Tandberg D: Glass in the hand and foot, JAMA 248:1872-1874, 1982.

25. White J and Duncan A: The comparative effectiveness of iodophor and hexachlorophene surgical scrub solutions, Surg Gynecol Obstet 135:890-892, 1972.

7 *Instruments and Suture Materials*

Basic Instruments
   Needle Holders
      Technique for handling needle holder
   Forceps and Skin Hooks
      Technique for handling forceps
   Scissors
      Technique for scissor tip control
   Hemostats

Knife Handles and Blades
Suture Materials
   Absorbable Suture Materials
   Non-Absorbable Suture Materials
   Wound Adhesives
Needle Types
References

It is not necessary to have large numbers of instruments and suture materials for emergency wound care. Wounds and lacerations can be managed with a few well-chosen instruments and a limited number of wound closure products. Although the type of instruments remains relatively constant, each wound requires careful planning in order to choose wound closure materials. Absorbable and nonabsorbable sutures as well as a variety of wound tapes and staples can be selected according to the specific patient problem. The following are guidelines for the selection of wound closure materials as well as the choice and proper handling of instruments. Tapes and staples are discussed in Chapter 13.

BASIC INSTRUMENTS

Wound care can be accomplished with the following set of instruments: needle holders, tissue forceps, skin hooks, suture scissors, dissection scissors, iris (tissue) scissors, hemostats, a knife handle, and appropriate knife blades. For simple lacerations that do not require sharp debridement or revision, a needle holder, forceps, and suture scissors will suffice. There is a bewildering variety of instruments currently available through the major suppliers of surgical instruments, but only the types and configurations of instruments necessary to manage wounds and lacerations are covered here. There are also numerous disposable instrument sets that meet the needs of many minor wound care problems.

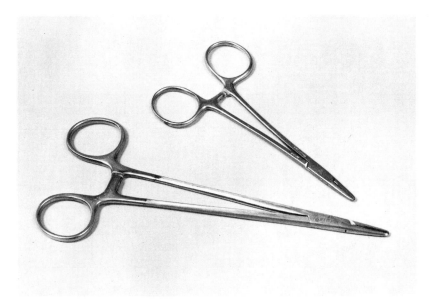

FIG. 7-1 Needle holders used in emergency wound care: 4½-inch and 6-inch Webster style needle holders with serrated carbide tipped jaws.

Needle Holders

Because most lacerations are closed with relatively small suture materials, the needle holder need not be bulky or large. A 4½-inch Webster needle holder with serrated carbide-tipped jaws can accommodate most curved suture needles (Fig. 7-1). Occasionally, large needles are used and an instrument such as a 6-inch Webster needle holder will be necessary.

Technique for Handling Needle Holder

Just as important as the choice of needle holder is the technique used for holding and arming it with the needle. Fig. 7-2 demonstrates the right and wrong way to hold the instrument during introduction of the needle into tissue. The rings are only used to clamp and unclamp the jaws by closing and releasing the locking mechanism. When introducing the needle into the skin, better precision can be gained by grasping the needle holder close to the jaws in the manner illustrated.

The needle holder is armed with the needle by closing the very tip of the jaws onto the body of the needle (Fig. 7-3). If the needle is pushed farther back into the jaws of the instrument, the curve of the body shaft will be flattened, significantly weakening the needle and making it susceptible to breakage. The needle itself is grasped at right angles, approximately one-third of the way down the body shaft from the swaged end to which the suture is attached.

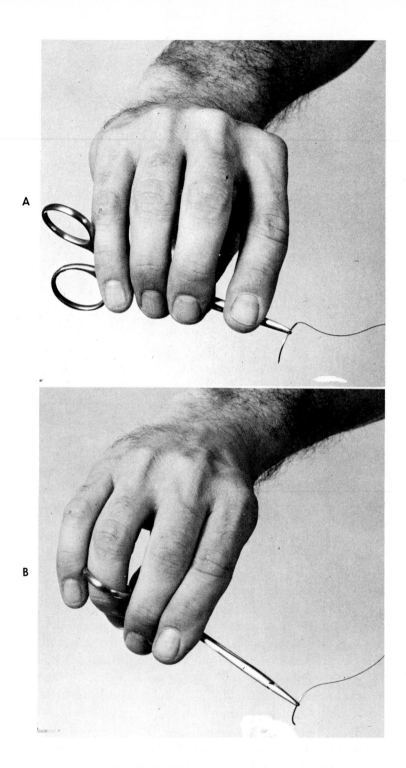

FIG. 7-2 Technique for properly holding the needle holder. **A,** The correct way allows for proper needle entry into the skin. **B,** The incorrect way—the finger holes are not used when introducing the needle holder into the skin.

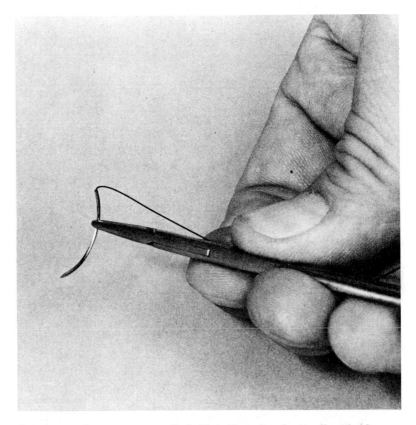

FIG. 7-3 Technique for arming a needle holder. Note that the needle is held approximately one-third of the way from the swage and is grasped at the very tip of the needle holder. The angle of the needle to the holder is exactly 90 degrees.

When placing a suture in a child or in any patient who is uncooperative or moving excessively, it is recommended that the third, fourth, and fifth fingers of the hand holding the needle holders be placed against the skin of the patient in order to brace the hand against sudden movement. As a result, when the patient moves, the operator's hand remains in the proximity of the wound edge and the suture can be placed more accurately.

Forceps and Skin Hooks

Grasping and controlling tissue with forceps or skin hooks during skin closure is essential to proper suture placement. However, whenever force is applied to skin or other tissues, inadvertent damage to cells can occur if an improper instrument or technique is used. Skin hooks are preferable to forceps because the "crushing" or "pincer" effect of forceps is eliminated. However, to use skin hooks properly, con-

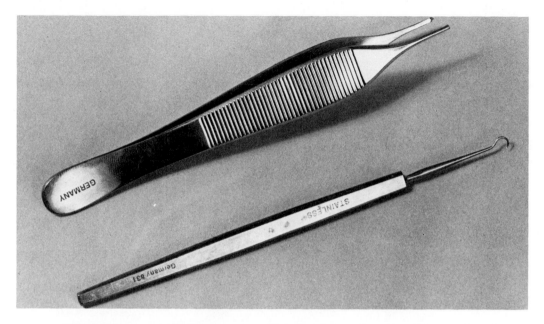

FIG. 7-4 Tissue grasping instruments: a 4¾-inch Adson, a forceps with fine teeth, and a standard plastic skin hook.

siderable skill and practice is required. Forceps are still widely used and are safe when proper technique is applied. The currently recommended forceps are 4¾-inch Adsons with small teeth (Fig. 7-4). Teeth decrease the need to apply excessive force to grasp and secure tissue. Forceps without teeth are to be discouraged because the flat surface of their jaws tends to crush tissue more easily.

Technique for Handling Forceps

When grasping tissue, the jaws of the forceps are never closed on skin. The epidermis and dermis are avoided in favor of the superficial fascia (subcutaneous tissue). By holding superficial fascia gently, the skin will be stabilized and inadvertent damage to the dermis will be avoided (Figs. 7-5 A and B).

Fig. 7-6 illustrates the correct and incorrect methods for handling forceps. The "pencil grasp" method allows for better control of the forceps and tends to diminish the amount of force delivered to tissue.

Skin hooks have the appearance of miniature retractors, but the hook portion has pointed tips to grasp dermis or superficial fascia. They are not recommended for piercing the epidermis, which creates an unnecessary puncture mark. Skin hooks are inserted directly into the wound and the hook portion is used to gain purchase on the dermis or superficial fascia. In this manner the epidermis is avoided.

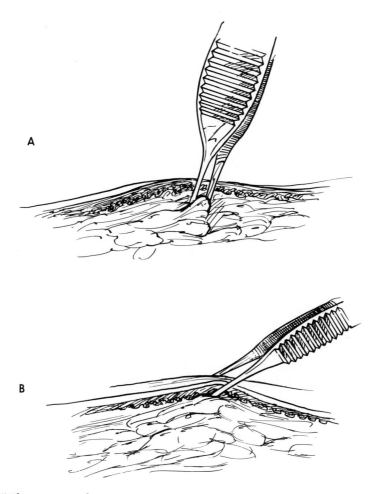

***FIG.* 7-5** The correct and incorrect way to grasp tissue with a forceps. **A,** The correct way is to grasp the tissue by the superficial fascia (subcutaneous tissue). **B,** The incorrect way to grasp tissue is by crushing the dermis and epidermis between the jaws of the forceps.

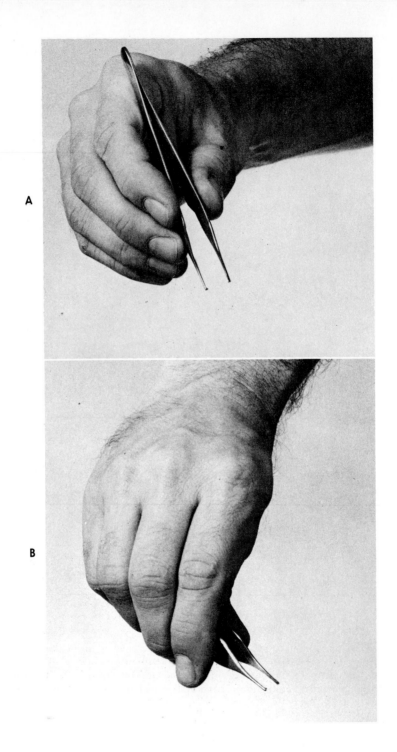

FIG. 7-6 The correct and incorrect way to hold the forceps manually. **A,** The forceps is held in the pencil grasp fashion as the correct technique. **B,** The incorrect technique is to grasp the forceps as illustrated.

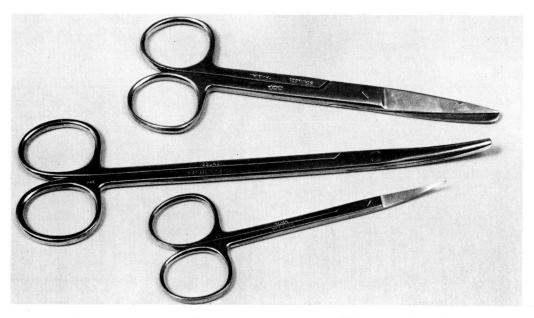

FIG. 7-7 Scissors. Top—all-purpose suture scissors; middle—Metzenbaum dissection scissors; bottom—curved iris or tissue scissors.

Scissors

There are three types of scissors that are useful in minor wound care: iris or tissue scissors, dissection scissors, and suture scissors (Fig. 7-7). Four-inch iris scissors, both curved and straight, are predominantly used to assist in wound debridement and revision. These scissors are very sharp and are appropriate in situations that require very fine control. They are, however, very delicate and are not recommended for cutting sutures. Occasionally during suture removal, however, when very small sutures have been used in the face area, iris scissors can be used for their removal.

For heavier tissue revision, as might be necessary for wound undermining, blunt-tipped 6-inch Metzenbaum dissection scissors are recommended. Iris scissors are too small and delicate for this task and the larger Metzenbaums can overcome this shortcoming.

Standard 6-inch, single blunt-tip, double-sharp suture scissors are most useful for cutting sutures, adhesive tape, sponges, and other dressing materials. Because of their size and bulk, these scissors are very durable and practical.

Technique for Scissor Tip Control

Whenever scissor-tip control is essential, such as cutting close to the knots of deep or dermal closures with absorbable sutures, the technique illustrated in Fig. 7-8 is

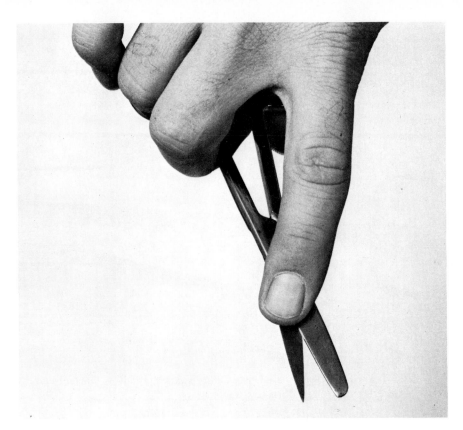

FIG. 7-8 Proper technique for tip control for scissors.

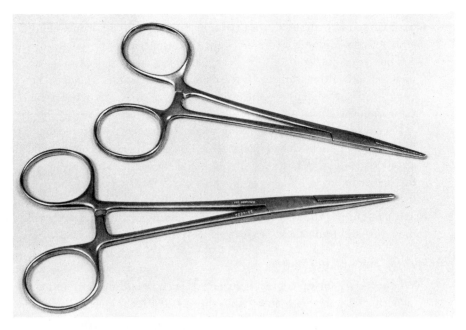

FIG. 7-9 Hemostats. Top—mosquito hemostat; Bottom—standard hemostat.

recommended. The tips of the scissors are brought gently down to the knot. Just prior to cutting, the tips are rotated slightly to avoid cutting the knot itself.

Hemostats

Hemostats have three functions in minor wound care. Originally, hemostats were designed to clamp small blood vessels for hemorrhage control. Another use is to grasp and secure superficial fascia during undermining and debriding wounds. Finally, this instrument is an excellent tool for exposing, exploring, and visualizing the deeper areas of a wound. Two types of hemostats are commonly used in wound care (Fig. 7-9). For general use, the standard hemostat is recommended. Finer work in small wounds is often best served by the 5-inch curved mosquito hemostat with fine serrated jaws.

Knife Handles and Blades

The choice of a knife handle can be limited to the #3 standard Bard/Parker®-style knife handle. Generally three blade configurations are necessary for a variety of tasks (Fig. 7-10). The #10 blade is not commonly needed in minor wound care but occasionally is helpful for larger excisions during wound revision. Very commonly used and quite versatile is the #15 blade. It is small and well suited for precise debridement and wound revision. This blade is also preferred for foreign-body excision as well as the intricate work necessary around eyes, lips, ears, and fingertips. The #11 blade is configured ideally for incision and drainage of superficial ab-

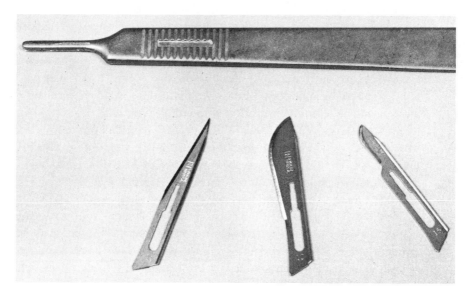

FIG. 7-10 Knife handle and #11 (left), #10 (middle), #15 (right) knife blades.

scesses. It can also be used to help remove very small sutures such as those that might be placed in the face.

SUTURE MATERIALS

There are several criteria that must be met before a particular suture can be used to close lacerations. A good suture must have appropriate tensile strength to resist breakage, good knot security to prevent unraveling, pliability and workability in handling, low tissue reactivity, and the ability to resist bacterial infection. Currently there are two main classes of suture materials: absorbable and non-absorbable. Each type has a variety of materials that meet these criteria.

Absorbable Suture Materials

Polyglycolic acid, PGA (Dexon®) currently enjoys widespread use as an absorbable suture material. PGA is a synthetic, braided polymer. When compared to plain or chromic catgut, PGA is much less reactive and is experimentally better able to resist infection from contaminating bacteria.[4] PGA has excellent knot security and maintains at least 50% of its tensile strength for 25 days.[9] The main drawback of PGA is that it has a high friction coefficient and "binds and snags" when wet. For this reason, some experience is required to properly pass this material through tissues and "seat" the throws during knotting.

Recently, the manufacturer has modified PGA (Dexon Plus®) by coating it with polaxamer 188, an agent that significantly reduces the friction and drag through tissues. Although handling has become easier with this modification, more throws (4 to 6) are required to prevent knot slippage than for plain PGA (3 to 4). The main uses of PGA are for single deep (dermal) closures of superficial fascia (subcutaneous tissue) in wounds as well as ligature of small bleeding vessels to effect hemostasis.

An older but less commonly used absorbable suture material is gut. Gut is an organic material manufactured from sheep intestines. A newer form of this suture is gut treated with chromium trioxide to retard absorption in tissues. When compared to PGA, plain gut and chromic gut appear to have inferior tensile strength and wound security.[6,9] The main use of chromic gut is to close lacerations within the oral mucosa. Wounds within the bounds of the oral cavity tend to heal rapidly and do not require prolonged suture support. Chromic gut is more rapidly absorbed than PGA on the oral mucosa and does not need suture removal.[5] Polyglactin-910, PG 910 (Vicryl®) is another braided synthetic polymer used for deep closures. It has similar dry tensile strength when compared to PGA, but maintains in vivo strength somewhat longer. On the other hand, PGA has greater knot security.

Two monofilament absorbable suture materials, polyglyconate (Maxon®) and polydioxanone (PDS®), which have been recently introduced, have some advantages over PGA and polyglactin-910. The main advantage of the new monofilaments is that they maintain their in vivo tensile strength longer than the braided materials.[3,8] They also appear to have greater knot security and lower friction coefficients, which can make them easier to work with in tissues. Because they are monofilaments, they enjoy the theoretic advantage of creating a lower potential for infection. These new materials have excellent characteristics and have the potential to replace older, braided sutures.

Non-Absorbable Suture Materials

Of all the non-absorbable suture materials, monofilament nylon (Ethilon®, Dermalon®) is the suture that is most commonly used in surface, percutaneous closure. The monofilament configuration makes it minimally tissue reactive and able to resist infection from experimental wound contamination when compared to braided suture material.[4] Nylon has tensile strength that ensures wound security. The main disadvantage of nylon is the difficulty in achieving good knot security. Because monofilaments have greater memory (the tendency to return to their packaged shape) than braided sutures, they tend to unravel if not tied correctly. Therefore, at least 4 to 5 carefully fashioned "throws" or knots are required to achieve a secure final knot.

The polymer polypropylene (Prolene®) is another non-absorbable monofilament. Polypropylene appears to be stronger than nylon and has better overall wound security.[9] It is also less reactive and is able to resist infection at least as well as nylon.[4] However, it has greater memory than nylon and is somewhat more difficult to work with. The main uses of polypropylene are for percutaneous and pull-out dermal closures.

A new and interesting monofilament suture material is polybutester (Novafil®).[2] Polybutester appears to be stronger than other monofilaments. This material does not have significant memory and therefore does not maintain its packaging shape like nylon and polypropylene do. For this reason it is reported to be easier to work with and has greater knot security. A unique feature of polybutester is that it has the capacity to elongate or "stretch" with increasing wound edema. Once the edema subsides, polybutester resumes its original shape.

Less commonly used for minor wound care problems are the braided, non-absorbable suture materials. These include cotton, silk, braided nylon, and multifilament dacron. Until the advent of synthetic fibers, silk was the mainstay of wound closure. It is the most workable of sutures and has excellent knot security. The usefulness and popularity of silk has declined, however, because of its propensity for causing tissue reactivity and infection.[4,9] Research has shown that like silk, the braided synthetics have a greater tendency to cause wound infection when exposed to contaminating bacteria.[1,4] These materials, however, have excellent workability and knot security. Because of the latter properties, braided sutures have some usefulness on the face where maximal control and precision are needed. The earlier removal time of facial sutures and the natural resistance of the face to infection make the chance of inflammation and infection developing almost negligible.

Wound Adhesives

A new approach to closing traumatic wounds in the emergency setting is by the use of a tissue adhesive. Tissue adhesives have been used for closing surgically made incisions, but only recently has one been reported to successfully close scalp lacerations.[7] In a study of 50 patients with clean, sharp traumatic lacerations that were less than 6 hours old and less than 6 centimeters in length, 49 were reported to have healed fully without developing infection or any other complication. One 3 mm dehiscence was noted that required no further treatment. The adhesive used was histo acryl, a biodegradable butyl-2-cyanoacrylate monomer. This compound does have its disadvantages. It generates heat during bonding that can potentially cause tissue damage and patient discomfort. It also bonds so rapidly (within 20 seconds) that revision of the closure is precluded once the edges are apposed. Clearly this method needs extensive investigation before it can be recommended for general use in traumatic wound care.

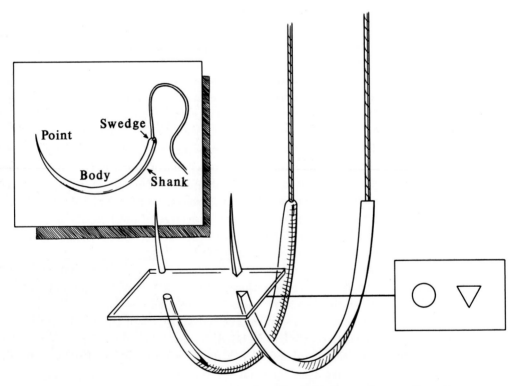

FIG. 7-11 Basic needle configurations: Left—the standard round, tapered needle; Right—the reverse cutting needle. Note that the sharp edge is on the convex portion of the needle.

NEEDLE TYPES

Like instruments and suture materials, there is a bewildering variety of needles manufactured for wound closure. However, the vast majority of wound closures can be accomplished with a limited number of needles. Curved needles have two basic configurations: tapered and cutting (Fig. 7-11). For wound and laceration care, the cutting needle is used almost exclusively. What are now commonly referred to as cutting needles are in fact reverse cutting needles. The needle is made in such a way that the outer edge is sharp so as to allow for smooth and atraumatic penetration of the skin and the inner portion is flattened so that the needle puncture wound is not inadvertently enlarged as the suture passes through the hole and the knot is tied.

Needles come in two grades, cuticular and plastic. These differ significantly in their usefulness for wound care. Cuticular needles are less expensive but noticeably less sharp than plastic grade needles. The increased sharpness of plastic needles allows the operator to better control entry and passage of the needle through tissues. Plastic needles are also less traumatic. Although they are more expensive, these needles are recommended for emergency wound and laceration repair. There is a bewildering number of code designations for needles. Cuticular needles can be recognized by the letters C (cuticular) or FS (for skin). Plastic grade needle codes usually start with the letter P.

References

1. Alexander J, Kaplan J, and Altemeier W: Role of suture materials in the development of wound infection, Ann Surg 165:192-199, 1967.
2. Bernstein G: Polybutester suture, J Dermatol Surg 14:615-616, 1988.
3. Bourne RB, Bitar H, and Andreae PR: In vivo comparison of four absorbable sutures: Vicryl®, Dexon Plus®, Maxon®, and PDS®, Can J Surg 31:43-45, 1988.
4. Edlich R et al: Physical and chemical configuration of sutures in the development of surgical infection, Ann Surg 177:679-687, 1973.
5. Holt G and Holt J: Suture materials and techniques, Ear Nose Throat J 60:23-30, 1981.
6. Howes E: Strength studies of polyglycolic acid versus catgut sutures of the same size, Surg Gynecol Obstet 137:15-20, 1973.
7. Morton RJ, Gibson MF, and Sloan JP: The use of tissue adhesive for the primary closure of scalp wounds, Arch Emerg Med 5:110-112, 1988.
8. Rodeheaver GT et al: Mechanical performance of monofilament synthetic absorbable sutures, Am J Surg 154:544-547, 1987.
9. Swanson N and Tromovitch T: Suture materials 1980s: properties, uses, and abuses, Int J Dermatol 21:373-378, 1982.

8 Decisions Before Closure—Timing, Debridement, and Consultation

Timing of Closure
   Primary Closure (Primary Intention)
   Secondary Closure (Secondary Intention)
   Tertiary Closure (Delayed Primary
     Closure)
     Technique for delayed primary closure
Wound and Laceration Exploration
   Techniques for wound exploration
Hemostasis
   Tourniquet Hemostasis
     Indications
     Technique for large-extremity
       tourniquet application

Technique for digital tourniquet
   application
Tissue Debridement and Techniques
   Debridement
     Technique for simple debris excision
     Technique for excision of damaged
      dermis
     Technique for full wound excision
Surgical Drains
Indications for Intravenous Antibiotic
   Therapy
General Guidelines for Consultation
References

Before repair of a wound or laceration is initiated, a thorough evaluation of the patient must be completed. Initial patient evaluation and stabilization is discussed in Chapter 1. After patient evaluation is completed, the next step is to perform a complete evaluation of the wound site and the surrounding or related anatomic structures. To carry this out, specific patient care decisions need to be made prior to wound closure, and they are determined by the answers to the following questions:

What is the proper timing of wound closure—primary, delayed, or open?
Which wounds need invasive exploration?
What are the appropriate measures to achieve wound hemostasis to facilitate exploration and repair?
What is appropriate tissue debridement?
What are the indications for immediate intravenous antibiotic administration?
When should consultation be obtained?

TIMING OF CLOSURE

Determining the time of injury is important to wound repair. The chance of developing a wound infection increases with each hour that elapses from the time of injury.[12] It has been traditionally believed that there is a "golden period" within which a wound or laceration can be safely closed primarily (primary intention). The exact length of that period is influenced by such factors as the mechanism of injury, anatomic location, and level of contamination. As a rough guideline, 6 to 8 hours from the time of injury is thought to be a safe time interval within which to repair the average uncomplicated laceration. However, this can vary from as little as 3 hours for heavily contaminated wounds of the foot to 24 hours for clean lacerations of the face. Determination as to whether a wound can be closed primarily is best made after wound preparation measures have been performed. As a general rule, if a wound cannot be adequately cleansed, irrigated, and debrided to appear clean and "fresh", then careful consideration has to be given to alternative methods of wound management. The methods of primary, secondary, and tertiary closure are described below (Fig. 8-1). Each discussion sets forth guidelines to assist in the decision concerning the timing of closure.

Primary Closure (Primary Intention)

Primary closure can only be done on lacerations that are relatively clean and minimally contaminated, with minimal tissue loss or devitalization. These wounds are most often created by shearing forces. They can be closed with sutures, wound tapes, or staples. Repair of these wounds is usually necessary within 6 to 8 hours from the time of injury on most regions of the body. For the feet, this period might be somewhat shorter, specially if the wound is deep. Hand lacerations also need careful assessment relative to the time of injury because they tend to have a higher rate of infection.[7,13] Wounds of the highly vascular face and scalp can often be sutured up to 24 hours after injury.[9] Because there are no hard and fast rules that govern every possible situation, the following recommendation is offered: any injury that can be converted to a fresh-appearing, slightly bleeding, non-devitalized wound, with no visible contamination or debris after aggressive cleansing, irrigation, and debridement, is a candidate for primary closure.

Secondary Closure (Secondary Intention)

Skin infarctions, ulcerations, abscess cavities, punctures, small cosmetically unimportant animal bites, and partial-thickness (dermal base preserved) tissue losses are often better left to heal by secondary intention. They are not closed with sutures and are allowed to gradually heal by granulation and eventual re-epithelialization. After an appropriate program of wound care, they can become candidates for later skin coverage, if necessary, by grafting. These wounds have a pronounced inflammatory response and are prone to significant wound contraction over time.

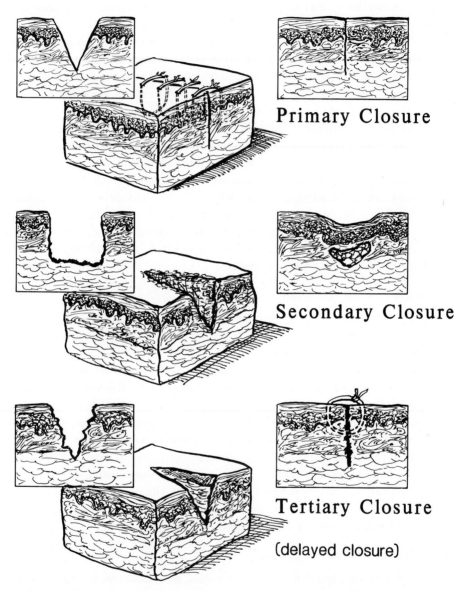

Primary Closure

Secondary Closure

Tertiary Closure

(delayed closure)

FIG. 8-1 Primary closure is accomplished by closing the wound with sutures at the time of presentation to the Emergency Department. Secondary closure occurs as a result of natural healing without intervention other than cleansing and debridement. Tertiary closure (delayed primary closure) is carried out approximately 4 to 5 days after the injury.

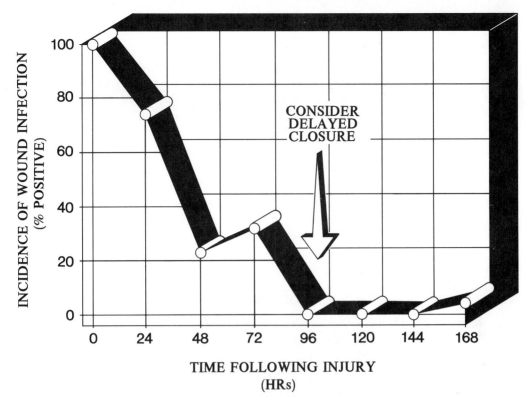

FIG. 8-2 Graph illustrating the incidence of wound infection risk after injury, and optimal timing of tertiary or delayed wound closure. (Adapted from R Edlich et al, *A manual for wound closure*, St Paul, Minn, 1979, Surgical Products Division, 3M Co.)

Tertiary Closure (Delayed Primary Closure)

There are some wounds that can be closed with sutures or tapes after being cleansed, debrided, and observed for 4 to 5 days.[2,8] These are wounds that are too contaminated to close primarily, but have not suffered significant tissue loss or devitalization. Wounds that fall into this category are often older, excessively contaminated with soil, feces, saliva or vaginal secretions, caused by human or animal bites (see Chapter 14 for detailed discussion of bite wounds), or the result of high-velocity missiles, such as bullets. Wounds created after exploration for and removal of non-inert foreign bodies are also candidates. The rationale for closure after four days is shown in Fig. 8-2, which illustrates the incidence of wound infection following delayed closure at varying times from the original injury.

Technique for Delayed Primary Closure

Cleanse, irrigate, and debride as much as possible during the initial encounter. Pack the wound with saline-moistened fine mesh or Xeroform® gauze. Cover the wound with bulky, absorbent gauze dressing. If no signs of infection or excessive discomfort become evident, uncover and inspect the wound after 4 to 5 days. If the wound appears clean and uninfected, then it can be closed with percutaneous skin closures or wound tapes. Dermal (deep) or subcutaneous sutures are usually avoided.

If the wound has accumulated some impeding granulation tissue over the 4-day period, it can be judiciously excised to permit better wound edge apposition. Occasionally, the wound is amenable to complete excision at this time to ensure the best cosmetic result. Often oral antibiotics are administered after initial care prior to delayed closure. Dicloxacillin or one of the first-generation cephalosporins are appropriate choices. Erythromycin can be given to patients who have a significant history of allergy to the penicillins. The choice of whether to give antibiotics or not is individualized depending on the patient.

WOUND AND LACERATION EXPLORATION

Surface wounds and lacerations require thorough inspection and direct exploration if necessary. It is important always to evaluate the functional status of the relevant nerves, tendons, arteries, joints, or other related structures of the wounded area and to remain suspicious for potentially occult, serious underlying structural damage. Although more specific information is included in other chapters and sections specific to special anatomic sites and problems, the following guidelines are offered as general indications for wound exploration:

Suspicion of a foreign body, particularly if it is potentially not inert, such as wood or plant material. Radiographs taken before exploration are particularly useful in revealing the presence of glass, gravel, and metallic foreign bodies. They are *not* helpful for finding organic debris and splinters.

Lacerations in the proximity of joint capsules.

Lacerations over tendons, specially if the functional testing of the hand is "normal." It is not uncommon to reveal serious partial tendon lacerations only by direct visualization. Unrepaired, partially lacerated tendons can undergo delayed rupture within 12 to 48 hours.

Scalp lacerations that are large or are caused by a significant force. Unrecognized skull fractures can be revealed by exploration and palpation of the skull through the wound.

Lip lacerations, if a tooth or fragment of a tooth cannot be accounted for. X-ray is another method to reveal missing teeth.

Lacerations of the upper eyelids can penetrate the orbital septum and sever the levator palpebrae muscle. The presence of periorbital fat upon exploration raises the possibility that one of those two injuries has occurred.

Techniques for Wound Exploration

Often the wound can be adequately exposed with a hemostat by separation of the wound edges. In other cases, the hemostat can be used to grasp the superficial fascia (subcutaneous tissue) of one wound edge while the tissue forceps is applied to the other edge to retract and gain exposure. If available, small self-restraining retractors (Mastoid or Wheatlander retractors) are recommended. Optimally, a second pair of hands can assist in the process, that is, an assistant can retract the wound with small Ragnell retractors or skin hooks.

If exposure is still not adequate, then a small wound extension incision can be made through the dermis with a knife handle and a #15 blade or with iris scissors. The extension begins at one wound end and should proceed parallel to structures such as nerves or tendons in the hand in order to minimize accidental injury (see Fig. 8-3). In other areas of the body, it is made parallel to the skin tension lines discussed in Chapter 2. Depending on the original orientation of the laceration this extension might create just a longer wound or a corner effect.

The superficial fascia (subcutaneous tissue) is not incised but is gently spread apart with forceps or tissue scissors, without damaging deeper functional structures, to reveal any suspected tendon or joint capsule injury, or foreign body.

HEMOSTASIS

Often wounds bleed actively, particularly during assessment and exploration. In addition to the problem of adequate wound visualization with active bleeding, hematomas can cause an increase in the rate of wound infection and delay the healing process.[1]

The simplest and most effective way to stop bleeding is by applying direct pressure to the wound with hand-held 4×4 sponges. Continuous pressure has to be applied for a minimum of 10 minutes. Because of the time involved, 4×4 sponges secured with an Ace wrap can be substituted if the wound is in an anatomic area that lends itself to wrapping. Mixing epinephrine 1:1000 with 5 mL of normal saline and applying a moistened sponge for five minutes to the wound will often suffice in cases where pressure fails. Epinephrine is, however, contraindicated for use on the fingers, toes, ears, penis, and tip of the nose. Packing the wound with the hemostatic agent Gelfoam® is another hemostatic strategy.

Direct clamping with a hemostat and a hand-tied ligature with an absorbable suture is reserved for larger, single bleeding vessels that can be directly visualized under optimal conditions of lighting, instrument preparation, and operator comfort. "Blind" clamping in a bleeding wound, in hopes of grasping the bleeder, is strongly discouraged. Unnecessary tissue damage can occur, particularly in areas where important structures like nerves and tendons are likely to be found.

Definitive hemostasis of the extremity can be achieved by the use of tourniquets

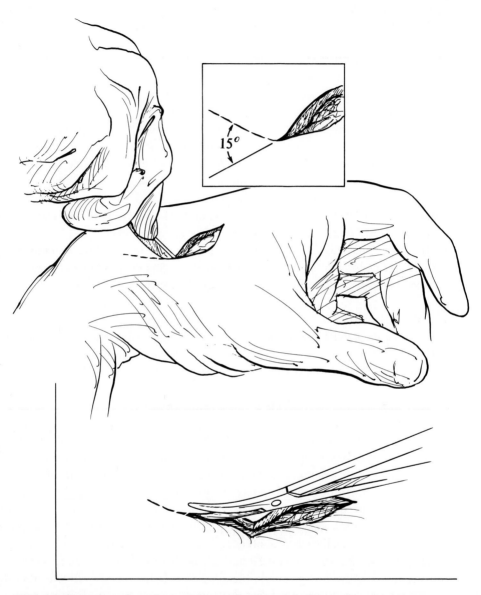

FIG. 8-3 Illustration of a technique to extend a wound for better deep-structure exploration and evaluation. Note that the incision is at a slight angle from the original axis of the wound and parallel to underlying structures.

with the strict observance of proper technique and the time limits of application. Complications of tourniquets include potential ischemia of the extremity, compression damage of blood vessels and nerves, and jeopardy to marginally viable tissues.[8]

Tourniquet Hemostasis
Indications

To more easily and correctly identify anatomic structures such as tendons, joint capsules, nerves, and vessels as well as to locate difficult-to-find foreign bodies. Debridement of marginally devitalized tissue is not carried out in a bloodless field because the distinction between exsanguinated and truely ischemic tissue cannot easily be made.

Technique for Large-Extremity Tourniquet Application

Prior to placement of a single-cuff sphygmomanometer, elevate the extremity. Firmly apply an elastic bandage by starting at the fingers or toes and proceeding proximally to the site of the anticipated site of cuff placement, preferably the upper arm or thigh. Inflate the cuff to a pressure higher than the patient's systolic pressure but do not exceed 250 mm Hg. Clamp the cuff tubing instead of closing the air release valve in order to prevent slow leakage of air and to ensure a rapid release method if needed. Remove the elastic bandage and proceed with the exploration. The purpose of the elastic bandage is to prevent venous back-flow bleeding.

Patient discomfort will become apparent by 30 to 45 minutes of cuff time, but hopefully the procedure will have been completed.[11] The maximum cuff inflation time is 1 hour.

Technique for Digital Tourniquet Application

Unfold a 4 × 4 gauze sponge to its fullest length and fold it in half so it appears to be an 8-inch band. Moisten that band with saline. Wrap the band firmly around the finger, starting at the tip and proceeding to the base. Stretch a Penrose drain around the base of the finger in a sling-like fashion and apply a hemostat to the drain to form a tight "ring" at the base of the finger. Remove the sponge wrapping. A Penrose drain can also be substituted for the gauze sponge wrap.

There are pre-formed rubber disposable tourniquets that "roll" onto the finger and exsanguinate it before coming to rest at the digit base. After use, they can be easily severed and released. These tourniquets are easier to apply and effective in most cases where the digit circumference can accommodate them.

The maximum allowable tourniquet time for a finger is 20 to 30 minutes.

TISSUE DEBRIDEMENT AND TECHNIQUES

Before actual suturing and knot-tying, the wound has to be made free of contaminants and devitalized tissue. Devitalized tissue can be recognized by its shredded, ischemic, blue or black appearance. Occasionally, these appearances can be misleading and true demarcation between viable and devitalized tissue cannot be made until 24 hours following wounding.[3] Therefore, one overriding principle of wound debridement is to spare as much tissue as possible immediately after the injury. Further excision and modification of the wound can be made at later interventions. If consultant surgeons are needed to perform wound revisions, they will be grateful for as much preserved tissue as possible.

Static skin tension plays an important role in wound edge debridement and revision. It is tempting to want to excise jagged wound edges to convert an irregular laceration into a straight one. If the wound is already gaping because of static tension, then debridement of tissue might increase the tension necessary to pull the straight edges together. The result might be worse than just closing the wound with minimal tissue removal. See Chapter 2 for further discussion of skin tension.

Debridement
Technique for Simple Debris Excision

Most debridement can be carried out by simple, judicious excision of debris-laden tissue, using tissue forceps and iris scissors (Fig. 8-4). Superficial fascia (subcutane-

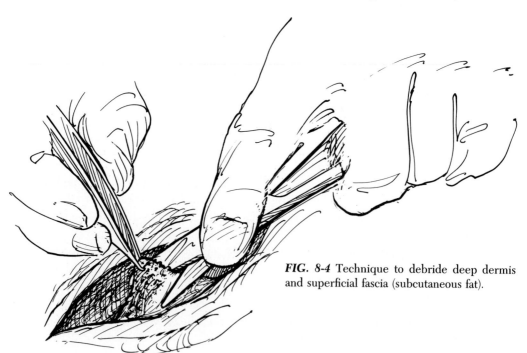

FIG. 8-4 Technique to debride deep dermis and superficial fascia (subcutaneous fat).

ous fat) under the dermis can be freely excised without any concern for cosmetic results. Soiled, devitalized fatty tissue is a fertile substrate for the growth of bacteria with subsequent development of infection.[6]

Technique for Excision of Damaged Dermis

More care has to be taken in debriding and excising epidermis and dermis. The best principle is to trim as little skin as possible, particularly on the face. It is preferable to replace small bits of wound edge in a jigsawlike pattern than to excise a ragged wound only to be left with a contracted scar that sinks below the plane of the epidermis during healing. Incident light that strikes a pitted scar calls attention to this noticeable cosmetic defect.

The proper method to trim a dermal wound edge is illustrated in Fig. 8-5. Iris (tissue) scissors or a #15 blade can be used. The wound edge is cut or incised at a

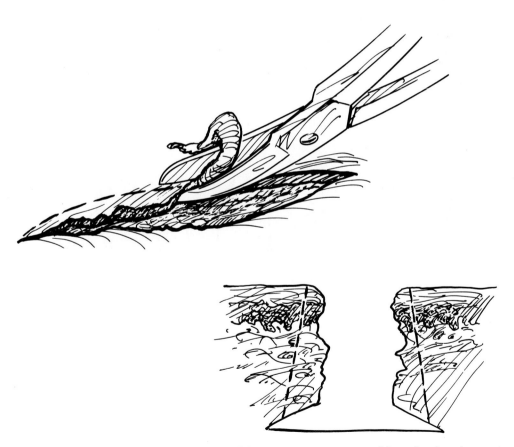

FIG. 8-5 Technique for excision by careful tissue scissor trimming of devitalized epidermis and dermis. Note the angle of excision that will facilitate wound-edge eversion during percutaneous closure.

slight angle so that the epidermal surface of the skin edge juts out slightly farther than the dermal portion. In this manner, when the wound is closed, it will naturally evert with the proper suture placement technique and resulting suture loop configuration.

Technique for Full Wound Excision

Full wound excisions are reserved for injuries in which all wound edges are devitalized and are obviously impossible to salvage. There must also be sufficient tissue redundancy in the anatomic location of the wound. If redundancy is inadequate, then excision will create a gap or defect that can only be closed under excessive

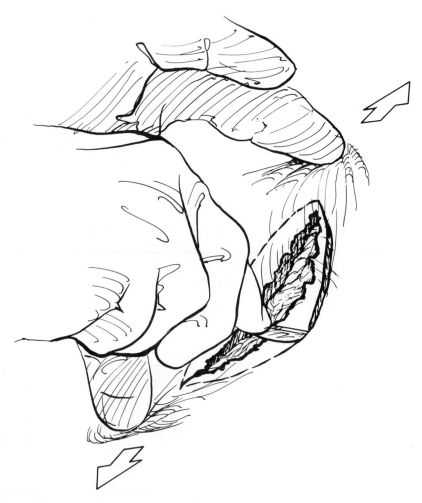

FIG. 8-6 Technique for initiating or "scoring" the epidermis and dermis prior to full wound excision. Note that the fingers are used to provide tension to the skin and the axis of the wound. This will facilitate easier application of the scalpel to the skin.

tension. Areas where there is sufficient tissue to accommodate excision include the chest, abdomen, arms, and thighs. Whenever there is doubt about this procedure, it is best to consult a surgical specialist.

Use the scalpel with a #15 blade to outline the tissue to be removed by partially incising or "scoring" the dermis (Fig. 8-6). Generally the excision is shaped like a long ellipse. In order to achieve proper closure without excessive tension the length of the ellipse should exceed the width by at least a 3 to 1 ratio. Once the ellipse is defined, use the scalpel or iris scissors or both in combination, to complete the excision (Fig. 8-7). The wound edges are incised at the same angle as described for dermal edge trimming. Not only do the edges have to be excised, but the excised tissue has also to be released from the superficial fascia (subcutaneous tissue). Considerable bleeding often ensues and hemostatic measures might have to

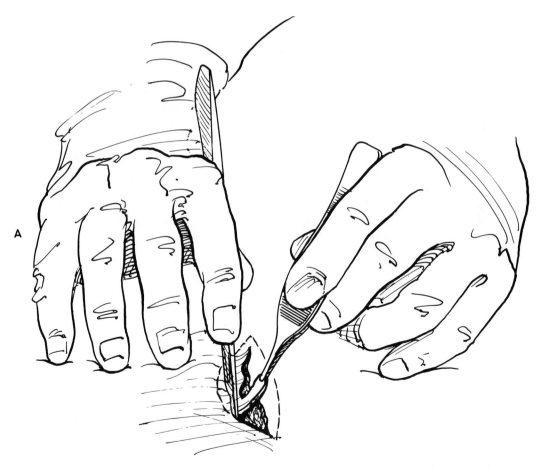

A

FIG. *8-7* Technique for full wound excision. **A,** The scalpel can be used to excise the wound complet.   *Continued.*

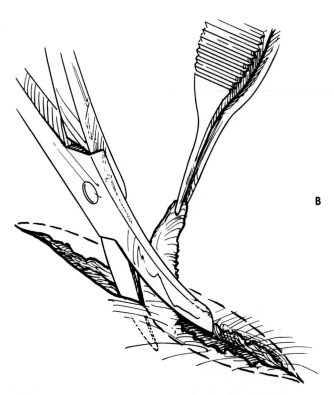

FIG. 8-7, cont'd B, Tissue scissors can be used to follow the original wound outline created by the "scoring" of the epidermis and dermis with the scapel blade.

be used before proceeding to closure. Excisions usually require both deep (dermal) and percutaneous sutures.

SURGICAL DRAINS

Surgical drainage in emergency care remains a controversial subject. Drains are indicated to remove large collections of pus or blood, or to assist in eliminating large pockets of dead space. Drains can act as retrograde conduits for contaminating bacteria from either the wound or skin. Under experimental wound conditions, sub-infective inoculums of bacteria have been shown to greatly increase the infection rate in drained versus undrained control wounds.[10] As a general rule, wounds that can be managed in an emergency department setting do not need drains.

Non-abscess wounds that are contaminated or complicated enough to consider the placement of a drain probably need to be evaluated by a consulting surgeon.

INDICATIONS FOR INTRAVENOUS ANTIBIOTIC THERAPY

For simple uncomplicated wounds and lacerations, there is no good clinical evidence that systemic antibiotics provide protection against the development of wound infection.[13,14] Often, however, the physician is faced with a wound or laceration that necessitates the consideration of immediate antibiotic coverage during or even prior to wound management itself. There is experimental evidence that antibiotic action rapidly decreases in effectiveness if it is not initiated within 3 hours of the injury.[12] Therefore, if intravenous antibiotics are thought necessary by the physician, they need to be administered without delay. The following are situations in which the immediate administration of intravenous antibiotics should be considered:

> Mutilating wounds, especially of the hand or foot (i.e., lawn-mower or chain-saw injuries).
>
> Grossly contaminated wounds with penetrating debris and "ground-in" foreign material.
>
> Lacerations in areas of lymphatic obstruction and lymphedema
>
> Extensive lacerations of the ear and its cartilaginous skeleton
>
> Suspected penetration of bone (open fractures), joints, or tendons.
>
> Amputation injuries, especially where replantation is a consideration.
>
> Extensive or distal extremity animal-bite wounds (See Chapter 14)
>
> Significant lacerations in patients with pre-existing valvular heart disease.
>
> Presence of disease or drugs causing immunosuppression or altered host defenses, e.g., diabetes

The initial intravenous antibiotic of choice is usually a first-generation cephalosporin such as cefazolin (Kefzol®, Ancef®). For penicillin-allergic patients, gentamicin is a reasonable alternative. Another alternative is ciprofloxacin (Cipro®), due to be released as an intravenous formulation in the United States in 1990. This drug has excellent gram-positive as well as gram-negative coverage. It is strongly recommended that a wound culture be taken prior to initiation of antibiotics in order to assist in later modification of therapy if necessary.

GENERAL GUIDELINES FOR CONSULTATION

Inevitably, physicians are faced with wounds, lacerations, and related problems that cause them to consider consulting a specialist. There are no hard and fast rules governing consultations. Each emergency physician has his or her own level of expertise, experience, and comfort. For example, some physicians will repair extensor tendon lacerations without difficulty, others would refer the patient to a specialist. Specific issues concerning special anatomic sites and wound problems are covered in the appropriate chapters and sections. The following are general guidelines for obtaining consultation:

> Extent of wound: Certain wounds can be technically managed by emergency physicians but the time necessary to close the wound would significantly impede the operation of the emergency department. If direct physician involvement time exceeds 30 to 60 minutes, then consultation might be considered.

Another option in this case is to call a colleague at your skill level to manage this problem so that care can continue in the department.

Complexity of wound: Some wounds can be repaired adequately by the emergency physician, but the patient would be better served by consultation and repair in a more controlled, surgical setting.

Physician uncertainty: If after a thorough wound evaluation and exploration the full extent of the injury cannot be revealed, a consultation is appropriate.

Large defects: Often some defects will require immediate coverage or grafting.

Elderly patients: Large lacerations that cannot be easily apposed without excessive tension often need grafting.

Surgical drainage: Large, complicated, or severely contaminated wounds might require the placement of surgical drains.

Hand and foot injuries: Flexor tendons, digital nerves, open fractures, amputations, and joint penetrations are best managed by a specialist (see Chapter 12).

Open fractures and joint penetration other than on the hand: A laceration over a fracture, even if the mechanism does not suggest contiguity between the two injuries, still technically constitutes an open fracture and a consultant should be called.

Compression (wringer injuries): Certain wounds can appear trivial but are caused by compression between two rollers (washing machine, industrial). Delayed, extensive, soft tissue and muscle damage can occur.

Injection injuries: Paint gun and grease gun injuries can appear as benign puncture wounds that hours later will lead to widespread tissue injury from the high-pressure jet of chemical that has penetrated the deep soft tissues.

Facial injuries: If the patient is significantly concerned about the cosmetic outcome of a wound repair, even though it might be technically uncomplicated, consultation is often obtained. Other indications for consultation for facial injuries are discussed in Chapter 11.

Suspected Brown Recluse spider or other arthropod bite: After the initial insult, local care to manage the tissue necrosis can be complicated.

Other venomous animals such as poisonous snakes.

Significant burns and electrical injuries are discussed in Chapter 16.

Wounds in patients who have serious underlying systemic disorders where wound healing will be less than optimal, e.g., severe peripheral vascular disease, diabetes, neutrophil, and other immunologic defects.

References

1. Altemeier W: Principles in the management of traumatic wounds and infection control, Bull NY Acad Med 55:123-138, 1979.
2. Dimick AR: Delayed wound closure: indications and techniques, Ann Emerg Med 17:1303-1304, 1988.
3. Edlich RF et al: Principles of emergency wound management, Ann Emerg Med 17:1284-1302, 1988.
4. Grossman J, Adams J, and Kunec J: Prophylactic antibiotics in simple hand lacerations, JAMA 245:1055-1056, 1981.
5. Haughey R, Lammers R, and Wagner D: Use of antibiotics in the initial management of soft tissue hand wounds, Ann Emerg Med 10:187-192, 1981.
6. Haury B et al: Debridement: an essential component of wound care, Am J Surg 135:238-242, 1978.
7. Hutton P, Jones B, and Law D: Depot penicillin as prophylaxis in accidental wounds, Br J Surg 65:549-550, 1978.
8. Lammers RL: Principles of wound management. In Roberts JR and Hedges JR, editors: *Clinical Procedures in Emergency Medicine*, Philadelphia, 1985, WB Saunders.
9. Losken HW and Auchinloss JA: Human bites of the lip, Clin Plast Surg 11:159-161, 1984.
10. Magee C et al: Potentiation of wound infection by surgical drains, Am J Surg 131:547-549, 1976.
11. Roberts JR: Intravenous regional anesthesia, J Am Coll Emerg Phys 6:261-264, 1977.
12. Robson M, Duke W, and Krizek T: Rapid bacterial screening in treatment of civilian wounds, J Surg Res 14:426-430, 1973.
13. Rutherford W and Spence R: Infection in wounds sutured in the accident and emergency department, Ann Emerg Med 9:350-352, 1980.
14. Thirlby R and Blair A: The value of prophylactic antibiotics for simple lacerations, Surg Gynecol Obstet 156:212-216, 1983.

9 Basic Laceration Repair—Principles and Techniques

Definition of Terms
   Bite
   Throw
   Percutaneous closure
   Dermal closure
   Interrupted closure
   Continuous closure
Basic Knot-Tying Techniques
Principles of Wound Closure

Layer Matching
Wound-Edge Eversion
   Techniques for wound edge eversion
Wound Tension
   Techniques for reducing wound
     tension
Dead Space
Closure Sequence and Style
References

Each wound and laceration has different technical requirements that have to be met in order to properly effect closure. By understanding the basic principles that underlie the technical requisites of wound care, lacerations and wounds can be closed with the best chance for an optimal result. During actual closure, every attempt is made to match each layer evenly and produce a wound edge that is properly everted. Of paramount importance is proper knot-tying technique to facilitate eversion and to prevent excessive tension on the wound edge. When necessary, dead space is closed and finally, sutures are spaced and sequenced to provide the best and most gentle mechanical support.

DEFINITION OF TERMS

Several techniques and maneuvers used in wound care are referred to by terms that can be confusing. These terms are defined below so that the reader thoroughly understands the material contained in this chapter.

Bite

A bite is the amount of tissue taken when placing the suture needle in the skin or fascia. The farther away from the wound edge that the needle is introduced into the epidermis, for example, the bigger the bite will be.

Throw

Each suture knot consists of a series of throws. A square knot is fashioned with two throws. Because of its tendency to unravel, several additional throws are necessary to secure the final knot when nylon is being used.

Percutaneous closure (Skin closure)

Sutures, usually of a nonabsorbable material, that are placed in skin with the knot tied on the surface are called percutaneous closures. They are also referred to as skin closures.

Dermal closure (Deep Closure)

Sutures, usually of an absorbable material, that are placed in the superficial (subcutaneous) fascia and dermis with the knot buried in the wound are called deep closures.

Interrupted closure

Single sutures, tied separately, whether deep or percutaneous, are called interrupted sutures.

Continuous closure (Running Closure)

A wound closure effected by taking several bites that are the full length of the wound, without tying individual knots, is a continuous or running suture. Knots are tied only at the beginning and end of the closure to secure the suture material.

BASIC KNOT-TYING TECHNIQUES

There are several knots that can be used to tie sutures during wound closure. The most common is the surgeon's knot (Fig. 9-1, A-G). The advantage of this knot is that the double first throw offers better knot security and there is less slipping of the suture material as the wound is gently pulled together during tying. The wound edges will remain apposed while the second and subsequent single throws are accomplished. The knot-tying sequence shown in Fig. 9-1 illustrates the proper instrument technique required to obtain a surgeon's knot. The instrument tie can be used for almost all knots, whether for deep or superficial closures.

Occasionally it is necessary to effect a hand tie. Hand ties in minor wound care are most useful for ligating vessels to achieve hemostasis. After a small bleeding vessel is clamped with the tip of a hemostat, an absorbable suture is brought around the vessel held by the hemostat and tied in the manner illustrated in Fig. 9-2. Because two hands are necessary for this tie, an assistant is often required to hold the hemostat and display the tie so that the vessel can be easily encircled with the suture.

Text continued on p. 110.

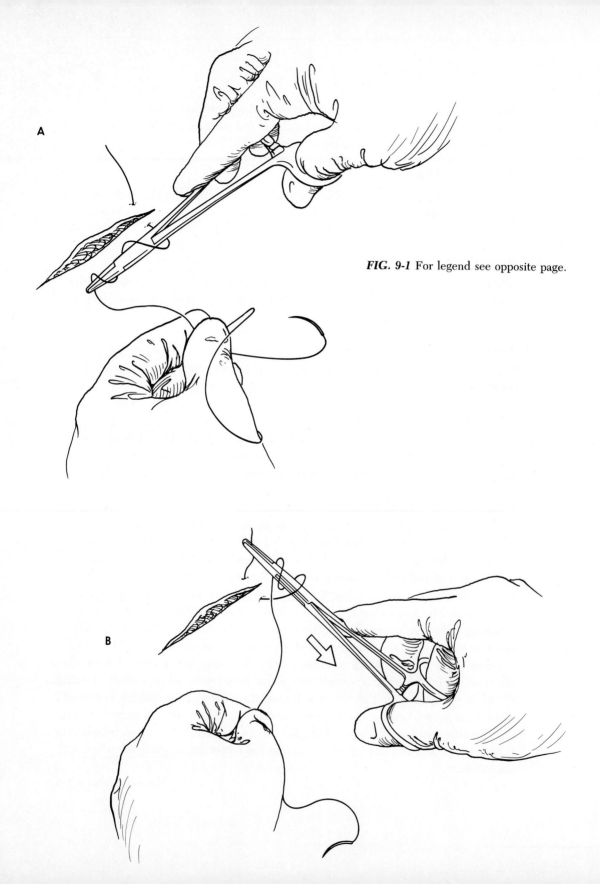

FIG. 9-1 For legend see opposite page.

C

D

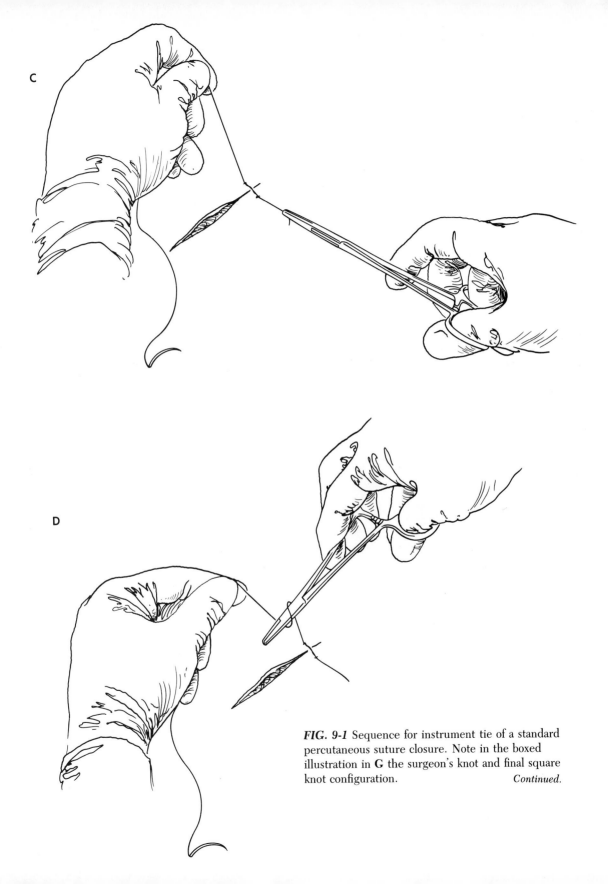

FIG. 9-1 Sequence for instrument tie of a standard percutaneous suture closure. Note in the boxed illustration in **G** the surgeon's knot and final square knot configuration. *Continued.*

E

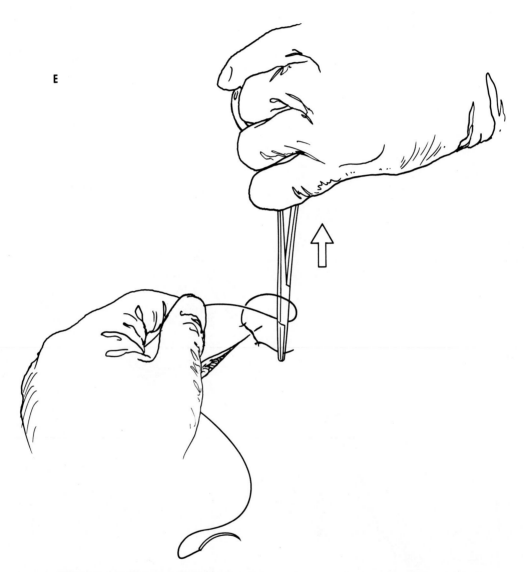

FIG. 9-1, cont'd Sequence for instrument tie of a standard percutaneous suture closure. Note in the boxed illustration in **G** the surgeon's knot and final square knot configuration.

F

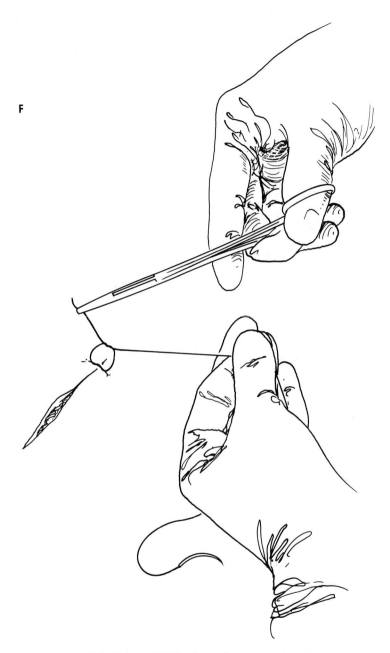

FIG. 9-1, *cont'd* For legend see opposite page.
Continued.

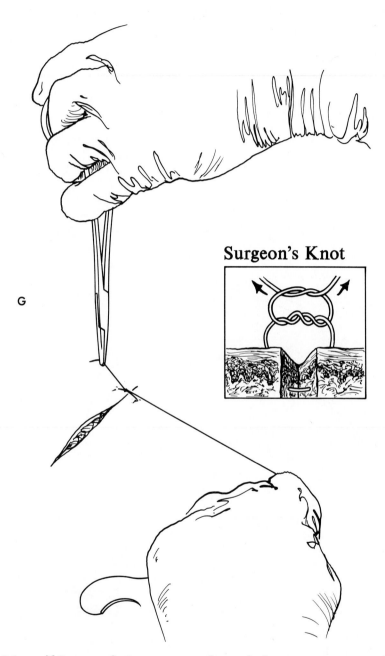

G

Surgeon's Knot

FIG. 9-1, cont'd Sequence for instrument tie of a standard percutaneous suture closure. Note in the boxed illustration the surgeon's knot and final square knot configuration.

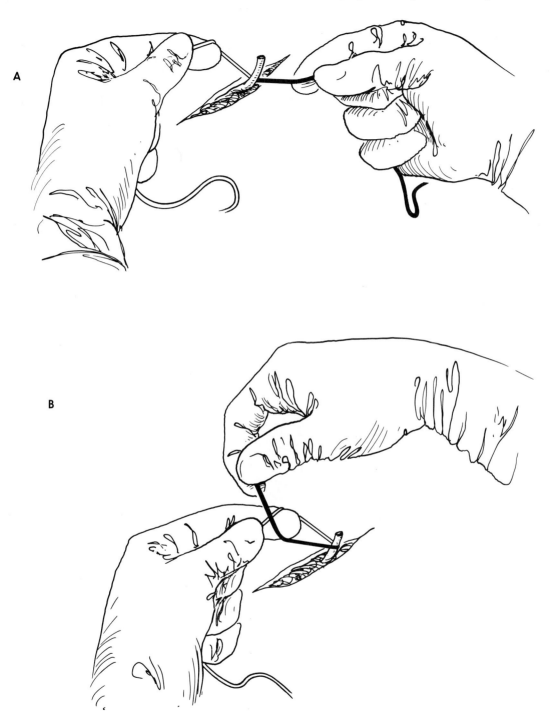

FIG. 9-2 Sequence for a two-handed tie of hemostat-clamped vessels for hemostasis.
Continued.

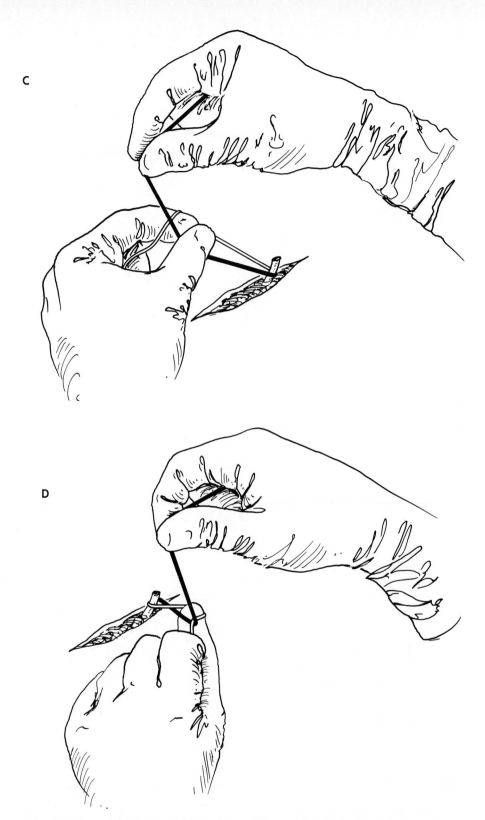

FIG. 9-2, *cont'd* Sequence for a two-handed tie of hemostat-clamped vessels for hemostasis.

E

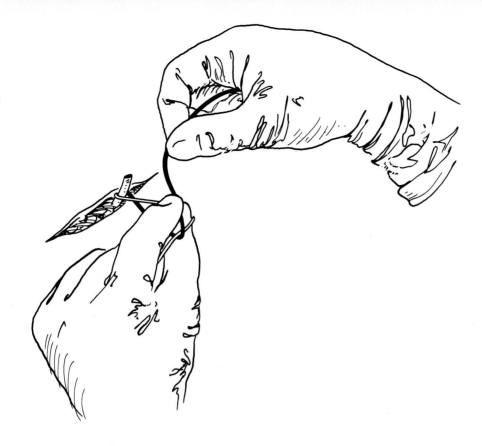

F

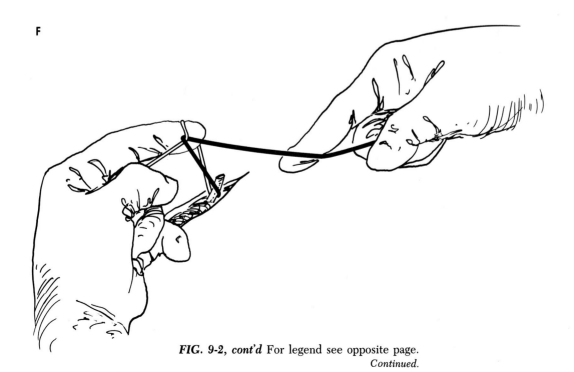

FIG. 9-2, *cont'd* For legend see opposite page.
Continued.

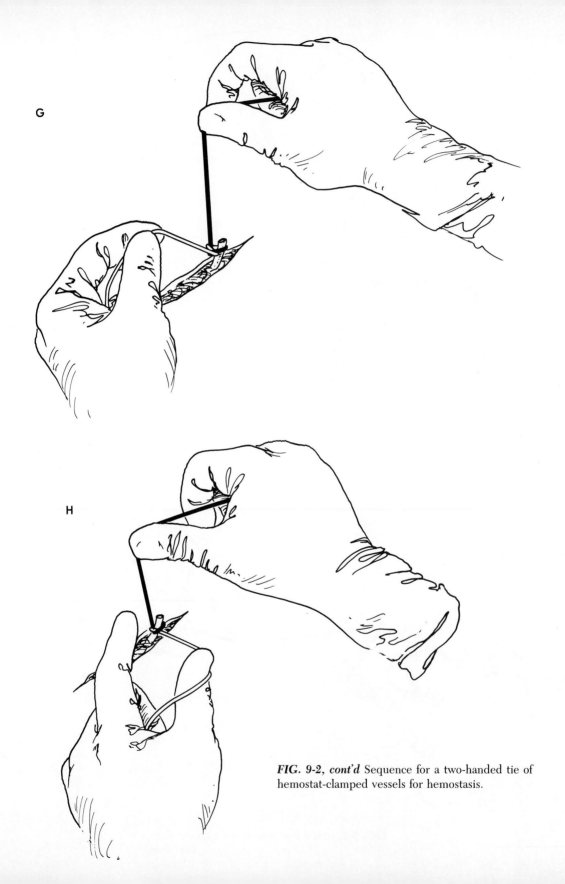

G

H

FIG. 9-2, *cont'd* Sequence for a two-handed tie of hemostat-clamped vessels for hemostasis.

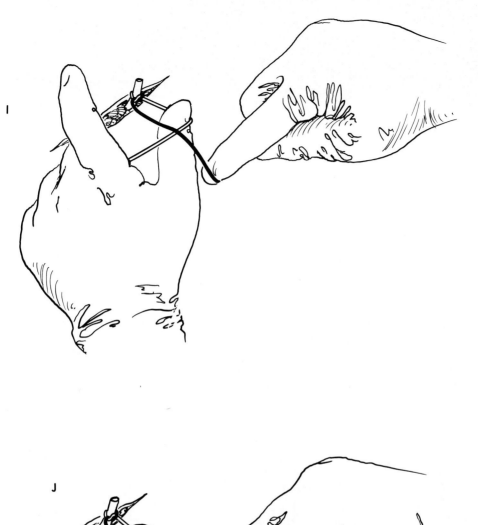

I

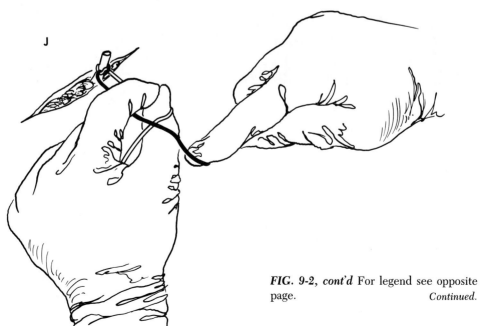

J

FIG. 9-2, *cont'd* For legend see opposite page. *Continued.*

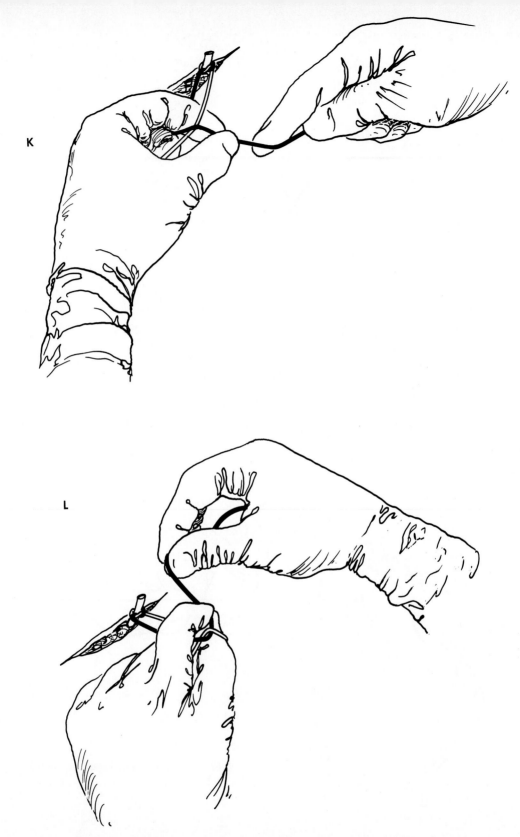

FIG. 9-2, *cont'd* Sequence for a two-handed tie of hemostat-clamped vessels for hemostasis.

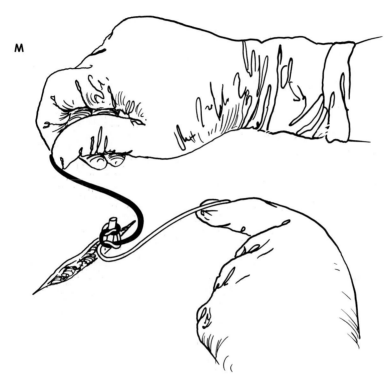

FIG. 9-2, cont'd For legend see opposite page.

PRINCIPLES OF WOUND CLOSURE

Layer Matching

When closing a laceration it is important to match each layer of a wound edge to its counterpart. Deep fascia, when opened traumatically, is closed to deep fascia. Superficial fascia has to meet superficial fascia. Finally, dermis to dermis will necessarily bring epidermis to epidermis. Failure to appose layers meticulously can cause improper healing with an unnecessarily large scar (Fig. 9-3).

Wound-Edge Eversion

Paramount to achieving a cosmetically acceptable scar is proper wound-edge eversion during the initial repair. Because of the normal tendency of scars to contract with time, a slightly raised wound edge above the plane of the normal skin will gradually flatten with healing and have a final appearance that is cosmetically acceptable (Fig. 9-4, *A* and *B*). Wounds that are not everted will contract into linear pits that will become noticeable cosmetic defects because of their tendency to cast shadows under incident light.

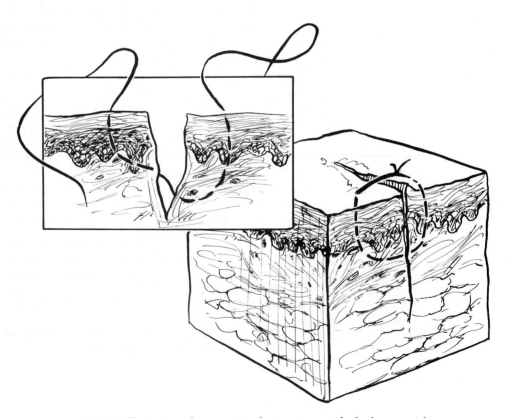

FIG. 9-3 Illustration of incorrect technique to provide for layer matching.

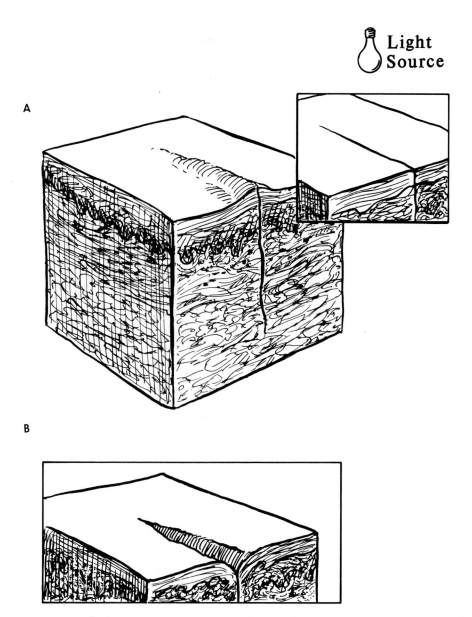

Light Source

A

B

FIG. 9-4 Wound edge eversion. **A,** Correct technique allows for a slight rise of the wound edges above the skin plane. These edges will eventually contract to flatten out at the skin plane. **B,** Wound edges that are not properly everted will contract below the skin plane and allow incident light to cause unsightly shadows.

Techniques for Wound-Edge Eversion

The key to achieving proper wound-edge eversion is to use the correct technique for introducing the needle into the skin and producing the proper suture configuration. As illustrated in Fig. 9-5, the point of the needle should pierce the epidermis and dermis at a 90-degree angle before it is curved around through the tissues. In order to ensure a 90-degree angle, the needle holder has to be held in the manner described in Chapter 7. It is mechanically very difficult to maneuver the needle correctly if the operator's fingers remain in the finger rings of the needle holder. Fig. 9-5 A, B, and C illustrates the correct and incorrect final configuration of an interrupted suture to achieve wound-edge eversion.

Vertical Mattress Suture. Another useful method for wound-edge eversion is the vertical mattress suture. This suture is placed by first taking a large bite of tissue approximately 1 to 1.5 cm away from the wound edge and crossing through the tissue to an equal distance on the opposite side of the wound. The needle is then reversed and returned for a very small bite (1 or 2 mm) at the epidermal/dermal edge in order to closely approximate the epidermal layer (Fig. 9-6). The vertical mattress suture is very helpful in areas of lax skin (elbow, dorsum of hand) where the wound edges tend to fall or fold into the wound. Another advantage of the vertical mattress suture is that it can act as a deep as well as superficial closure all in one suture. Some wounds are not deep enough to accommodate a separate, absorbable suture but still need some deep support to close dead space. This technique can meet that need.

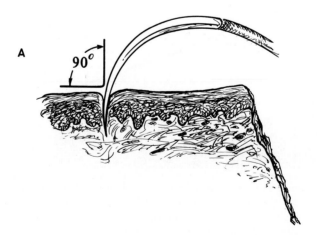

FIG. 9-5 Technique for proper wound edge eversion. **A,** The suture needle is introduced at a 90-degree angle to the epidermis.

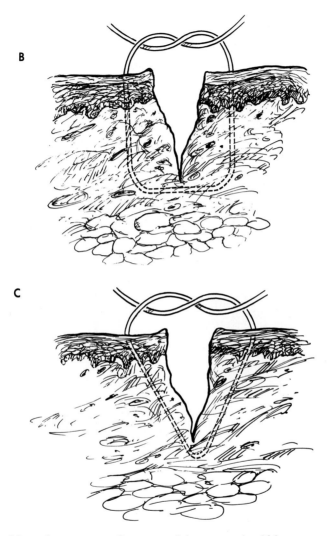

FIG. 9-5, *cont'd* **B,** The proper configuration of the suture should be square or bottle shaped. It is recognized that this configuration is difficult to achieve in actuality; however, this figure illustrates the correct principle. **C,** The incorrect technique of needle placement and suture configuration will lead to wound edge inversion, which will lead to "pitting" of the eventual scar.

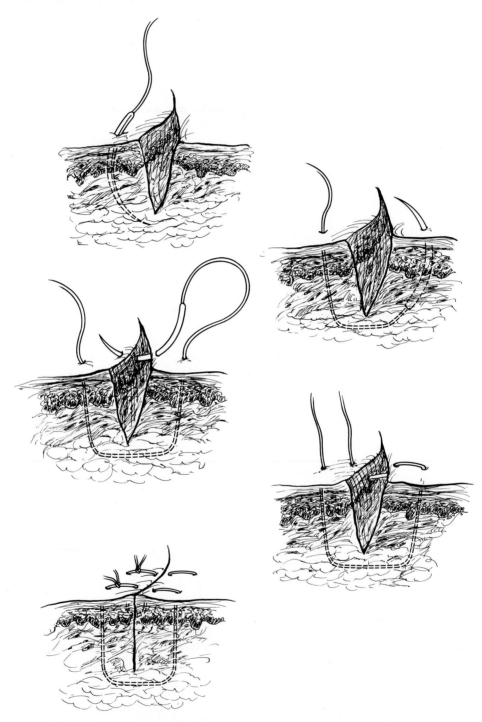

FIG. 9-6 Technique for a vertical mattress suture. Note that the second bite barely passes through the dermis to provide meticulous apposition of the epidermal edges.

Horizontal Mattress Suture. Another technique, the horizontal matress suture, can also be used to achieve wound edge eversion (Fig. 9-7). The needle is introduced into the skin in the usual manner and is brought out at the opposite side of the wound. A second bite is taken approximately .5 cm adjacent to the first exit and is brought back to the original starting edge, also .5 cm from the initial entry point. The knot is tied leaving an everted edge.

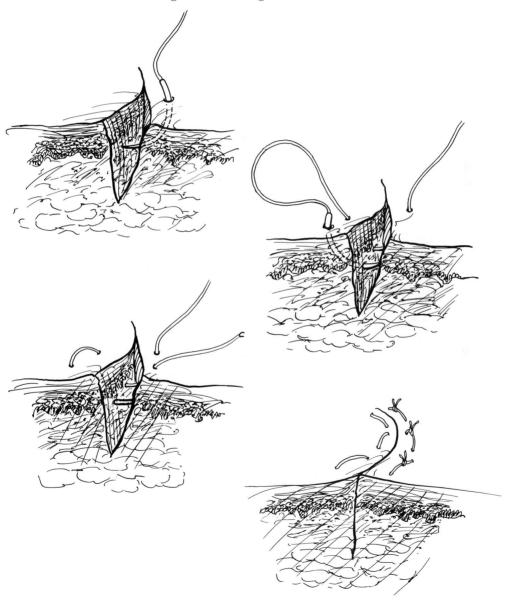

FIG. 9-7 Technique for placing a horizontal mattress suture.

Wound Tension

Whenever wound edges are brought together by suturing, there is inevitable tension created in the tissue within the suture loop. It is very important to minimize tension in order to preserve capillary blood flow to the wound edge. Excessive force exerted on the tissue will lead to ischemia and possibly cause some degree of cellular necrosis.[1] Necrosis provokes a more intense inflammatory response with the eventual formation of an irregular, cosmetically unacceptable scar. When tying knots, the first throw is crucial. As the wound edges are brought together, they are allowed to just barely touch. Bringing the edges together more forcibly by making the first throw too tight will promote ischemia. Wound edges tend to become slightly edematous after repair; therefore, a small amount of slack between them will disappear. The addition of edema to a suture line that is already too tight can be disastrous.

Techniques for Reducing Wound Tension

Several techniques can reduce wound tension. Proper placement of deep closures to bring the dermis close together before suture closure will reduce final wound edge tension. Fig. 9-8 illustrates the method for placing and tying deep closures. To start this suture, the needle is placed in the wound itself and the bite starts in the superficial fascia, close to the underside of the dermis. Take as little fat as possible into the suture loop. The needle is then brought through the dermis. At this point, the needle has to be rearmed with the needle holder. The needle is then introduced into the dermis of the matching opposite wound edge and carried down into the superficial fascia to complete the second bite.

Crucial to this technique is that both the trailing and leading portions of the suture remain on the same side of the portion of the suture that crosses from dermis to dermis. In this manner, when the knot is tied, it will be buried. If the trailing edges are on opposite sides of the dermal suture crossing, the knot will be pushed superficially and will interfere with epidermal healing. Three or four throws are adequate to secure the knot, and the suture ends are cut close to the knot itself, leaving no more than 2-mm "tails." The temptation to place numerous deep closures must be resisted. These sutures act as foreign bodies and can potentiate infections.[2] Therefore, place only as many sutures as are necessary to accomplish the task of reducing wound tension.

Wound Undermining. Another technique for reducing tension is wound undermining. Undermining will release the dermis and superficial fascia from its deeper attachments, allowing the wound edge to be brought together with less force. Anatomic areas where undermining is useful include the scalp, forehead, and lower legs, particularly over the tibia where the skin is under a great deal of natural tension. Caution has to be exercised in deciding to undermine because this procedure can spread bacteria into deeper tissues as well as create a deeper, larger dead space.

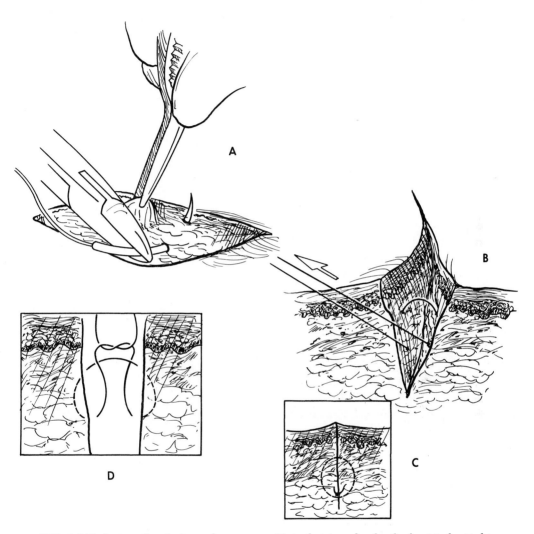

FIG. 9-8 Technique for placing a deep suture. Note that in order for the knot to be tied in the appropriate manner, the leading and trailing edges of the suture should be on the same side of the loop or the cross stay of the suture. See text for complete description of technique. Correct technique is illustrated in parts **A, B,** and **C.** Incorrect knot placement is shown in part **D.**

The technique for undermining is illustrated in Fig. 9-9, *A*. For most minor wound care problems, the proper tissue plane is between the dermis and the superficial fascia (subcutaneous tissue). Metzenbaum dissection scissors (or for smaller wounds, an iris scissors) or a hemostat can be inserted parallel to the underside of the dermis within the superficial fascia. The instrument is gently spread to create a

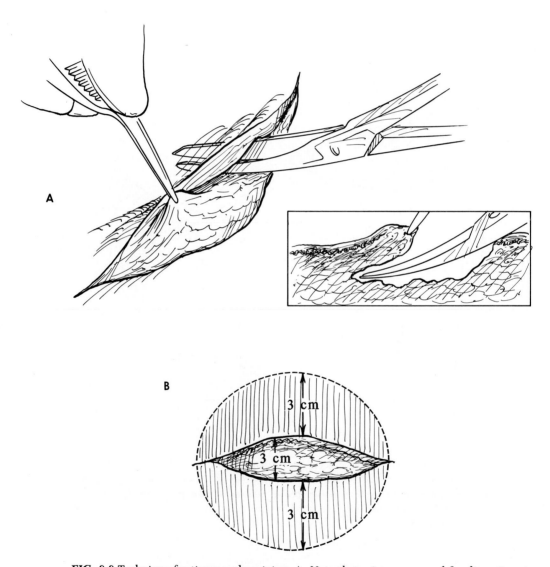

FIG. 9-9 Technique for tissue undermining. **A,** Note that scissors are used for dissection at the dermal superficial fascia level. Tissue spreading is preferred to cutting the sharp edges. **B,** The zone of undermining is illustrated.

plane of dissection. Actual cutting is kept to a minimum to prevent excessive bleeding. A general rule is to undermine a wound from end to end, to a distance from the wound edge that approximates the extent of "gapping" of the wound edges. In other words, if a wound gaps open 3 cm from edge to edge, then undermining is carried out to 3 cm under the dermis, perpendicularly away from the wound edge. A common mistake in using this technique is to fail to include the wound ends. Fig. 9-9, *B* illustrates the proper zone of undermining during dissection.

Placing more sutures closer together will also reduce wound tension (Fig. 9-10). Mechanically, a greater number of sutures will lessen the total force exerted on

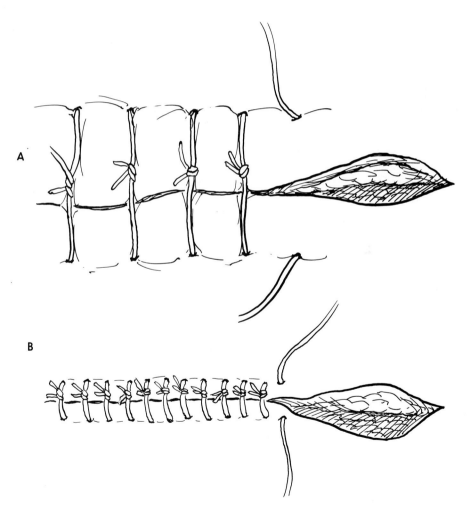

FIG. 9-10 A technique for reducing wound tension. **A,** A few sutures, placed far apart and far from the wound edges, will increase wound tension. **B,** More sutures placed closer together and closer to the wound edges will reduce tension.

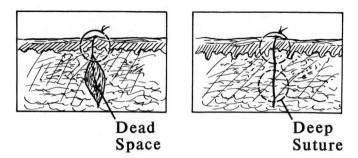

Dead Space   Deep Suture

FIG. 9-11 Example of dead space and a two-layered closure to obliterate that space.

each suture, thereby reducing potential tissue compression. One has to keep in mind, however, that sutures act as foreign bodies and can potentiate infection. Therefore, when closing a wound a balance has to be struck between the number of sutures used and the effect desired.

Dead Space

In the past it was axiomatic that no open or dead spaces should be left behind during wound closure. These spaces tend to fill with hematoma and can act as potential sites for wound infection (Fig. 9-11). Hematoma formation in these areas can also delay wound healing. There is experimental evidence, however, that suture closure of these spaces, when they are contaminated with bacteria, will increase the chance of wound infection.[2] Therefore, it is recommended that deep closures only be used to close dead space in clean, minimally contaminated wounds. Even in these cases, because suture material acts as a foreign body as few sutures as possible should be used.

Closure Sequence and Style

Students learning wound care often ask how close together sutures should be placed. As a general rule, sutures are placed just far enough from each other so that no gap appears between the wound edges. As a general guideline, the distance between sutures is equal to the bite distance from the wound edge (Fig. 9-12). The great variability of lacerations, however, dictates that experience will rapidly teach the practitioner the proper distances at which sutures should be placed to close the wound.

The final appearance of a suture line should be neat and organized. The knots are aligned to one side of the laceration. In addition to appearing orderly, knots are placed away from the wound edge to prevent a further inflammatory response that can be provoked by an increased amount of foreign material over the healing surface.

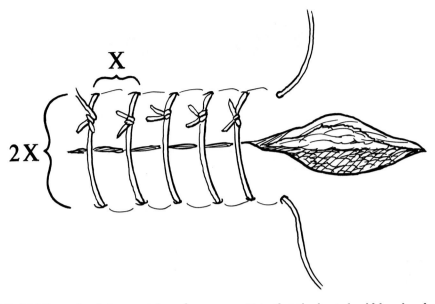

FIG. 9-12 Example of closure style and sequence. Note that the knot should be placed evenly on one side of the wound. Knots directly over the wound will increase inflammation and scar tissue formation.

References

1. Crikelair G: Skin suture marks, Am J Surg 96:631-639, 1958.

2. Edlich R et al: Technique of closure: contaminated wounds, J Am Coll Emerg Phys 3:375-381, 1974.

10 Complicated Lacerations and Wounds: Problems and Solutions

Long, Straight Lacerations
   Description
   Technique for the continuous
      over-and-over (running) suture
Beveled Edges
   Description
   Technique for closure of a beveled
      edge
Medium-Deep Lacerations
   Description
   Technique for closure of medium-deep
      lacerations
Pull-out Dermal Closure
   Description
   Technique for the pull-out dermal
      closure
Corners and Uncomplicated Flaps
   Description
   Technique for closing a corner
Complicated Flap (Partial Avulsion)
   Lacerations
   Description
   Technique for preparing and repairing
      a complicated flap
   Technique for closure of flaps with
      non-viable edges: the V-Y closure
   Technique for closure of a wound with
      a completely non-viable flap
Geographic Lacerations

Description
Technique for closure of geographic
   wounds
Wounds with Tissue Loss
   Description
   Technique for converting a triangle to
      an ellipse
   Technique for closing a circular or
      irregular defect
"Dog Ear" Deformities
   Description
   Technique to close a "dog ear"
Parallel Lacerations
   Description
   Technique for closure of parallel
      lacerations
Thin-Edge, Thick-Edge Wound
   Description
   Technique for closure of a thin-edge,
      thick-edge wound
Laceration in an Abrasion
   Description
   Technique for closure of a laceration in
      an abrasion
Aged Skin
   Description
   Techniques for closing wounded aged
      skin
References

The majority of lacerations and wounds are straightforward and can be closed with the basic techniques described in Chapter 9. Because of the complexity of wounding forces, materials and configurations, and host factors, some wounds require alternate closure techniques to appose the tissues in an optimal manner. The following are descriptions of some of the more complicated wound problems that can be encountered in a wound care setting. Techniques for "solving" these "puzzles" are suggested below.

LONG, STRAIGHT LACERATIONS
Description

Lacerations, usually caused by simple shearing forces, can be quite long, and therefore time-consuming to close. They are often caused by slash wounds from a knife or glass. The continuous "over-and-over" (running) suture technique can be used when time is a factor. Wounds over 5 cm in length can be considered for this technique. The time saved is beneficial to the person repairing the wound, because he or she can return quickly to other duties. The drawbacks to this technique are that if one loop of the suture breaks or is imperfectly positioned, then the whole process has to be repeated. Another technique that is gaining favor in emergency wound-care settings for long, straight lacerations is wound stapling. See Chapter 13 for indications and techniques.

Technique for the Continuous Over-and-Over (Running) Suture

The technique for continuous over-and-over suturing is demonstrated in Fig. 10-1, A. The closure is started with the standard technique of a percutaneous interrupted suture, but the suture is not cut after the initial knot is tied (Fig. 10-1, A). The

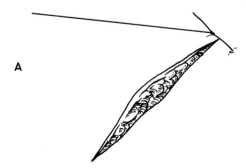

A

FIG. 10-1 Technique for continuous over-and-over suture (running suture). Note that the needle bites are made at an angle of 45 degrees to the axis of the wound. By taking bites at this angle, the cross stay of the suture at the skin surface will be at an angle of 90 degrees to the wound axis. See text for complete description of technique.   *Continued.*

B

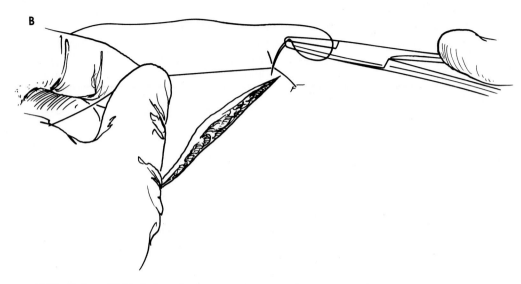

FIG. 10-1 cont'd Technique for continuous over-and-over suture (running suture). Note that the needle bites are made at an angle of 45 degrees to the axis of the wound. By taking bites at this angle, the cross stay of the suture at the skin surface will be at an angle of 90 degrees to the wound axis. See text for complete description of technique.

needle is then used to make repeated bites, starting at the original knot by making each new bite, through the skin, at an angle of 45 degrees to the wound direction (Fig. 10-1, *B-F*). The cross-stays of suture, on the surface of the skin, will be at an angle of 90 degrees to the wound direction. The final bite is per made at an angle of 90 degrees to the wound direction to bring the suture out next to the previous bite exit (Fig. 10-1, *G*). The final bite is left in a loose loop. The loop acts as a free end of suture for knot tying. The first throw of the final knot is made by looping the suture end held in the hand around the needle holder, then grasping the free loop (Fig. 10-1, *H*). The first throw is snugged down to skin level (Fig. 10-1, *I*). The knot is completed in the standard instrument-tie manner with several more throws at skin level (Fig. 10-1, *J* and *K*).

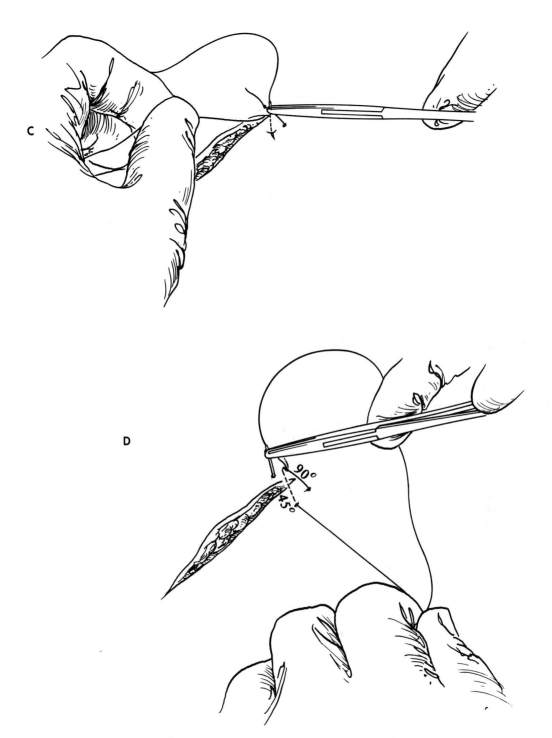

FIG. 10-1 cont'd For legend see opposite page.
Continued.

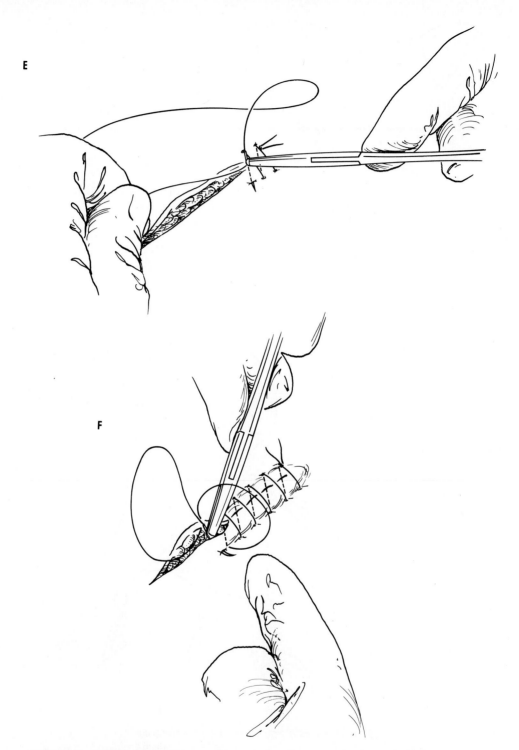

FIG. 10-1 cont'd Technique for continuous over-and-over suture (running suture). Note that the needle bites are made at an angle of 45 degrees to the axis of the wound. By taking bites at this angle, the cross stay of the suture at the skin surface will be at an angle of 90 degrees to the wound axis. See text for complete description of technique.

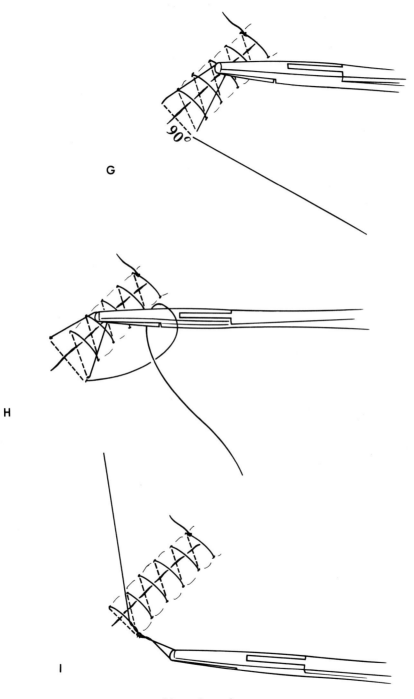

FIG. 10-1 cont'd For legend see opposite page.
Continued.

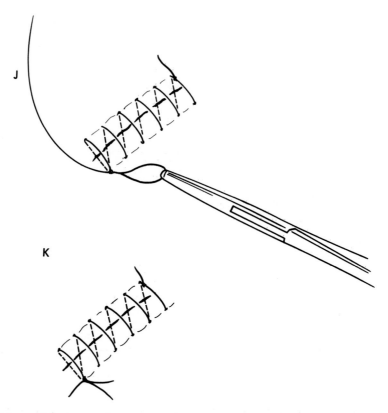

FIG. 10-1 cont'd Technique for continuous over-and-over suture (running suture). Note that the needle bites are made at an angle of 45 degrees to the axis of the wound. By taking bites at this angle, the cross stay of the suture at the skin surface will be at an angle of 90 degrees to the wound axis. See text for complete description of technique.

BEVELED EDGES
Description

A very common problem in layer matching is the beveled-edge laceration. Beveled edges are created when the striking angle of the wounding object is not perpendicular. The angle and force, however, is not acute enough to create a true flap deformity.

Technique for Closure of a Beveled Edge

A common misconception about the repair of this wound is that a larger bite is taken from the thin edge of the laceration than from the bigger edge. In fact, the opposite technique is the solution to proper layer matching. The technique for

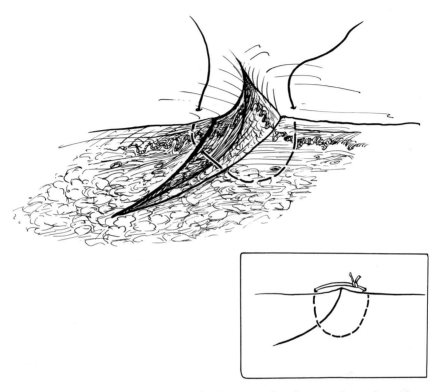

FIG. 10-2 Technique for closing a beveled edge. Note that there is a larger bite taken on the larger wound edge. There is a smaller bite taken on the flap portion of the wound edge.

closing a beveled laceration is illustrated in Fig. 10-2. By taking unequal bites as shown, the edge will be brought into correct apposition with the opposite edge. The horizontal mattress technique can also be effective in this setting.

MEDIUM-DEEP LACERATIONS

Description

Some lacerations are deep but not deep enough to technically permit the proper placement of dermal (deep) supporting sutures. If these lacerations were closed with superficial skin closures alone, the wound might not be adequately supported and potential dead space could be left behind.

Technique for Closure of Medium-Deep Lacerations

The simplest and most effective technique is the use of the vertical mattress suture (see Fig. 9-6). Vertical mattress sutures are made with both deep and superficial percutaneous bites. In some cases simple interrupted percutaneous (skin) closures can be alternated with the vertical mattress sutures to achieve the same effect.

PULL-OUT DERMAL CLOSURE

Description

A favorite technique of plastic surgeons is the pull-out dermal stitch using a non-absorbable suture material such as polypropylene. This suture material is stiffer and stronger than nylon and allows for easier removal.[3] The newer non-absorbable suture material, polybutester (Novafil®), is particularly useful for this technique.[1] This technique is limited to straight lacerations less than 4 cm long because the suture would be too hard to extract at removal time. Children have naturally higher skin tension, so this technique is thought by some to be superior for that age group because it prevents suture marks. In spite of this fact, pull-out dermal closure has no distinct advantage over percutaneous closure when final wound and scar appearance is compared.[4] Another use for this technique is for closure of lacerations over which splinting materials or plaster will be placed. It can also be used in patients who are at risk for keloid formation so as to prevent keloid formation at the needle puncture sites.

Technique for the Pull-Out Dermal Closure

Prior to placement of a pull-out dermal closure the superficial fascia (subcutaneous tissue) has to be adequately apposed with absorbable suture to bring the dermis close to approximation. The actual closure is begun by passing the needle of 4-0 or 5-0 polypropylene 1 to 1.5 cm from the wound end through the skin and bringing it out parallel to and through the plane of the dermis. Subsequent bites are made, as illustrated (Fig. 10-3) parallel to the dermis at a depth of 2 to 3 mm into the dermis. Each bite should "mimic" the other with regard to bite size and dermal depth on each side of the wound until the "tail" is brought out at the opposite end of the wound. The beginning and final "tail" can be secured by wound tape. In the face, this suture can remain in place for up to 7 days. This technique is often used in conjunction with wound taping to accurately match dermal and epidermal layers.

The suture is removed merely by pulling on one end with forceps or a needle holder and sliding the suture out of the dermal layer.

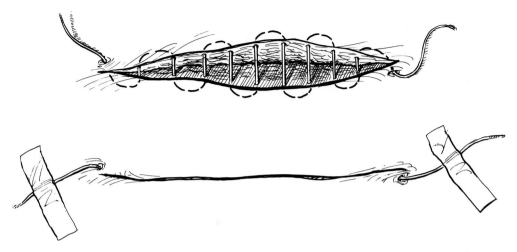

FIG. 10-3 Technique for pull-out dermal closure. See text.

CORNERS AND UNCOMPLICATED FLAPS

Description

Many wounds are irregular and jagged, with corners that need to be secured during closure. Corners and flaps are particularly vulnerable because they receive their blood supply only from an intact base. Improper suturing of the tip of a corner can compromise an already tenuous vascularity.

Technique for Closing a Corner

A simple technique is demonstrated in Fig. 10-4 to secure a corner without interrupting the small capillaries at the tip. The technique used is the half-buried horizontal mattress suture. The suture is introduced percutaneously, through the skin in the non-corner portion of the wound. The needle is brought through the dermis and then passed *horizontally* through the corner dermis and brought back to the same plane of dermis on the opposite side of the non-corner portion. Finally, it is led out through the epidermis. The key to this suture is that the flap portion of the suture passes horizontally through the dermis and not vertically through both the epidermis and dermis. Once the tip is in place with the corner stitch, then the remainder of the flap can be closed with interrupted percutaneous or half-buried horizontal mattress sutures, which should be placed far enough from the tip to allow for unrestricted dermal circulation.

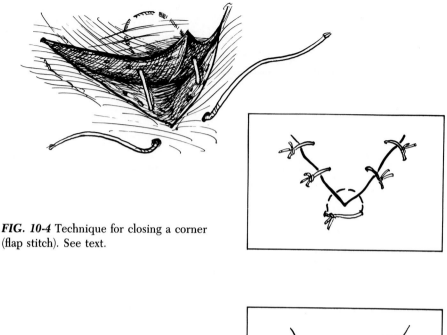

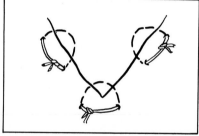

FIG. 10-4 Technique for closing a corner (flap stitch). See text.

A single corner stitch can encompass several corners of stellate lacerations by capturing all of the corners of flaps (Fig. 10-5) until the final percutaneous re-exposure is completed to tie the knot. The corner suture is one of the most useful suture techniques in emergency wound and laceration care for complex wound closure.

COMPLICATED FLAP (PARTIAL AVULSION) LACERATIONS
Description

Complicated flap lacerations are essentially corners in which the dermis has undergone significant separation from the superficial fascia (subcutaneous tissue). The vascular supply of a complicated flap is even more tenuous because it derives from only its intact dermal portion. A general rule is that the flap base should exceed flap length by a ratio of 3:1.[2] Flaps with lower ratios are less likely to survive. The rule varies according to anatomic site and other considerations. Obviously, a long,

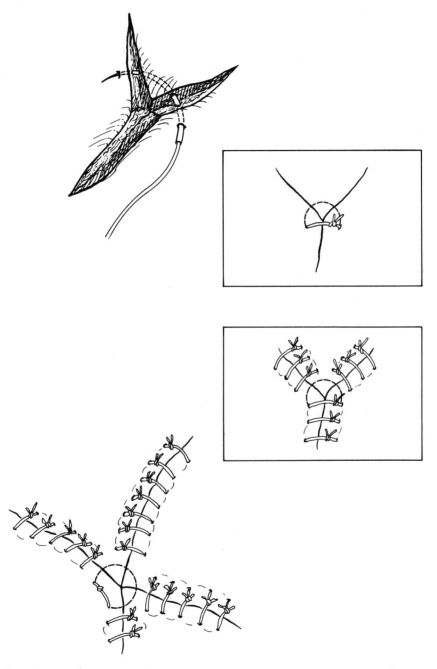

FIG. 10-5 Technique for using the corner stitch to close a stellate or multi-flap laceration.

narrow-based flap is in greater jeopardy than a short, broad-based one. Flaps that are distally based, opposite to the natural cutaneous arterial flow, and that rely solely on venous backflow for oxygen and nutrients are particularly tenuous. The repair technique has to be meticulous, gentle, and dictated by the condition of the flap, the width of the total wound, and the anatomic location.

Technique for Preparing and Repairing a Complicated Flap

Excessive fatty superficial fascia (subcutaneous tissue) on the underside or dermal part of the flap can impair healing when it is secured to its base with sutures. A raw dermal surface is preferable to damaged fat when the flap is replaced in the laceration defect. In this sense, flaps are similar to grafts. In order to improve the chance of flap survival during early healing, it is best to remove the excessive fat from the

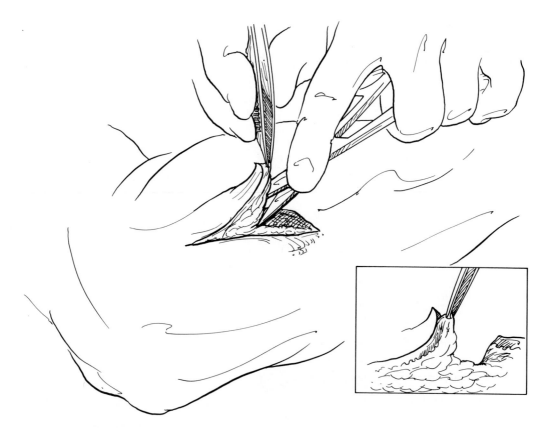

FIG. 10-6 Technique for defatting the base of a flap in order for better union and vascularization to occur after suture anchoring. Fat is removed at the dermal-superficial fascia plane.

flap before suturing. The technique is illustrated in Fig. 10-6. Iris scissors can be used to trim the fat until only a fresh or tissue surface remains.

If the flap is otherwise in good condition with viable edges, then the initial suture is the half-buried mattress suture described above for corner closure. The remainder of the flap can be closed with the same suture technique for the corner closure with simple interrupted percutaneous sutures.

Technique for Closure of Flaps with Non-Viable Edges: the **V-Y** Closure

Often flaps will have damaged edges that are not viable, in which case the edges can be excised to create a smaller but more viable flap. Fig. 10-7 illustrates how this flap is then secured by converting a V-closure to a Y-closure to accommodate the smaller amount of tissue available. With iris scissors, the edges of the flaps are trimmed back to viable tissue. The remaining flap, however, will not be large enough to accommodate the resultant defect. By using a modified corner stitch technique, the flap tip can be brought together with the wound edges in a Y-configuration. The remainder of the wound is closed with small-bite percutaneous interrupted sutures.

Technique for Closure of a Wound with a Completely Non-Viable Flap

In this case, closure can be achieved by "ellipsing" the flap (Fig. 10-8) and completely closing the wound by following the 3:1 ratio rule for ellipse closure (see Chapter 8). In some cases there is insufficient tissue redundancy so ellipsing will not be feasible, and the wound has to be considered for open healing (secondary intention) or grafting.

GEOGRAPHIC LACERATIONS
Description

One of the most challenging wounds is the "geographic laceration," a wound that can be irregular in both configuration and depth. These lacerations are caused by differential forces occurring at the same time to create a complex wound. Closure requires some creativity.

Technique for Closure of Geographic Wounds

The first principle is to appose the natural geographic points (Fig. 10-9). After that, simple percutaneous interrupted sutures might suffice, but a creative mix of different techniques and suture sizes might ultimately be required. It is not uncommon to use 5-0 and 6-0 non-absorbable sutures in the same wound to accommodate the different tissue thicknesses and "anchoring" capacities. Closure techniques may appear unorthodox, but for traumatic wounds, the maxim "whatever works" should be followed in order to obey basic closure principles and achieve the best possible result.

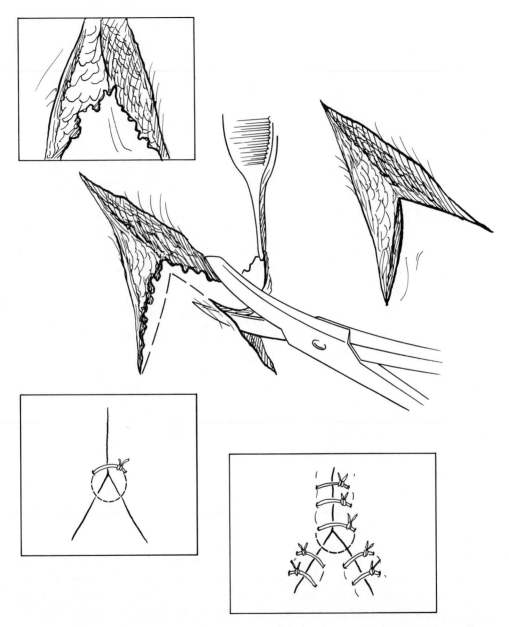

FIG. 10-7 Technique for closure of flaps with nonviable edges: the **V-Y** closure. Note that the edges of the flap are excised. The remaining flap will not be large enough to fill the defect; therefore, a corner stitch is placed to close the wound as a **Y** instead of its original **V** configuration.

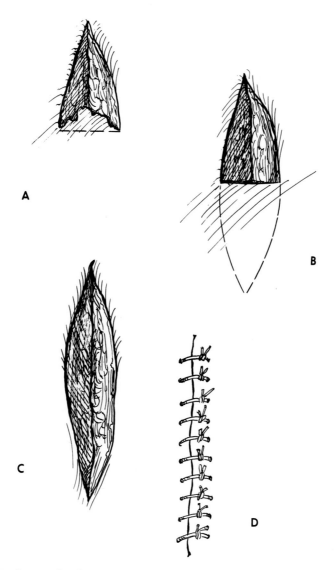

FIG. 10-8 Technique for closure of the wound with a completely nonviable flap. In this case, a complete ellipse can be fashioned and then closed primarily.

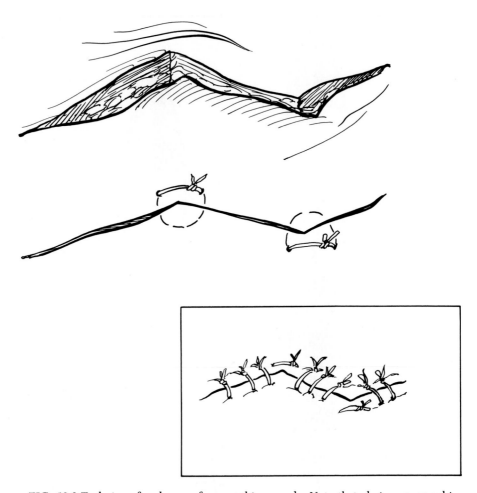

FIG. 10-9 Technique for closure of geographic wounds. Note that obvious geographic points are apposed first with either simple percutaneous sutures or corner sutures.

WOUNDS WITH TISSUE LOSS
Description

When tissue is lost through the primary wounding event or after debridement, the following questions have to be asked:

Is the tissue loss partial- or full-thickness? Full-thickness losses are identified by the complete loss of dermis. Superficial fascia (subcutaneous fat) will "show" through the wound. Partial-thickness losses are identified by the raw appearance of underlying dermis without its covering epidermis. Partial-thickness losses, especially when intact dermal elements are visible, heal quite well without aggressive intervention.

If the the defect is full-thickness, does it need repair or grafting? Generally, any resultant full-thickness defect, even after repair attempts are made, that remains 1 to 2 cm^2 in area or less, can be left to heal by open healing (secondary intention). This rule can apply to wounds on finger tips as well.

What defects warrant grafting? Generally, full-thickness gaps or defects that are greater than 2 cm^2 in area need to be considered for grafting. Whenever questions about the possibility of grafting arise, a consultation with a specialist is recommended. Some defects can be closed primarily, without grafting, and suggested techniques are described below.

Technique for Converting a Triangle to an Ellipse

If a defect is configured as a triangle, then conversion of that defect to an ellipse can be made by extending the "defect" by excision to include the opposite intact triangle (see Fig. 10-8, *B* to *D*). If the basic 3:1 length-to-width rule (described in Chapter 8, under wound excision) can be maintained during this process, then the whole defect can be closed with a few dermal (deep) supporting sutures and a line of percutaneous sutures with the result of a simple, single suture line. Occasionally, undermining may be required to bring the wound edges together to reduce wound-edge tension. Again, there must be sufficient tissue redundancy to perform this closure successfully.

Technique for Closing a Circular or Irregular Defect

The simplest way to close this defect is to turn it into an ellipse as illustrated in Fig. 10-10. If the defect is too great, the technique of a double V-Y closure can be used. In this case, the defect is covered by two sliding pedicle flaps created by a scalpel as illustrated in Fig. 10-11. It is crucial not to disturb the fascial attachments of the flaps, for that is from where the blood supply is to come. Only incise the dermis to allow the flaps to move forward on their vascular base into the gap.

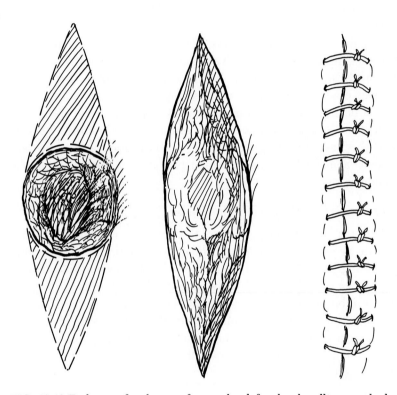

FIG. 10-10 Technique for closure of a circular defect by the ellipse method.

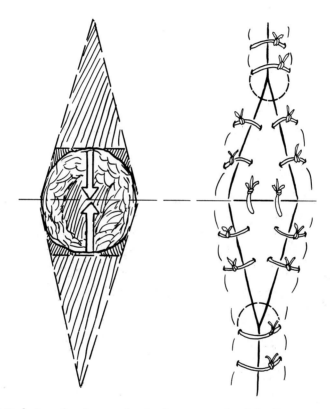

FIG. 10-11 Technique for closure of a circular or irregular defect by advancing flap pedicles to effect a double **V-Y** closure. (Adapted from Zukin D and Simon R: Emergency wound care: principles and practice, Rockville, Md, 1987, Aspen Publishers Inc.)

"DOG-EAR" DEFORMITIES
Description

Trying to evenly close a laceration, particularly if it has a curving configuration, can lead to bunching of one of the wound edges as the suture closure proceeds. One edge of the wound can become redundant and can lead to the creation of a "dog ear."

Technique to Close a "Dog Ear"

To correct this problem, an incision is made with a #15 blade, beginning at the end of the wound and at a 45-degree angle from the direction of the laceration on the side of the redundancy (Fig. 10-12). The redundant tissue flap is excised along an imaginary line that directly corresponds with the incision. The remaining portion of tissue then fits the new configuration of the laceration-incision and is appropriately sutured. The final outcome is a slightly angulated wound with a "hockey-stick" appearance.

PARALLEL LACERATIONS
Description

Two or more parallel lacerations that are in close proximity are often the result of self-inflicted wounds on the wrists or forearms. They are usually superficial but because of the nature of the anatomic site, these wounds can result in significant injuries to the underlying flexor structures of the wrist. Careful functional testing of nerves and tendons and wound exploration is often necessary prior to closure.

Technique for Closure of Parallel Lacerations

After close inspection and exploration to rule out tendon or nerve damage, there are several methods for closing parallel lacerations without compromising the blood supply to the tissue "strips" between lacerations. Some wounds can be closed with the horizontal mattress suture, modified to cross all lacerations (Fig. 10-13, A). Wound tapes are particularly effective if the lacerations are superficial (Fig. 10-13, B). Finally, the alternating percutaneous approach can be used if the vascular supply of the tissue will not be compromised (Fig. 10-13, C).

THIN-EDGE, THICK-EDGE WOUND
Description

When differential forces are applied to skin, a wound can be created in which the thickness of one edge is markedly different from the other wound edge. In order to properly appose the two edges, simple percutaneous interrupted sutures will often not suffice. The "thin" edge has to be elevated to meet the appropriate layers of the full-thickness edge.

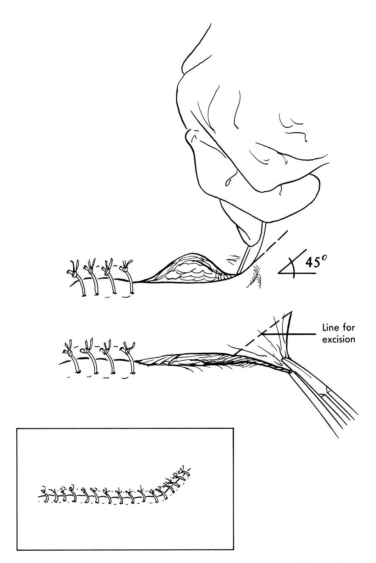

FIG. 10-12 Technique for closure of redundant tissue or a "dog ear." Note that the incision is made approximately at an angle of 45 degrees from the original axis of the wound. See text for complete description of technique.

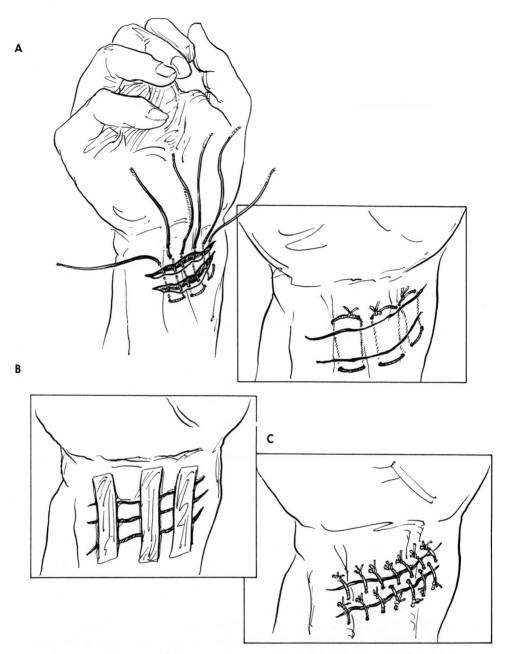

FIG. 10-13 Note the three techniques for closure of parallel lacerations. **A,** The horizontal mattress technique is used to cross all lacerations for closure. **B,** Wound tapes can be used to close these lacerations. **C,** If the island of tissue is wide enough, alternating sutures can be used on each laceration. However, it is necessary to be very careful not to compromise vascular supply when using this technique. (Adapted from Zukin D and Simon R: Emergency wound care: principles and practice, Rockville, Md, 1987, Aspen Publishers Inc.)

Technique for Closure of a Thin-Edge, Thick-Edge Wound

One technique for matching uneven layers is to use the vertical mattress suture previously described in Chapter 9. Another technique is to use the half-buried horizontal suture in the manner shown in Fig. 10-14.

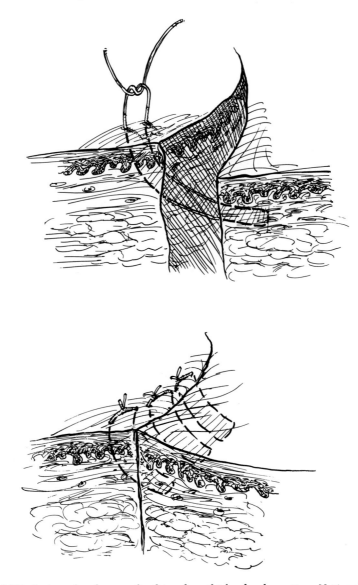

FIG. 10-14 Technique for closure of a thin-edge, thick-edge laceration. Notice that the horizontal mattress technique is used; however, one portion is buried and not brought through the opposite side of the wound surface.

LACERATION IN AN ABRASION
Description

Another complex wound is the loss of surface skin accompanied by a laceration in the defect.

Technique for Closure of a Laceration in an Abrasion

The laceration can be repaired by using the deep (dermal) closure with the knot buried under the wound surface. The technique is described in Chapter 9. Once the laceration is closed (Fig. 10-15), the defect can be managed by allowing it to close by secondary intention or grafting, depending on whether it is a partial- or full-thickness loss.

AGED SKIN
Description

People with older, thinner skin are subject to large avulsions of skin even if the traumatic forces involved are minor. The skin usually separates at the dermal/superficial fascia (subcutaneous layer). The skin is thin, friable, and does not hold sutures well. Patients taking large doses of chronic corticosteroids have similar skin biomechanics that result in similar disruptions.

Techniques for Closing Wounded Aged Skin

It is very important not to close elderly, friable skin under tension. Attempts to do so can risk the already tenuous vascularity of the skin and result in a large area of

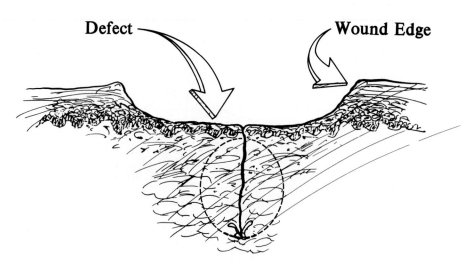

FIG. 10-15 Technique for closure of a laceration within a deep abrasion. Note that the deep-suture technique is used and the abraded surface is avoided.

tissue loss. If the wound cannot be brought back together properly without undue tension, it is best to leave a gap for later grafting. Under these conditions a consultation with a specialist is recommended.

If the wound edges can be apposed easily, the simplest method to close friable, elderly skin is to use wound tapes. Applying the tapes is technically not difficult, but because of their adherence, they need to be removed very carefully in order not to disrupt the delicate, early collagenous bonds of healing.

Another closure method is to appose the edges with horizontal mattress sutures (see Fig. 9-7). The configuration of this suture allows for maximal "gathering" of tissue minimal "tearing" forces are applied.

References

1. Bernstein G: Polybutester suture, J Dermatol Surg 14:615-616, 1988.
2. Grabb WC: Introduction to the clinical aspects of flap repair. In Grabb WC and Myers MB, editors: Skin flaps, Boston, 1975, Little, Brown and Co.
3. Swanson NA and Tromovitch TA: Suture materials, 1980s: properties, uses, and abuses, Int J Dermatol 21:373-378, 1982.
4. Winn HR, Jane JA, and Rodeheaver GT: Influence of subcuticular sutures on scar formation, Am J Surg 133:257-259, 1977.

11 *Special Anatomic Sites*

Scalp
  Preparation for Closure
    Scalp closure: uncomplicated
      lacerations
    Scalp closure: galeal lacerations
    Scalp closure: compression lacerations
      with irregular margins
    Scalp closure: avulsion or "scalping"
      lacerations
    Aftercare
Forehead
  Preparation for Closure
    Uncomplicated lacerations
    Complex lacerations: multiple small
      flaps, lacerations, and abrasions
      ("windshield injury")
    Complex lacerations: ragged-edge
      lacerations, large flaps, and tissue
      defects
    Aftercare
Eyebrow and Eyelid
  Preparation for Closure
    Closure of extramarginal lid lacerations
    Closure of intramarginal lid lacerations
    Closure of eyebrow lacerations
    Aftercare
Cheek or Zygomatic Area
  Preparation for Closure
    Closure of uncomplicated cheek
      lacerations
    Deep or through-and-through
      lacerations
    Aftercare
Nasal Structures
  Preparation for Closure

Skin lacerations
Mucosal and cartilage wounds
Septal hematoma
Lacerations with bone involvement
Aftercare
Ear
  Preparation for Repair
    Uncomplicated lacerations
    Lacerations involving cartilage
    Perichondral hematoma
    Aftercare
Lips
  Preparation for Closure
    Uncomplicated lacerations
    Complicated and through-and-through
      lacerations
    Aftercare
Oral Cavity
  Preparation for Repair
    Buccal mucosal and gingival lacerations
    Tongue lacerations
    Aftercare
Perineum
  Preparation for Closure
    Lacerations of the penis and scrotum
    Lacerations of the introitus
    Aftercare
Knee
  Aftercare
Lower Leg
  Aftercare
Foot
  Aftercare
References

Table 11-1 *Suggested Guidelines for Suture Material and Size for Body Region*

Body Region	Percutaneous (Skin)	Deep (Dermal)
Scalp	5-0/4-0 Monofilament[1]	4-0 Absorbable[2]
Ear	6-0 Monofilament	—
Eyelid	7-0/6-0 Monofilament	—
Eyebrow	6-0/5-0 Monofilament	5-0 Absorbable
Nose	6-0 Monofilament	5-0 Absorbable
Lip	6-0 Monofilament	5-0 Absorbable
Oral mucosa	—	5-0 Absorbable[3]
Other parts of Face/Forehead	6-0 Monofilament	5-0 Absorbable
Trunk	5-0/4-0 Monofilament	3-0 Absorbable
Extremities	5-0/4-0 Monofilament	4-0 Absorbable
Hand	5-0 Monofilament	5-0 Absorbable
Extensor tendon	4-0 Monofilament	—
Foot/Sole	4-0/3-0 Monofilament	4-0 Absorbable
Vagina	—	4-0 Absorbable[3]
Scrotum	—	5-0 Absorbable[3]
Penis	5-0 Monofilament	—

1. Non-absorbable monofilaments:
   Nylon: Ethilon, Dermalon
   Polypropylene: Prolene
   Polybutester: Novafil
2. Absorbable materials for dermal and fascial closures
   Polyglycolic Acid: Dexon, Dexon Plus
   Polyglactin 910:   Vicryl
   Polydioxanone: PDS (monofilament absorbable)
   Polyglyconate: Maxon (monofilament absorbable)
3. Absorbable materials for mucosal and scrotal closure
   Chromic Gut
   Polyglactin 910:   Vicryl

Although the wound closure principles and suture techniques discussed in Chapters 9 and 10 can be applied to all lacerations and wounds, several areas of the body have unique anatomic considerations that require special attention. Particular emphasis is placed on the face because of cosmetic concerns that are focused on this area. Initial management and wound closure are crucial to eventual scar formation and the final appearance of the injury. Table 11-1 is the reference guide for choice of suture material and size for each anatomic region of the body.

SCALP

The scalp extends anteriorly from the supraorbital ridges to the external occipital protuberance posteriorly, as shown in Fig. 11-1. Laterally the boundaries are the

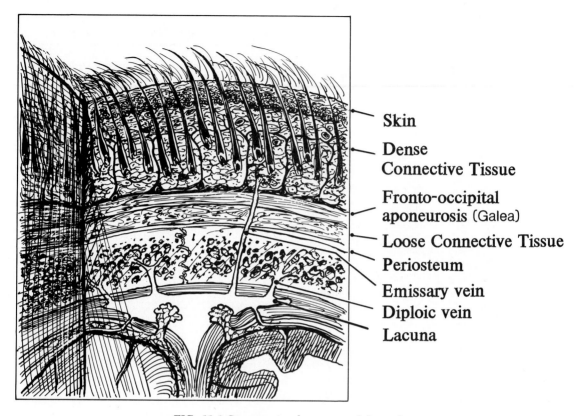

FIG. 11-1 Cross-sectional anatomy of the scalp.

temporal lines. The epidermis and dermis are densely covered with hair. Ragged lacerations are often closed without regard to cosmesis under the assumption that hair will hide the scar. However, the majority of all males will experience some balding in their lifetime, a fact that must be taken into consideration during wound closure.

Underlying the dermis is a dense layer of connective tissue that corresponds to the superficial fascia. This layer is richly invested with arteries and veins. Although this profuse vascularity protects against the development of infection, the denseness of the connective tissue tends to hold vessels open when the scalp is lacerated. For this reason, even small lacerations can cause considerable bleeding, even leading to hypovolemia and hypotension.

The next layer is the aponeurosis or galea aponeurotica. It is a dense tendon-like structure that covers the skull and inserts into the frontalis muscle of the forehead anteriorly and into the occipitalis muscle posteriorly. Failure to repair large, horizontal lacerations of the aponeurosis can cause the frontalis muscle to contract asymmetrically, which can cause a significant cosmetic deformity of the forehead.

Deep to the aponeurosis is a layer of loose connective tissue. This layer acts as a potential space because of its loose attachments. Blood and bacteria can easily spread from a laceration of the skin through this space. Significant injuries can cause extensive sub-aponeurotic (subgaleal) hematoma. Beneath the loose connective tissue layer is the pericranium or periosteum of the skull itself.

Preparation for Closure

Because of the propensity of the scalp to bleed profusely, hemorrhage control is necessary prior to attempts at closure. Trying to suture a bleeding scalp wound can be unnecessarily difficult and frustrating. Gross contaminants, if present, should be removed immediately with a brief cleansing or irrigation. The wound is then covered with sterile, saline-moistened sponges and compressed with an elastic bandage. This bandage can be left in place for 30 minutes to an hour. After compression, significant bleeding will usually have been brought under control. Occasionally, suture ligation is needed after clamping of a large vessel if pressure does not suffice. After pressure bandage removal and wound evaluation have been performed, an anesthetic should be administered. Repair can then take place under more controlled conditions. Because scalp lacerations frequently occur in intoxicated patients, the strategy of waiting for hemostasis has the added benefit of allowing the patient to "settle down" before any attempts at intervention are made.

Anesthesia for scalp wounds can be accomplished by the direct or parallel wound technique using lidocaine with epinephrine. This solution will further control bleeding if necessary. Visual inspection and digital palpation of large wounds is recommended in order to identify galeal or bone injuries. The pericranium, or periosteum, is frequently injured during trauma. Injuries to this layer can often be seen or palpated through a laceration. Because of its close adherence to the bone, any disruption of the pericranium can be mistaken for a skull fracture. Whenever this suspicion is raised, skull films are recommended to rule out a true fracture even though an actual break is often not found.[5]

Hair removal prior to closure is only necessary if it interferes with the actual closure and knot tying. Hair is not usually contaminated with high levels of bacteria and can be easily cleansed with standard wound-preparation solutions.[8] In a study of 68 patients with traumatic scalp lacerations, no wound infections were documented in patients whose hair had not been removed prior to closure.[7] If removal is necessary for mechanical reasons, then clipping with scissors or shaving with a recessed blade razor will suffice.[4] Shaving at skin level can increase the chance for wound infection.[1,10]

It is not uncommon for scalp lacerations to be accompanied by large hematomas underlying the wound. These hematomas are potential sources for infection and must be removed prior to wound closure.

Scalp Closure: Uncomplicated Lacerations

Uncomplicated, shearing lacerations can be closed with a single percutaneous layer of nonabsorbable 5-0 or 4-0 monofilament nylon, staples, or absorbable chromic gut suture. The latter material is often preferred for children because suture removal becomes unnecessary. Some practitioners find this strategy to be equally effective for adults. The most common suture closure method is the percutaneous interrupted technique. Staples are useful for long, time-consuming lacerations; stapled wounds heal the same as those treated with other closure methods.[6,9] Occasionally, a layer of dermal (deep) absorbable sutures is necessary initially to approximate the wound edges prior to the use of final percutaneous sutures.

Scalp Closure: Galeal Lacerations

Because the galea is a key anchoring structure for the frontalis muscle, large frontal lacerations need to be separately repaired with 3-0 or 4-0 absorbable sutures to prevent a serious cosmetic deformity from developing. If the frontalis muscle loses its anchoring point at the muscle-galeal junction along the frontal scalp line, then contraction of that muscle will become asymmetric and noticeable to the patient and any observer. Closure of large galeal lacerations in other areas of the scalp is also recommended to prevent excessive scar formation because the galeal gap fills excessive collagen tissue by secondary intention under the percutaneous closure line.

Scalp Closure: Compression Lacerations with Irregular Margins

Often lacerations of the scalp are caused by blunt rather than sharp shearing forces. The wound and its edges are irregular and macerated. Simple closure with percutaneous, interrupted sutures can be difficult under these conditions. The scalp does not have excessive tissue redundancy, so debridement has to be kept to a minimum or else the wound cannot be approximated without abnormally high tension. Fortunately, the rich vascularity of the scalp will allow for eventual successful healing even if less than optimal tissues are brought together. Therefore, after judicious wound-edge trimming, the horizontal mattress suture technique is recommended to approximate the remaining edges (Fig. 11-2).

Compression injuries can result in complex, stellate lacerations. Once again, judicious debridement is advised. The corner closure (flap) technique described in Chapter 10 will often approximate all of the corners and flaps in one suture. The remainder of the repair is carried out with simple percutaneous or half-buried mattress sutures.

Scalp Closure: Avulsion or "Scalping" Lacerations

High-speed forces that are delivered in a tangential manner to the scalp can cause large flaps or complete loss of portions of the scalp. Associated intracranial injury

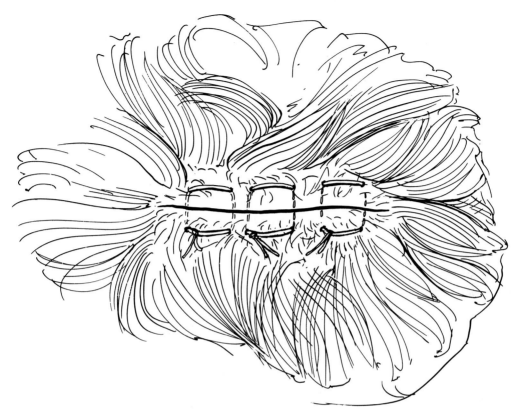

FIG. 11-2 Horizontal mattress suture technique for closure of scalp wounds with uneven or macerated edges.

can also occur. These wounds are best managed by a consultant. Preserved portions of complete scalp avulsions, like other amputated parts, are wrapped in saline moistened gauze, placed in a plastic bag, and cooled over ice. It is possible that they might be reimplanted in the defect by using grafting or microvascular anastamoses techniques.

Aftercare

After repair, it is often necessary to place a temporary (24-hour) light-pressure compression wrap with an elastic bandage over the scalp dressing to prevent recurrence of wound hematoma. The patient can be instructed to remove the bandage after the recommended compression period and leave the gauze dressing in place. (See Chapter 17 for scalp dressing techniques.) Scalp sutures are left in place for 6 to 8 days for adults and 5 to 7 days for children. Gentle bathing of the scalp can commence 24 hours after closure.

FOREHEAD

The forehead is a common site of injury in both children and adults. It is also of paramount cosmetic importance because of its visibility. Three principles govern the initial repair of a forehead injury:

1. Skin tension lines that parallel skin creases play a major role in the outcome of any laceration. A laceration that is perpendicular to dynamic skin tension lines tends to heal with a more visible scar than one that is parallel to these lines (see Chapter 2).
2. The forehead has little excess tissue to permit extensive revisions and excisions. The temptation to excise ragged wounds has to be carefully assessed or resisted. A small defect can inadvertently become larger by over-aggressive repair efforts.[2] It is often best to preserve as much tissue as possible just by "tacking down" ragged tissue tags so that later cosmetic revisions can be made when conditions are more favorable.
3. Whenever possible, as few dermal (deep) absorbable sutures as possible are placed in order to prevent excessive tissue reaction and eventual increased scar formation.

Preparation for Closure

Anesthesia for small or single lacerations of the forehead can be accomplished by the direct or parallel injection techniques, using an anesthetic with adrenalin to decrease bleeding. Large or multiple lacerations often are best managed by the forehead block (see Chapter 5). This block reduces the number of needle sticks and prevents distortion of the tissues to allow for more accurate wound edge approximation.

Once anesthesia is achieved, the wound can be explored for any bony abnormality or foreign-body. Radiographs are recommended when the suspicion for either is raised. Surprisingly large pieces of glass can be discovered under small and innocuous-appearing wounds. After gentle scrubbing with a sponge, irrigation, and debridement with the tip of a #11 blade, most foreign material should have been removed. Foreign material occasionally remains despite these efforts and will often slough off with the eventual loss of the wound crust or with the natural turnover of the epidermis. Any remaining permanent material can be surgically removed at a later date. It must be emphasized, however, that every effort is made to remove potential tattooing objects at the time of the first repair. When in doubt, consultation with a specialist should be considered.

Uncomplicated Lacerations

Most lacerations can be closed with the simple percutaneous technique using a 6-0 monofilament nonabsorbable suture. Deeper lacerations require placement of a few supporting dermal (deep) 5-0 absorbable sutures prior to placement of the percutaneous layer. The percutaneous technique in any laceration should be performed by taking small bites (close to the wound edge) with several sutures rather than large bites with few sutures. This technique will reduce wound-edge tension and allow for more accurate wound edge apposition.

Complex Lacerations: Multiple Small Flaps, Lacerations, and Abrasions ("Windshield Injury")

One of the most dramatic injuries is the multiple abrasion-laceration that occurs after the forehead strikes a large, flat surface. The anesthetic of choice is the forehead block. Flaps that are smaller than 5 mm are closed with single 6-0 percutaneous nonabsorbable sutures (Fig. 11-3). Larger flaps can be closed by using the corner technique. Partial-thickness abrasions and shallow gouges (less than 5-10 mm wide and 1-2 mm deep) can be left to heal by secondary intention. Other lacerations are

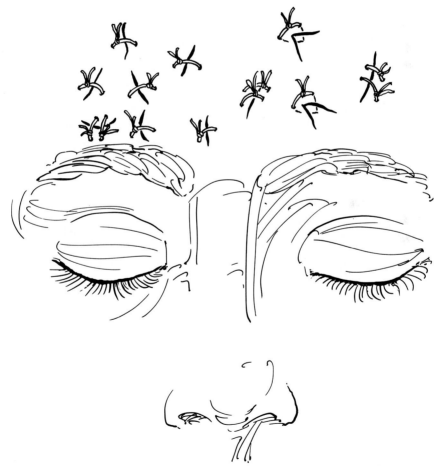

FIG. 11-3 Small abrasions/lacerations, caused by the "windshield" injury, can often be closed by using simple, single, percutaneous sutures or single corner sutures.

closed as necessary with percutaneous sutures. A petroleum-based antibiotic ointment, such as Neosporin, applied three times a day will suffice as a dressing. Again, because of cosmetic concerns, a consultant might be helpful, especially if the flaps and gouges are larger and more complex.

Complex Lacerations: Ragged-Edge Lacerations, Large Flaps, and Tissue Defects

Ragged and macerated edges can be trimmed as described in Chapter 8. If the unevenness or maceration is not extensive, then complete excision is an option if the laceration is parallel to the skin tension lines and there is sufficient tissue redundancy. Lacerations perpendicular to skin tension lines have less tissue redundancy and cannot tolerate wide excision. Once again, the principle of tissue preservation has to be kept in mind when considering excision. Large flaps are prone to what is known as the "trap-door" phenomenon in which congestion and lymphedema lead to unsightly bulging of the flap after repair. These injuries are best managed by a consultant. Finally, tissue defects (greater than 1-2 cm) with edges that cannot be brought together without tension are best managed by a consultant.

Aftercare

Facial lacerations usually do not require dressings. Daily application of Neosporin ointment is recommended for protection and to allow for easier suture removal (by reducing crusting). Facial sutures are removed within 3 to 5 days to prevent suture mark formation. Larger lacerations (larger than 2 cm) are supported by wound tapes for one week after suture removal.

EYEBROW AND EYELID

The eye and periorbital tissues are susceptible to serious injury by relatively minor trauma. Fig. 11-4 illustrates various structures that must be checked for damage before repair proceeds. Should any of the important anatomic parts in the following discussion be involved, immediate referral to a consultant is recommended.

Lacerations of the medial aspect of the eye can injure the tear duct apparatus (lacrimal canaliculus and nasolacrimal duct) or the medial palpebral ligament at the medial canthus. Copious tears running down the cheek of the patient is a sign of possible tear duct injuries. A laceration of the medial palpebral ligament will displace the lid apparatus laterally and requires meticulous reapposition and repair to restore the position of the lid. The levator palpebrae muscle is responsible for maintaining the eyelid in its normal position when open. Interruption of the muscle will cause traumatic ptosis. Injury to the muscle is suspected when periorbital fat can be seen to extrude from a laceration of the upper lid. Failure to recognize this condition and failure to perform proper repair will lead to permanent ptosis and an inability to open the eye fully.

Close inspection of the eye itself is necessary to rule out a hyphema, corneal abrasions, and foreign bodies. Of these injuries, hyphema is the most serious. It is

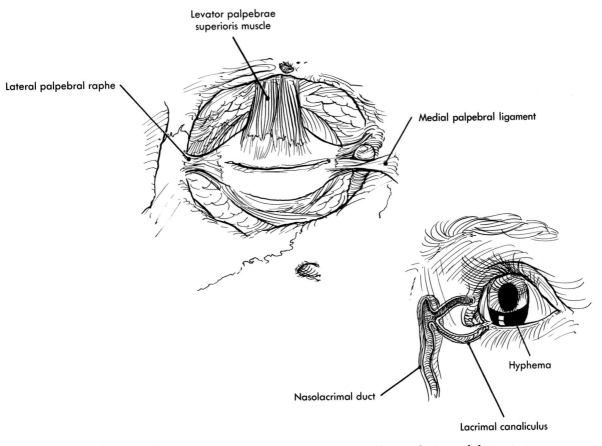

Levator palpebrae
superioris muscle

Lateral palpebral raphe

Medial palpebral ligament

Hyphema

Nasolacrimal duct

Lacrimal canaliculus

FIG. 11-4 Illustration of important anatomic structures that can be injured during eye trauma. The integrity of these structures must be confirmed prior to the closure of any laceration (see text).

caused by a direct blow to the eye and is recognized by a blood layer in the anterior chamber of the eye in patients in the upright position. In patients who are supine, blood will distribute evenly in the anterior chamber over the iris and give the iris a different color from the opposite iris. The patient will also complain of decreased vision in the affected eye.

Preparation for Closure

It is best to deliver an anesthetic to the eyelid by direct wound infiltration, using a small 27- or 30-gauge needle. Adrenalin-containing anesthetics are not necessary. For the eyebrow, the same technique is used, but adrenalin in the anesthetic can be useful to control minor bleeding. Special care is taken not to introduce cleansing agents into the eye itself in order to prevent unnecessary corneal damage. Polax-

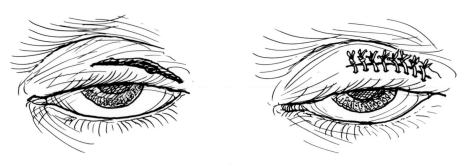

FIG. 11-5 Extramarginal lacerations of the upper lid are usually horizontal and can be closed with a simple row of percutaneous closures.

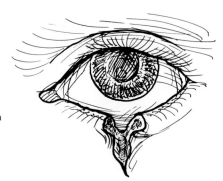

FIG. 11-6 A vertical, intramarginal lid laceration is best left to a consultant to repair.

amer 188 or povidone-iodine solution (not a detergent-containing solution) diluted 1:10 with saline are the cleansing agents of choice.[3] Inadvertent spilling of these preparations can be prevented by holding a folded 4 × 4 sponge over the closed eyelid margin to absorb free solution.

One important point to remember is not to shave the hair from the lid margin or brow because of the unpredictability of hair regrowth in this location.

Closure of Extramarginal Lid Lacerations

Extramarginal lacerations are usually horizontal and occur most commonly in the upper lid. If extramarginal lacerations are simple and superficial, they can be repaired with a single layer of 6-0 nonabsorbable suture material as illustrated in Fig. 11-5. No dressing is applied. These lacerations heal well enough so that scars become virtually unnoticeable with time.

Closure of Intramarginal Lid Lacerations

Intramarginal lacerations involve the lid margin and, like lip lacerations, require extremely careful repair to ensure proper alignment. Intramarginal injuries as shown in Fig. 11-6 are probably best left to a consultant for repair.

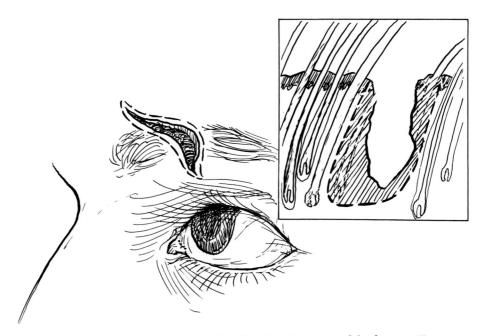

FIG. 11-7 Most eyebrow lacerations can be closed without tissue debridement. However, if macerated or devitalized tissue must be removed, it is important to excise this tissue parallel to the hair shaft. This excision technique will prevent an unsightly cosmetic defect.

Closure of Eyebrow Lacerations

Simple, uncomplicated eyebrow lacerations can be closed with a 6-0 or 5-0 nonabsorbable monofilament. Occasionally one or two dermal (deep) closures are necessary to approximate the superficial fascia. Great care is taken to properly align the brow margins to prevent a cosmetic deformity.

If the laceration has particularly ragged or macerated edges, then trimming or careful excision can be carried out. A basic principle to observe is that any debridement has to be parallel to the brow hair shafts (see Fig. 11-7). Failure to observe this principle can lead to an unnecessary defect following the repair.

Aftercare

No dressing is necessary for lid or brow lacerations. A daily, light application of Neosporin is recommended. Sutures are removed in 3 to 5 days in both children and adults.

CHEEK OR ZYGOMATIC AREA

There are two major structures underlying the cheek area, just anterior to the ear, that can be injured by penetrating lacerations. These are the parotid gland and the facial nerve (see Fig. 11-8). If the parotid gland is injured, salivary fluid can be seen

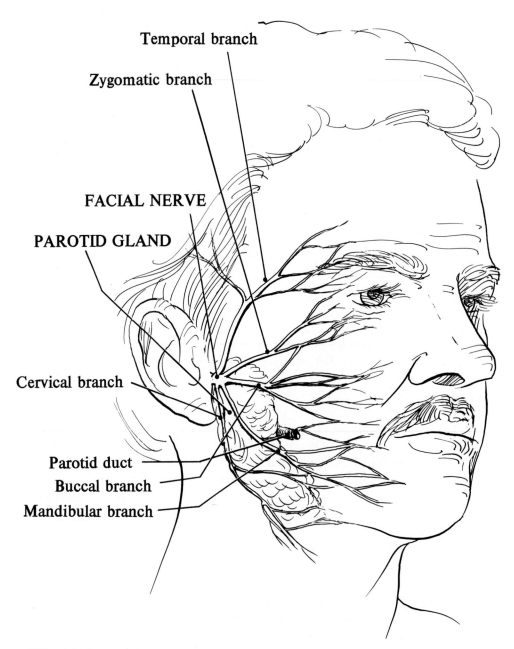

FIG. 11-8 The parotid gland and facial nerve underlie the zygomatic and cheek areas. Any lacerations anterior to the ear must be carefully assessed for injuries to the various branches of the facial nerve, parotid gland, or parotid duct.

leaking from the wound. Inspection of the inside of the mouth will often reveal bloody fluid coming from the opening of the parotid duct located on the buccal mucosa of the cheek at the level of the upper second molar tooth.

Lacerations of this region can also injure the facial nerve. It is necessary to test all five branches of the nerve to ensure that each one is intact. The temporal branch is tested by having the patient contract his or her forehead and elevate the brow. The function of the zygomatic branch is observed by having the patient open and shut his or her eyes. The act of sniffing with flaring of the nasal alae is also evidence for preserved function of that branch. Both buccal and mandibular branches innervate the lips during the acts of smiling and frowning. Finally, the cervical branch is tested by having the patient shrug his neck through contraction of the platysma muscle.

Preparation for Closure

The cheek is anesthetized and cleansed in the standard manner described above and in Chapters 5 and 6. Again, care is taken to avoid spilling cleansing solutions onto the eye itself.

Closure of Uncomplicated Cheek Lacerations

Standard percutaneous technique using 6-0 monofilament will close most lacerations. One important point to remember is that many people have natural creases in the skin of the cheek and face. These creases have the same importance cosmetically as the vermilion border of the lip. Proper alignment of them has to be given special attention. Often the initial percutaneous suture is placed to align with the crease before proceeding with the remainder of the closure.

Deep or Through-and-Through Lacerations

Complex lacerations that travel deep into the soft tissues of the cheek or those that penetrate the oral cavity are at risk for injuring the parotid gland or facial nerve as mentioned above. If neither of these structures is injured, repair can proceed. If there is any doubt, then a consultant is required. The oral cavity portion of a penetrating laceration is closed first with 5-0 chromic gut suture. If the oral portion of the laceration is less than 2 cm in length and is not gaping, it can be left open. The external wound is re-irrigated and closed with 6-0 monofilament.

Aftercare

Dressings are usually unnecessary for lacerations in this area. Daily application of Neosporin will allow for easier percutaneous suture removal at the 3-5 interval for children and adults. A recent controlled study of intraoral lacerations suggests that there is some benefit to administering oral penicillin VK 4 times daily for 5 days as prophylaxis against infection.[11] Erythromycin may be considered as an alternative.

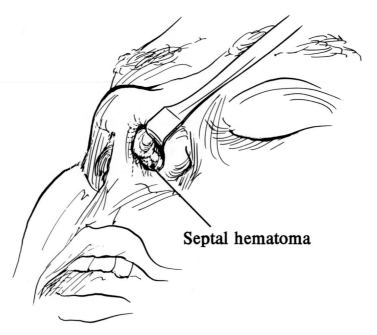

Septal hematoma

FIG. 11-9 Illustration of a septal hematoma in the area of the anterior nasal septum. Failure to drain this hematoma will lead to septal necrosis and collapse.

NASAL STRUCTURES

The nose is composed of both a bony and a cartilaginous skeleton. Like the ear, direct blows to the nose can cause the formation of a hematoma that compresses the cartilaginous septum (see Fig. 11-9). If not drained, this hematoma can lead to collapse through pressure necrosis of this important structure. Lacerations of the nose are common and are often associated with fractures. Radiographs do not always identify fractures and palpation remains a more sensitive indicator of bone injury and displacement.

Preparation for Closure

Prior to preparation and closure, the nose is inspected for the injuries mentioned above. Septal hematoma is recognized by its bluish, bulging appearance in the area of Kiesselbach's plexus (anterior septal area). The preferred method of examination is with a nasal speculum and an appropriately powerful light source. Penlights and otoscopes might be inadequate.

Anesthesia of the nose is best accomplished by the direct infiltration technique with a 27- or 30-gauge needle, using an agent without adrenalin. Nasal blocks are difficult to achieve and are usually reserved for major repairs. Cleansing of the nose is carried out by using povidone-iodine solution and saline irrigation.

Skin Lacerations

Most skin lacerations can be repaired with 6-0 nonabsorbable percutaneous mono-filament sutures. Sutures are placed with small bites because nasal skin tends to invert. The skin is also easily torn, so great care has to be taken to avoid creating excessive tension. Complex and irregular skin wounds have to be handled carefully. Since there is little redundancy of nasal skin, debridement has to be minimal. The best strategy is to "tack down" small tags or flaps percutaneously. Later revision can be carried out if necessary.

Mucosal and Cartilage Wounds

When the nasal mucosa is lacerated by penetration it has to be repaired with an absorbable suture such as a 5-0 polyglycolic acid suture. Deep or penetrating wounds can involve one of the many cartilaginous plates of the nasal skeleton. Placement of sutures in the cartilage is not necessary during repair. Closing the skin and mucosa over the cartilage will ensure adequate healing. Complete coverage of cartilage is mandatory because of its tendency to develop chronic chondritis if exposed. Avulsion and mutilating injuries of either the skin or cartilage are best managed by a consultant.

Septal Hematoma

Hematoma over the septal cartilage is drained with a hockey-stick or crescent-shaped incision as shown in Fig. 11-10. The incision is always made in the dependent portion of the hematoma. To prevent re-accumulation, an anterior nasal pack is placed with Vaseline gauze and the patient is referred to a consultant within 24 to 48 hours for inspection. When packing is placed, antibiotics are often recommended to prevent sinus infection. Amoxicillin or Bactrim are reasonable choices.

Lacerations With Bone Involvement

Lacerations of the skin over non-displaced nasal fractures without penetration and mucosal involvement can be closed using the previously described techniques. Complex lacerations with fracture displacement, mucosal injury from bone fragmentation, or extensive cartilage involvement are best managed by a consultant.

Aftercare

Dressings are optional for nasal lacerations. Often a simple Bandaid will suffice. The percutaneous sutures are removed in 3 to 5 days in both children and adults. Antibiotics are not recommended for any nasal laceration unless packing is placed.

EAR

The ear consists of a cartilaginous skeleton covered by tightly adherent skin with little intervening superficial fascia (subcutaneous tissue). One of the consequences of this fact is that a direct blow to the ear can cause a hematoma to form, usually in

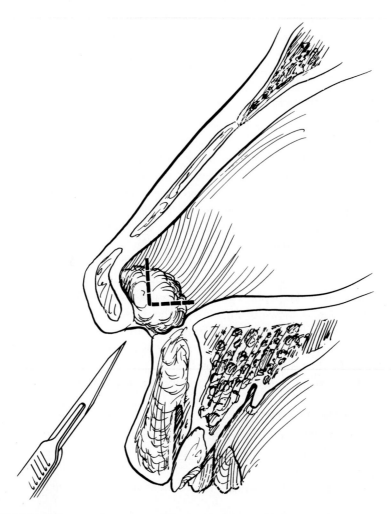

FIG. 11-10 Technique to drain a septal hematoma. A #11 blade is used to create a "hockey-stick" incision as illustrated. Following drainage, the nose is packed with Vaseline gauze. (Adapted from Zukin D and Simon R: Emergency wound care: principles and practice, Rockville, Md, 1987, Aspen Publishers Inc.)

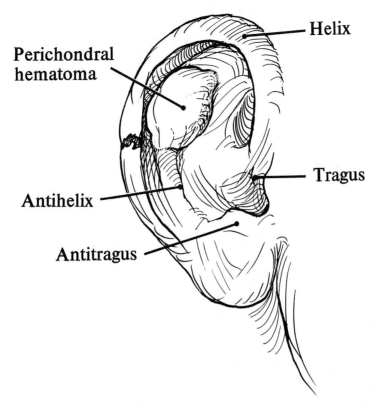

Helix

Perichondral
hematoma

Tragus

Antihelix

Antitragus

FIG. 11-11 Anatomy of the external ear. Note the presence of perichondral hematoma. Perichondral hematoma formation can occur following blunt trauma to the ear and can accompany lacerations.

the area of the antihelix, with a resultant breakdown of the cartilage caused by pressure between the skin and cartilage, as seen in Fig. 11-11. The eventual result is the well-known "cauliflower" ear.

Preparation for Repair

In addition to inspecting the external ear for hematoma formation and cartilage injury, the internal canal and tympanic membrane are visualized to complete the examination. Blunt injuries to the ear can cause perforations of the tympanic membrane. The most significant injury that can accompany lacerations to the ear is a basilar skull fracture, which can be recognized by hemotympanum or Battle's sign (ecchymosis of the mastoid area).

Small, uncomplicated lacerations to the ear can be anesthetized by direct infiltration with a 27- or 30-gauge needle using an anesthetic solution without adrenalin. The needle is carefully introduced between the skin and the cartilage, and only a small amount of anesthetic is deposited in order to minimize distortion of the wound edges. For large, complex lacerations and wounds, the ear block described in Chapter 5 can be used. Cleansing is carried out with povidone-iodine solution and irrigation. Because of the complicated topography of the ear, cotton-swab applicators can be particularly useful for cleansing.

Uncomplicated Lacerations

Simple lacerations of the helix and lobule that do not involve cartilage can be closed with interrupted or running 6-0 nonabsorbable monofilament suture (see Fig. 11-12). To prevent wound-edge inversion, small 1-2 mm bites are taken. If debridement is necessary, it should be kept to a minimum to prevent exposure of the cartilage. There is little redundancy of ear skin. Like the nose, cartilage exposure can lead to chronic chondritis and increased deformity of the ear. Sutures are removed 5 days after repair.

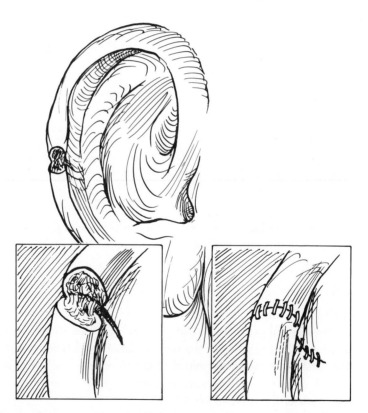

FIG. 11-12 Simple non-cartilaginous lacerations of the ear are closed with either interrupted or running percutaneous skin sutures.

Lacerations Involving Cartilage

Sharp, shearing lacerations that penetrate cartilage can be managed by carefully apposing the skin overlying the cartilaginous interruption. The skin is sufficiently adherent and supporting so that sutures do not have to be placed through the cartilage itself to bring together the lacerated cartilage edges. Sharp, through-and-through lacerations can be managed in a similar manner.

Irregular wounds that involve cartilage have to be managed while two principles are kept in mind. Debridement must be kept to a minimum and no cartilage must be left exposed. If cartilage is exposed and the skin cannot be brought together over it without undue tension, then it can be debrided conservatively to match the skin and cartilage edges. No sutures are placed in the cartilage (as shown in Fig. 11-13, A and B). Complex cartilage injuries require consultation.

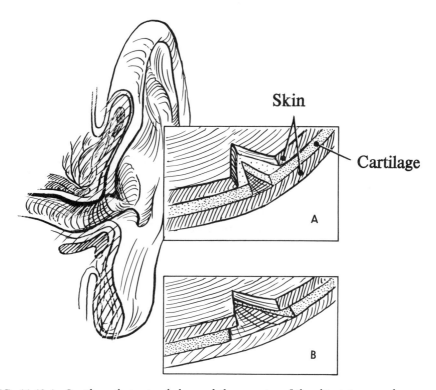

FIG. 11-13 A, Cartilage that extends beyond the margins of the skin injury can be trimmed back, by using tissue scissors, to ensure complete coverage both anteriorly and posteriorly by skin. **B,** Skin is closed with simple percutaneous sutures. No sutures are necessary for the cartilage. (Adapted from Zukin D and Simon R: Emergency wound care: principles and practice, Rockville, Md, 1987, Aspen Publishers Inc.)

Perichondral Hematoma

When a perichondral hematoma is present, it has to be adequately drained. A small incision is made over the hematoma and the hematoma is evacuated from the space between the perichondrium and the cartilage. Placement of a small rubber drain is optional. After drainage, a mastoid dressing is placed as described in Chapter 17. The dressing is removed in 24 hours and is inspected for re-accumulation. More often than not, complex lacerations and hematomas of the ear are best cared for by or under the guidance of a consultant.

Aftercare

Because the ear is difficult to dress it is often left open. If there is any question of possible perichondral blood accumulation after the patient is discharged, then a mastoid dressing is recommended (see Chapter 17). Sutures are removed after 4 to 5 days for adults and 3 to 5 days for children. When cartilage is involved or a septal hematoma has been drained, antibiotic prophylaxis is recommended. Choices include dicloxacillin, a first-generation cephalosporin, or amoxicillin with clavulanate, and erythromycin for the penicillin-allergic patient. Uncomplicated, non-cartilaginous injuries do not require antibiotics.

LIPS

Lacerations of the lip can cause devastating cosmetic defects if not properly and meticulously repaired. A misalignment by as little as 1 mm of the vermilion border, or "white line," can be easily noticed by the casual observer. It is also a defect that cannot easily be revised after primary healing has taken place. Other important anatomic structures include the mucosal border (the portion of the lip that divides the intra- and extra-oral portion of the lip) and the underlying orbicularis oris muscle. Each of these structures requires careful and exact apposition to achieve the best structural and cosmetic result. Vertical through-and-through lacerations will often violate all three of these structures.

Preparation for Closure

Although the mouth is replete with bacteria, and a lip laceration will not remain clean during the repair procedure, cleansing is only carried out to remove gross debris and dirt. If any teeth are broken, then a careful search is made in the wound for teeth fragments. Retained tooth particles can cause marked inflammation and infection leading to a complete breakdown of any attempted repair. Whenever a portion of a tooth cannot be located, a lateral radiograph of the face using soft-tissue technique will reveal the missing fragment.

Anesthesia for lip repairs is best accomplished by either an infra-orbital nerve block for the upper lip or a mental nerve block for the lower lip (see Chapter 5). Direct infiltration of the laceration can be used but excessive injection will cause distortion of the lip and create difficulties when attempting to properly align wound edges.

Uncomplicated Lacerations

Most lip lacerations usually do not require extensive revision or debridement. The key to closure is proper alignment of the anatomic structures listed previously. If the vermilion border is violated and the laceration is superficial, then the repair begins by placing the first suture exactly through that border on each side of the wound (Fig. 11-14). Once alignment is judged to be appropriate, then the remainder of the wound is closed with 6-0 nonabsorbable monofilament sutures. If the mucosal border is violated, it also is aligned meticulously. As a general rule, if the laceration extends beyond the mucosal border into the oral cavity, then 5-0 absorbable suture, such as chromic gut, is used to close that portion. Polyglactin 910 (Vicryl) is preferred by some authorities because it does not "stiffen" as much as gut.

Complicated and Through-and-Through Lacerations

Unlike many other structures of the face, the lip can be revised and significant portions of devitalized tissue, up to 5 mm of each wound edge, can be excised. Considerable judgment is required to deal with these cosmetic problems in image-conscious patients who have high expectations for excellent results.

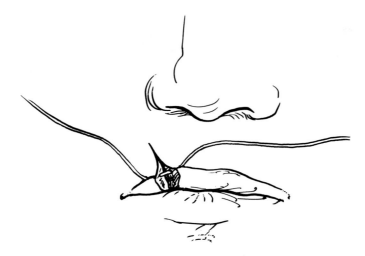

FIG. 11-14 The major goal when closing any lip laceration is to align the appropriate borders. Illustrated in this figure is the initial suture placement and alignment of the vermilion border. Once the vermilion border or "white line" is aligned, then the remainder of the laceration is closed.

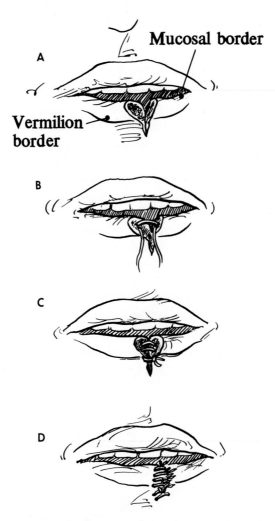

FIG. 11-15 A, Demonstration of a through-and-through laceration of the lip involving orbicularis oris muscle. **B,** Closure of the orbicularis oris muscle is carried out by using absorbable deep sutures such as polyglycolic acid. **C,** Once the orbicularis oris muscle is approximated, the vermilion border or "white line" is approximated. **D,** The remainder of the laceration is closed with simple percutaneous monofilament nylon sutures.

Repair of a vertical through-and-through laceration is illustrated in Fig. 11-15. The orbicularis oris muscle is carefully reapproximated with deep 5-0 absorbable suture material like polyglycolic acid. The vermilion border is approximated next using a simple 6-0 nonabsorbable suture monofilament. The remainder of the repair proceeds as described in the section on uncomplicated lacerations.

Aftercare

No dressing is placed on the lips. The patient is reminded not to bring excessive pressure to bear on the suture line while the sutures are in place. Rinsing the mouth after eating is recommended to prevent small particulate matter from penetrating the suture line. The extra-oral sutures are removed after 4 to 5 days in adults and 3 to 5 days in children to prevent the formation of suture marks. Antibiotics are recommended as discussed above for penetrating lacerations through the cheek into the oral cavity. Penicillin and erythromycin (for penicillin-allergic patients) are recommended choices.

ORAL CAVITY

The oral cavity consists of several structures, each of which requires separate considerations during management and repair. These are the buccal mucosa, gingiva, teeth, salivary glands and ducts, tongue, mandible, and the alveolar ridge of the maxillary bone. Injuries to the oral cavity can be a potential threat to airway patency.

Preparation for Repair

Other than airway considerations, the most important part of the evaluation of the oral cavity is the determination of the integrity of salivary structures, bone, and teeth. Visual inspection as well as palpation is necessary to complete the examination. Particularly troublesome are teeth, fragments of which must be accounted for if possible. They can easily lodge in the mucosa and the deep tissue of the lip where they can cause severe inflammation and infection if not removed prior to closure. If there is any question about the location of a tooth or fragment, radiographs of the soft tissues should be performed.

Teeth are often loosened by trauma to the oral cavity. Minimal loosening, as determined by gentle "rocking" of the tooth between the examining fingers, will usually reverse without intervention. Marked loosening or subluxation with an accompanying fracture of the alveolar ridge needs to be repaired with dental stabilization.

Intact teeth can also become avulsed. These teeth can be replaced in an anatomically intact socket but the prognosis for salvage decreases with each minute that passes. After 30 minutes the prognosis for salvage is low. Even if the periodontal ligament survives and the tooth reattaches, later root-canal intervention will be necessary to deal with the sequelae of the loss of neurovascular supply. Consultation with an oral surgeon or dentist is appropriate in these matters.

Buccal Mucosal and Gingival Lacerations

As a general rule, lacerations of either structure will heal without repair if the wound edges are not widely separated. These lacerations are usually 1 to 2 cm or less. Larger, gaping, or flap lacerations can be closed with 5-0 chromic gut or Vicryl

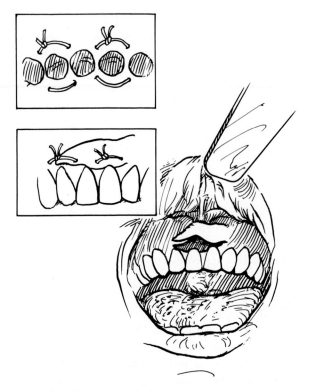

FIG. 11-16 Illustration of avulsion of gingival/mucosal tissue. The technique to close this injury is illustrated. The sutures are brought around the teeth and through the avulsed tissue flap. (Adapted from Zukin D and Simon R: Emergency wound care: principles and practice, Rockville, Md, 1987, Aspen Publishers Inc.)

permucosally. Only enough sutures are placed to appose the wound edges. The oral cavity tissues heal remarkably fast and do not require extensive repair. The patient is instructed to eat soft food and to rinse his or her mouth gently after each meal.

Occasionally, a flap of tissue will be created during injury to the gingiva overlying the mandibular or maxillary ridge. Because of the lack of support by thin supporting tissues, the gingival flap cannot be easily sutured. A technique illustrated in Fig. 11-16 demonstrates how sutures are brought circumferentially around teeth to provide the necessary anchor for the repair. 4-0 or 5-0 chromic gut or Vicryl can be used.

Tongue Lacerations

Repairing a lacerated tongue can be challenging. Lacerations of 1 cm or less that do not gape widely when the tongue is extended will heal without intervention. The key to the repair of larger lacerations is to gain the confidence of the patient. With frightened children this is often difficult and the patient might be best served in a surgical setting where an anesthesic can be delivered. In other cases an assistant is required to gain control of the tongue with dry gauze sponges (for traction). Another technique is to place two 2-0 silk sutures through the side borders (with prior anesthetizing of the two sites) of the tongue to accomplish the same end. The assistant stabilizes the retention sutures during repair. Always ensure that a bite block has been fashioned to prevent injuring the assistant or the operator. The tongue heals rapidly and can be closed with an absorbable suture like 5-0 chromic, polyglycolic acid or Vicryl.

Aftercare

For the first 2 or 3 days after repair of an intra-oral laceration, soft foods and liquids are recommended. Rinsing the oral cavity after eating is also helpful.

PERINEUM

Injuries to the perineum, i.e., penis, scrotum, and female introitus, can involve important structures that will need special attention. During the examination of wounds of the perineum, the urethra, corpora, testicles, and rectum must be assessed. Blood coming from the urethral meatus or difficulty urinating suggests urethral injury. The shaft of the penis is covered by very thin skin; violation of the corpora cavernosa or spongiosum often accompanies lacerations of the penis. The testicle is covered with a capsule-like fibrous covering called the tunica albuginea. Interruption of the corpora or tunica requires repair by a specialist. Most labial lacerations are uncomplicated but occasionally the female urethra or rectum is involved.

Preparation for Closure

Wounds to the perineum are prepared with a cleansing agent and are irrigated with saline as previously described. Uncomplicated lacerations can be anesthetized directly with lidocaine or bupivacaine. Care is taken not to use adrenalin-containing solutions for anesthetizing the penis because of potential ischemia due to constriction of end-arteries.

Lacerations of the Penis and Scrotum

Because the skin of the penis is so thin, lacerations are closed with a single layer of nonabsorbable suture like 5-0 nylon. Closure of the scrotal skin is carried out with chromic gut. Healing takes place rapidly and removal of sutures from the rugated skin, which can be difficult, is unnecessary.

Lacerations of the Introitus

Lacerations of the labia can involve the deeper supporting muscles. If that is the case, closure has to take place in two layers to ensure reapproximation of the muscles. The skin over the labia majora can be closed with a nonabsorbable material like nylon or polypropylene. The labia minora is covered with mucosa and can be closed with absorbable material. Uncomplicated lacerations of the vagina, unless they are extensive, will heal without sutures. Extensive or complex wounds are best referred to consultants.

Aftercare

Dressings for the genital area are hard to fashion. Gauze sponges supported by an athletic supporter are an option for men. Perineal pads are suggested for women. Hygiene of the genital area is important and daily gentle cleansing with soap and water is acceptable. Neosporin applied after bathing and before dressing application is recommended. Sutures of the penis are removed in 7 to 10 days for adults and 6 to 8 days for children.

KNEE

The knee is important because of the important structures that can be damaged following a laceration. The peroneal nerve, patellar tendon, medial and lateral collateral ligaments, and patella all have to be tested for function and integrity before repair. Of particular importance is the joint space itself. If penetration is suspected, then 50 cc of normal saline with a few drops of methylene blue are injected into the joint, in a sterile fashion, at a site distant from the laceration. Arthrocentesis technique is used. If the capsule is violated, then the dye will leak out of the laceration. For more subtle injuries, fluorescein dye can be used with an ultraviolet light detection lamp.

Uncomplicated, non-penetrating lacerations are closed with monofilament nylon after local anesthetic infiltration. Occasionally deep (dermal) sutures are required using an absorbable material. Penetrating injuries require consultation.

Aftercare

The key to good healing of knee lacerations is proper immobilization and elevation for several days. Crutches can be used for at least 48 to 72 hours if the extensor surface of the knee is involved or the wound is extensive. Knee flexion can be reduced by the application of a bulky dressing. Sutures are removed in 10 to 14 days in adults and 8 to 10 days for children.

LOWER LEG

The most vexing consideration with lower leg lacerations is the significant tension that occurs at the wound edge. Skin overlying the tibia is under a higher natural tension than most other regions of the body. Fig. 11-17 illustrates a technique for approximating the wound edges with as little tension as possible. 4-0 monofilament nylon is passed through sterile cotton-retaining pledgets obtained from the operat-

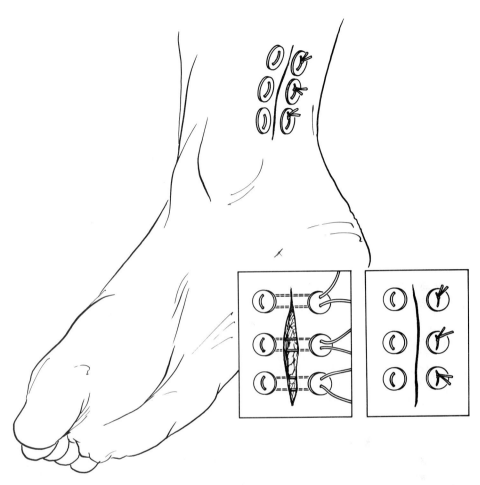

FIG. 11-17 Because of the high tension usually associated with lacerations in the lower leg (shin area), sterile cotton pledgets can be used as support for 3-0 or 4-0 monofilament nylon sutures as illustrated. (Adapted from Zukin D and Simon R: Emergency wound care: principles and practice, Rockville, Md, 1987, Aspen Publishers Inc.)

ing room. This technique allows for even distribution of tension along the wound edge without tearing. This pledget technique is particularly useful for older and thinner skin.

Aftercare

Elevation is an important element for lacerations and wounds of the lower leg. Dependent edema should not be allowed to develop. Sutures are removed after 8 to 12 days for adults and 6 to 10 days for children. Tape support for one week after suture removal is recommended.

FOOT

The foot is anatomically complex and has similarities to the hand. Complete lacerations to the tendons need to be repaired as they are in hands. Partial lacerations of extensor tendons can be treated with primary skin closure and splinting. Consultation is recommended under these circumstances. Anesthesia for the plantar surface of the foot is best carried out by a posterior tibial nerve or sural nerve block, described in Chapter 5. Occasionally this method of administering anesthesia needs to be supplemented by local infiltration. Superficial dorsal lacerations are closed with 4-0 or 5-0 monofilament nylon. Lacerations of the plantar surface, or sole, can be closed with 3-0 monofilament. Lacerations of the web spaces between the toes have the same significance as lacerations of web spaces of the hand. There are no crucial structures passing through these areas and repair of the skin alone should suffice.

Aftercare

Like any lower-extremity injury, elevation is an important adjunct to care. Crutches are useful, particularly for wounds on the plantar surface. Sutures are removed in 10 to 12 days for adults and 8 to 10 days for children.

References

1. Cruse P and Foord R: A five year prospective of 23,649 surgical wounds, Arch Surg 107:206-209, 1973.
2. Duschoff IM: About face, Emerg Med. Nov 1974, pp. 25-77.
3. Edlich RF et al: Principles of wound management, Ann Emerg Med 17:1284-1302, 1988.
4. Edlich R et al: Technical factors in the prevention of human wound infection. In Simmons R and Howard R, eds: Surgical Infectious Diseases, New York, 1982, Appleton-Century Crofts.
5. Fullarton GM et al: An evaluation of open scalp wounds, Arch Emerg Med 4:11-16, 1987.
6. George TK and Simpson DC: Skin wound closure with staples in the accident and emergency department, J Royal Coll Surg (Edin), 30:54-56, 1985.
7. Howell JM and Morgan JA: Scalp laceration repair without prior hair removal, Am J Emerg Med 6:7-10, 1988.
8. Pecora D, Landis R, and Martin E: Location of cutaneous microorganisms, Surgery 64:1114-1117, 1968.
9. Roth JH and Windle BH: Staple versus suture closure of skin incisions in a pig model, Can J Surg 31:19, 1988.
10. Seropian R and Reynolds B: Wound infections after preoperative depilatory versus razor preparation, Am J Surg 121:251-254, 1971.
11. Steele MT et al: Prophylactic penicillin for intraoral wounds, Ann Emerg Med 18:847-852, 1989.

12 *The Hand*

Initial Treatment
Patient History
Terminology
Examination of the Hand
   Nerve Testing
      Motor function
      Sensory function
   Tendon Function
      Extensor function
      Flexor function
Circulation
Radiography
Wound Exploration
Selected Hand Injuries and Problems
   Uncomplicated Lacerations

Fingertip Injuries
   Blunt/crushing injuries
   Nail removal technique
   Shearing injuries
   Avulsion injuries
Tendon Lacerations
Nerve Injuries
Amputated Parts
Paronychia
Felon
Pressure Injection Injuries
Antibiotics for Hand Wounds
   Dressings and Aftercare
References

A thorough understanding of the structure and function of the hand is essential to its care, even for seemingly minor injuries and problems. The complexity and relative density of important structures make the hand particularly vulnerable to injury with the attendant risk of serious, permanent impairment. Each anatomic structure and functional unit of the hand should be assessed, and with the use of conventional terminology, information concerning the examination can be properly recorded in the medical record and communicated to others. Problems that are appropriately managed by emergency wound-care personnel are discussed in the text that follows. Where there is any doubt concerning the proper course of management, every attempt is made to initiate an appropriate consultation.

INITIAL TREATMENT

Before a thorough and careful examination of a patient with an injured hand can take place, certain preparatory steps have to be taken. Except for the most trivial injuries, the patient is best managed by placing him or her on a stretcher upon arrival at the medical care facility. Hand injuries are often painful and provoke anxiety. Placing the patient in a supine position will prevent unexpected vasovagal syncope. The recumbent position will more easily allow for placement of the hand in an elevated position to decrease the swelling that occurs following injury.

Any rings or constricting jewelry are removed to prevent ischemia of a digit. Most rings can be removed by using a lubricant and applying gentle, persistent traction. Ring removal from swollen fingers can be carried out by using a specially designed ring cutter and spreading the ring open with two Kelly clamps applied to the edges of the cut portion. Reassure patients who are concerned about damaged rings that jewelers can restore rings to their original condition. Another method for the removal of rings is illustrated in Fig. 12-1. Umbilical tape or O-silk suture can be firmly wrapped around the finger and passed under the ring with a small forceps. The ring is extracted as the tape or suture is unwound proximally to the ring.

Most patients attempt to bandage the injured hand before proceeding to a medical care facility. These hastily fashioned, unsterile dressings should be carefully removed. Until treatment can be administered, sterile sponges moistened with normal saline should be applied, followed by a 2-inch or 3-inch gauze wrap. Any active bleeding will require manual pressure with gauze sponges. Only rarely is an extremity tourniquet needed to stop excessive hemorrhage.

If the wound is grossly contaminated with soil or other debris and if there will be a delay before treatment is administered, the hand is gently cleaned with a wound-cleansing agent followed by irrigation with normal saline. The chance of infection increases with each passing hour from the time of injury to repair. Early cleansing and irrigation can extend this safe period.

It is a common but unsupported practice to soak hand injuries in a wound-cleansing solution before repair. Although soaking is believed to loosen debris and help kill contaminating bacteria, there is no scientific evidence to support these beliefs.[21] In addition, wound-cleansing solutions containing detergents can experimentally be demonstrated to have toxic effects on healthy, non-injured tissues within the wounds.[3,7,22] Brief extremity immersion is recommended only to help remove gross soil and debris from the area surrounding the wound.

PATIENT HISTORY

There are certain key historical facts that help determine the timing and choice of repair, as well as other supportive treatment. As previously discussed, how much time has elapsed from the time that the injury was sustained will influence the decision of when to repair the wound. Clean wounds that are caused by shearing forces can probably be safely repaired up to 8 to 10 hours post-injury. Wounds caused by tension and compression mechanisms are more vulnerable and should be considered for closure sooner. Severely contaminated wounds, or those caused by mutilating forces, are best left for consultation and possible delayed closure. This decision is made based on individual cases.

A seemingly innocuous mechanism of injury is the puncture wound of the hand. Although the entry point is quite small and innocent-appearing, special care has to be taken not to miss a transected nerve or tendon. In addition, the possibility of a

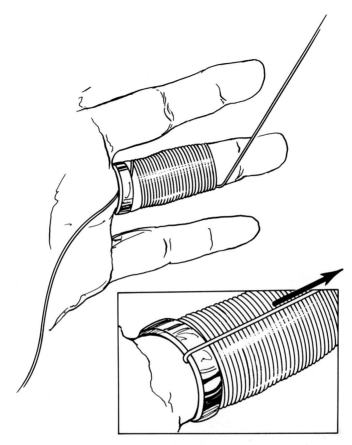

FIG. 12-1 Illustration of the technique to remove a ring by finger-wrapping with large silk suture or umbilical tape. Note that the suture is begun distally over the distal interphalangeal (DIP) joint and brought back to the ring. The tailend portion of the wrap is brought under the ring, usually with a small hemostat. The removal of the ring is begun by unraveling the wrap and tugging on the string that is proximal to the ring portion. As it unravels, the ring will gently travel forward distally over the finger.

foreign body being retained in a puncture wound has to be considered and radiography should be carried out when the suspicion is raised.

Other historical points of importance are the patient's hand dominance, history of prior hand deformities, profession, and hobbies. Although these considerations are seemingly not as important for patients with emergency lacerations and wounds, a simple matter of a mismanaged fingertip injury can significantly affect an activity like playing the guitar. For the guitar player, every step is taken to preserve the nail matrix. Preservation attempts might not be so necessary for an individual who does not require this anatomic part for either a job function or hobby.

Finally, any allergies the patient may have should be verified from a patient's history. Many drugs are given to patients with hand injuries. These drugs include tetanus toxoid, local anesthetics, pain medications, and a variety of antibiotics.

TERMINOLOGY

In order to properly document and communicate information about injuries of the hand and fingers, knowledge of the conventional terminology is required. All lacerations and wounds can be accurately located by the use of appropriate terms. For example, a ½-inch laceration on the back of the index finger at the first knuckle is accurately described as "a 1-cm superficial laceration of the index finger on the dorsal surface at the proximal interphalangeal joint (PIP)." Figs. 12-2 and 12-3 illustrate the various descriptive landmarks and joints. The back of the hand is the dorsal surface, while the palmar side is the palmar or volar surface. Common landmarks of the palm are the thenar and hypothenar eminence. The digits are best remembered and recorded, when necessary, as the thumb, index, middle, ring, and little finger. Each segment of the finger is named for the underlying bony phalanx. Although the

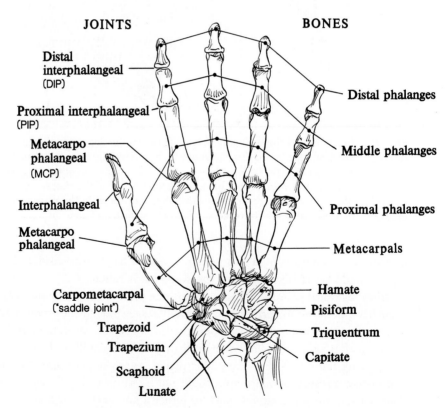

JOINTS

Distal interphalangeal (DIP)

Proximal interphalangeal (PIP)

Metacarpo phalangeal (MCP)

Interphalangeal

Metacarpo phalangeal

Carpometacarpal ("saddle joint")

Trapezoid

Trapezium

Scaphoid

Lunate

BONES

Distal phalanges

Middle phalanges

Proximal phalanges

Metacarpals

Hamate

Pisiform

Triquentrum

Capitate

FIG. 12-2 Descriptive anatomy of the joints and bones of the hand.

joints are descriptive of their location, it is the convention to use the abbreviations noted in Fig. 12-2.

Instead of using terms like inside and outside or medial or lateral, the sides of the hands and fingers are referred to as radial or ulnar. This convention eliminates the confusion elicited by the other terms. Any injury to any surface on the side of the hand or finger corresponding to the radius is so described. For example, a laceration of the side of the little finger is either radial or ulnar depending on whether it is on the side of the ulna or the radius; see Fig. 12-3.

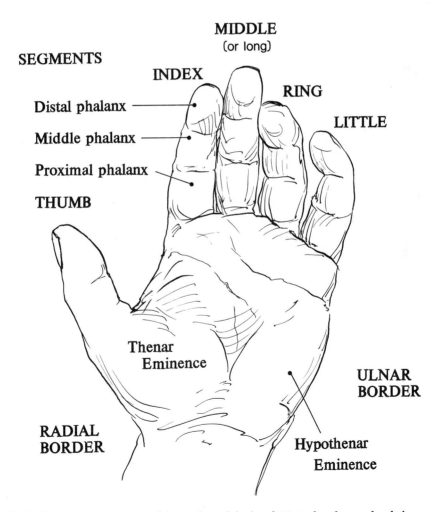

SURFACE ANATOMY
(Volar Surface)

FIG. 12-3 Descriptive anatomy of the surface of the hand. Note the ulnar and radial borders.

EXAMINATION OF THE HAND

The actual examination of the injured hand consists both of careful inspection of the wound and thorough functional testing. Nerve function is evaluated by assessing both motor and sensory components. The integrity of tendons can most often be determined by specific functional maneuvers. However, because tendons are often only partially severed and function is preserved, direct visualization by exploration is frequently necessary. In emergency wounds, circulation is so profuse that severed, bleeding vessels that travel in neurovascular bundles are often better indicators of nerve injury than actual threats to perfusion of the hand or finger. When necessary, radiographs are obtained to assist in the examination to rule out either fractures or foreign bodies. Finally, there is no substitute for exploration and direct visualization to discover structural damage of any type.

Nerve Testing
Motor Function

There are three major nerves responsible for both motor and sensory function of the hand. The radial nerve innervates the extrinsic muscles of the forearm that are responsible for extension of the wrist and fingers. This nerve does not innervate any muscle within the confines of the hand itself. The motor function of this nerve is tested by having the patient dorsiflex his or her wrist and fingers against a resisting force such as the examiner's hand. Intact motor strength, as provided for by an intact radial nerve, should prevent the examiner from overcoming the dorsiflexed wrist when a good deal of counterforce is applied.

In addition to the flexor carpi ulnaris and part of the flexor digitorum profundus, the ulnar nerve innervates most of the intrinsic muscles of the hand itself, including all of the interossei muscles and little and ring finger lumbricals. The motor portion of this nerve is responsible for the ability of the fingers to spread and close in a fan-like manner. A specific test for ulnar motor function is to have the patient abduct his index finger away from the middle finger, as shown in Fig. 12-4. This test is carried out by asking the patient to place his or her hand on a table or other hard surface, ulnar side down. The patient is asked to point the second digit toward the ceiling against an opposing force from the examiner. The first interosseous muscle, in the web space between the thumb and index finger, if properly functioning, can be palpated as it contracts. Fanning all fingers is a rapid indicator of ulnar nerve function.

The median nerve provides motor innervation to wrist flexors, the flexor digitorum superficialis, part of the flexor digitorum profundus (shared with the ulnar nerve), and the remaining intrinsic muscles of the hand, most notably those of the thumb that are responsible for opposition. Opposition to some degree is also mediated by the adduction component of the interossei as supplied to the ulnar nerve. Therefore, in order to properly test the median function, the hand is laid on its dor-

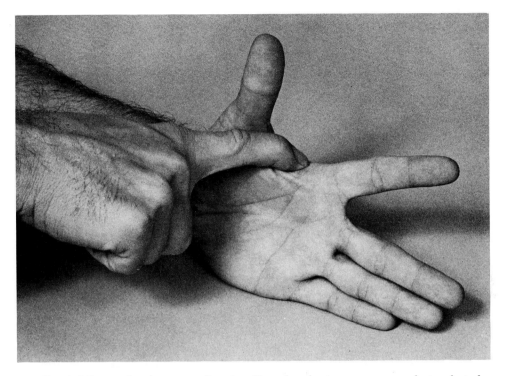

FIG. 12-4 Testing for ulnar nerve function. Note that the interosseous muscle is palpated as the index finger is forcibly abducted.

sal surface on a table. The patient is then asked to point the thumb directly at the ceiling, as shown in Fig. 12-5. The testing maneuver is completed by having the patient oppose his or her thumb toward the tip of the little finger while keeping the thumb pointed upward. A properly made ring consisting of the thumb and little finger should be hard to break by the examiner if the median nerve is intact.

Sensory Function

There are a variety of stimuli that can be delivered to the skin of the hand to test sensory function. Gross touch with a blunt object is the easiest but least specific. It can be useful, however, for rapid screening to assess the possibility of nerve damage especially when comparison testing is done between the injured and noninjured hands. If there is a nerve injury, the patient will often be able to report a difference in feeling. Pinprick stimulus is the most commonly used modality for testing. Pinprick is useful when alternated with blunt stimulus. In a complete nerve transection, the patient cannot tell the difference between a blunt and a sharp stimulus. Pinprick testing, nevertheless, is difficult to assess on the fingertips, espe-

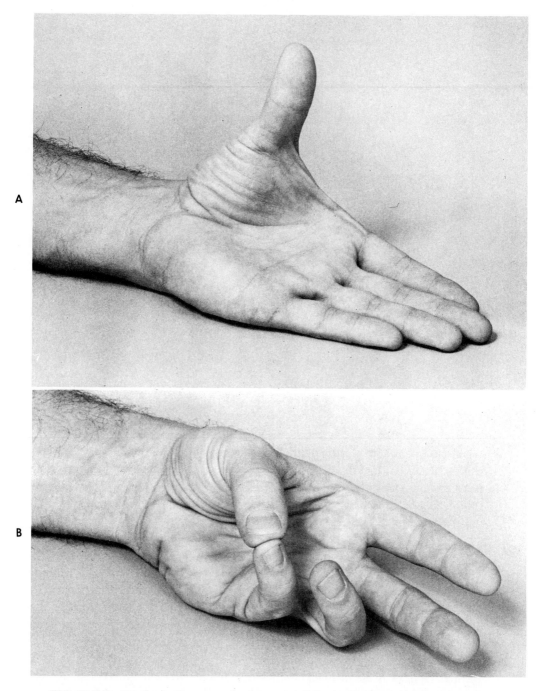

FIG. 12-5 Testing for median nerve function. **A,** While the hand is laid on a flat surface, the thumb is forcibly extended directly toward the ceiling. **B,** The thumb is apposed to the little finger to form a tight ring. This ring should not be easily broken by the examiner.

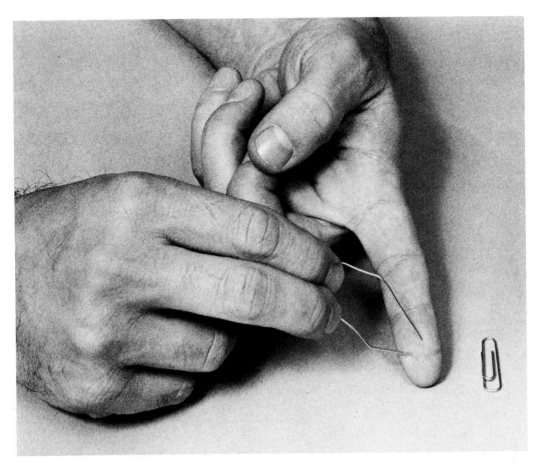

FIG. 12-6 Technique for testing sensory nerve function by two-point discrimination. A paper clip is bent in a manner to provide variable distance stimuli. See text for description.

cially in a manual laborer whose finger pads are covered with thick calluses.

A more accurate method of assessing sensory function is two-point discrimination.[10] A paper clip can be fashioned so that two ends can be opened or closed to varying distances from each other, as demonstrated in Fig. 12-6. A patient with a normally innervated fingertip should be able to distinguish two simultaneously delivered stimuli 6 mm or less apart. Most patients can tell a difference down to 3 mm. When identification of separate stimuli is reported by the patient at 8 mm apart or more, the examination is clearly abnormal.

Of the major nerves, the radial nerve provides the least important sensory innervation to the hand. This nerve supplies sensation to the radial portion of the dorsum of the hand, the dorsum of the thumb, and the proximal portion of the dorsal side of the second and third digits and half of the ring finger, as seen in Fig. 12-7.

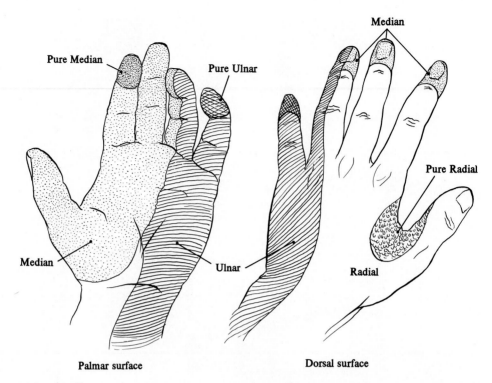

FIG. 12-7 Illustration of the distribution of the three major nerves providing sensory innervation of the hand. Note the areas of pure median, ulnar, and radial sensation.

To rapidly test gross radial sensory function, a stimulus is supplied to the first web space, an area of pure radial distribution.

Sensory distribution of the ulnar nerve includes the dorsal and volar surfaces of the ulnar side of the hand, the entire fifth digit, and the ulnar half of the fourth digit. To test an intact sensory component of the ulnar nerve, an appropriate stimulus is delivered to the area of purest ulnar distribution, the tip of the fifth digit.

The remainder of the hand is innervated by the median nerve. The radial side of the palm and volar surfaces of the thumb, index, middle, and radial half of the ring fingers comprise the area of sensory distribution. As depicted in Fig. 12-7, it is important to note that median nerve innervation extends to all of the fingertips of the thumb, index, and middle fingers, including the dorsal portion of the distal phalanges. Pure median sensation can be found at the tip of the index finger.

More common than injuries to the major nerves are injuries and lacerations to the digital nerves that lie within the hand itself. There are four digital nerves for each digit. The two palmar nerves, seen in Fig. 12-8, are the largest and most important. Sensation to the palmar surface as well as the dorsum of the fingertip is

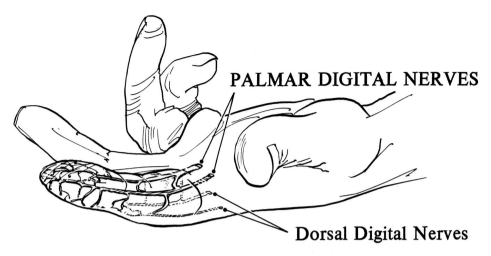

PALMAR DIGITAL NERVES

Dorsal Digital Nerves

FIG. 12-8 Note that each digit is supplied by four digital nerves. The palmar digital nerves predominate and provide the majority of the sensation to the volar aspect of the finger and finger tip proximal to the DIP. The nail bed is often included in the palmar digital nerve distribution.

carried through these two nerves. A laceration or puncture wound to the palmar or dorsal surfaces of the hand or to any individual digit requires careful sensory testing of the digits distal to the injury. As previously described, a variety of stimuli can be used for sensory testing. The most accurate method of detecting a nerve injury in this setting is the two-point discrimination test. In spite of attempts at objective testing, however, it is not uncommon for a patient to report a subjective loss of feeling. Even though stimulus testing is inconsistent or does not clearly document the loss, this subjective loss has to be taken seriously, and, if there is any doubt, consultation with a hand specialist is recommended.

Tendon Function

Tendon function can be difficult because of the number and complexity of the tendons to be tested. The following is a discussion of some of the general principles behind tendon function and testing. Table 12-1 contains a complete listing of each of the musculotendinous units in the hand and of their related nerve control.

Extensor Function

Extensor tendon function can be simply tested by having the patient extend his or her fingers against the force of the examiner (Fig. 12-9). Although this maneuver appears to be easy enough, there are complexities of the tendon anatomy than can cause confusion when interpreting the results of the exam. The wrist itself has three main extensor tendons that are responsible for proper extension at the wrist. If

Table 12-1 *Components of Hand Function*

Joint/Action	Musculotendinous Unit	Nerve Control
WRIST		
Flexion	Flexor carpi radialis	Median
	Palmaris longus	Median
	Flexor carpi ulnaris	Ulnar
Extension	Extensor carpi radialis	Radial
	Extensor carpi ulnaris	Radial
Radial deviation	Extensor carpi radialis	Radial
	Flexor carpi radialis	Median
Ulnar deviation	Extensor carpi ulnaris	Radial
	Flexor carpi ulnaris	Ulnar
METACARPOPHALANGEAL		
Flexion	Interosseous	Ulnar
	Lumbrical	Median/Ulnar
Extension	Extensor digitorum communis	Radial
	Extensor indicis proprius	Radial
	Extensor digiti minimi	Radial
Abduction	Dorsal interossei	Ulnar
Adduction	Volar interossei	Ulnar
PROXIMAL INTERPHALANGEAL		
Flexion	Flexor digitorum sublimis	Median
Extension	Interossei	Ulnar
	Lumbricals	Ulnar/Median
	Extensor digitorum communis	Radial
	Extensor indicis proprius	Radial
	Extensor digiti minimi	Radial
DISTAL INTERPHALANGEAL		
Flexion	Flexor digitorum profundus	Median/Ulnar
Extension	Same for proximal interphalangeal joint	
THUMB-CARPOMETACARPAL		
Flexion/Adduction	Adductor pollicis	Ulnar
	Flexor pollicis brevis	Ulnar
	Dorsal interosseous	Ulnar
	Flexor pollicis longus	Median
Extension/Abduction	Extensor pollicis longus	Radial
	Extensor pollicis brevis	Radial
	Abductor pollicis longus	Radial
	Abductor pollicis brevis	Median
Opposition	Abductor pollicis brevis	Median
	Flexor pollicis brevis	Median
	Opponens pollicis	Median

Table 12-1 *Components of Hand Function—cont'd*

Joint/Action	Musculotendinous Unit	Nerve Control
THUMB METACARPOPHALANGEAL		
Flexion	Flexor pollicis longus	Median
	Thenar intrinsics	Median/Ulnar
Extension	Extensor pollicis brevis	Radial
THUMB INTERPHALANGEAL		
Flexion	Flexor pollicis longus	Median
Extension	Extensor pollicis longus	Radial

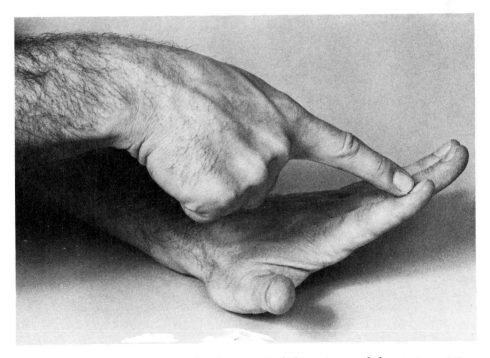

FIG. 12-9 Testing the extensor tendon function. Each finger is extended against a resisting force. This force should not be easily overcome.

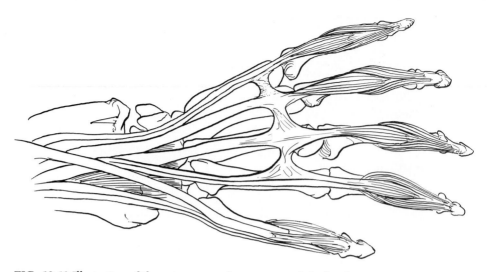

FIG. 12-10 Illustration of the extensor tendon anatomy of the hand. Note in particular the cross-linkages of extensor tendons at the distal metacarpal level. Severance of a extensor tendon proximal to these cross-linkages can give the examiner the false sense that the affected digit can be extended because of the help that cross-linkage provides through the adjacent tendon.

these tendons are cut, the wrist can be extended by the finger extensors but with far less force and can be easily overcome by the examiner. The thumb is served by an abductor and two extensor tendons. If one is cut, the second can still function. Each finger has one main extensor tendon responsible for extension with power. The second and fifth digits, however, have small accessory tendons that can weakly extend these fingers if the main extensors are knocked out of action.

Another anatomic point that can possibly cause misinterpretation in the examination for extension of the digits is that as extensor tendons cross the wrist, they flatten out and interconnect with other extensors over the dorsum of the hand (Fig. 12-10). Weak extension of an injured digit can occur by the action of the adjacent interconnecting tendon. These interconnections also can prevent severed extensor tendons from slipping back into the forearm after they are cut. This anatomic property of extensors makes anastomosis easier for extensors than for flexor tendons because the two severed ends can be readily retrieved during repair.

Whenever there is doubt about extensor tendon function, careful exploration has to be carried out through the laceration itself. Extensor tendons are quite superficial and can be easily identified with proper and gentle exposure. A key factor to remember is that the position of the hand at the time of examination and exploration may be different from the position of the hand during injury. If that should be the case, then the actual laceration to the tendon may be at a location away from

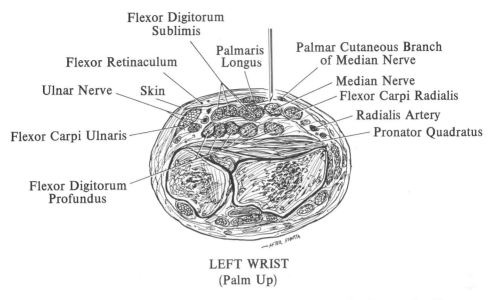

Flexor Digitorum Sublimis

Palmaris Longus

Flexor Retinaculum

Palmar Cutaneous Branch of Median Nerve

Ulnar Nerve   Skin

Median Nerve
Flexor Carpi Radialis

Radialis Artery

Flexor Carpi Ulnaris

Pronator Quadratus

Flexor Digitorum Profundus

— AFTER SOBOTTA

LEFT WRIST
(Palm Up)

FIG. 12-11 Cross-sectional anatomy of the wrist. Note in particular the superficial location of the median nerve. Any visible tendon laceration, such as to the palmaris longus, has to raise the suspicion of an injury to the median nerve.

the laceration on the skin. Therefore, active flexion/extension of the finger to cause the tendon to slide back and forth is encouraged during the exploration.

Flexor Function

The thumb has only one flexor tendon, but the index, middle, ring, and little fingers have two main flexor tendons. The volar surface of the wrist is a complex and vulnerable area, replete with important structures. As illustrated in Fig. 12-11, the median nerve lies just deep and radial to the palmaris longus, the most superficial tendon. Even trivial-appearing lacerations to the wrist can cause serious tendon and nerve damage.

The flexor tendons to each finger are paired. The flexor digitorum profundus tendons are responsible for power and mass action such as is needed for gripping. These tendons run deep to the flexor digitorum sublimis tendons, but at the level of the middle phalanx, the profundus splits through the sublimis and goes on to attach to the distal phalanx (Fig. 12-12). In order to test profundus function, the action of the sublimis tendon has to be blocked by holding each digit, one at a time, in extension at the middle phalanx (Fig. 12-13). The patient is then asked to flex the distal phalanx, which now can only be accomplished through the action of the profundus. Sixty degrees of flexion is normal during this maneuver.

The flexor digitorum sublimis tendons are responsible for the positioning of the

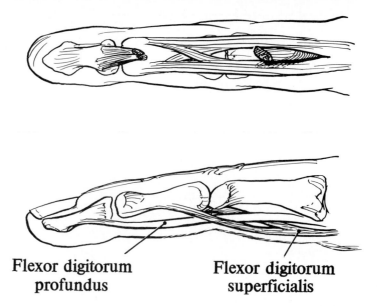

Flexor digitorum profundus

Flexor digitorum superficialis

FIG. 12-12 Note the relationship of the flexor digitorum profundus to the flexor digitorum superficialis. The profundus splits through the superficialis, which is attached on the middle phalanx. The profundus attaches to the distal phalanx.

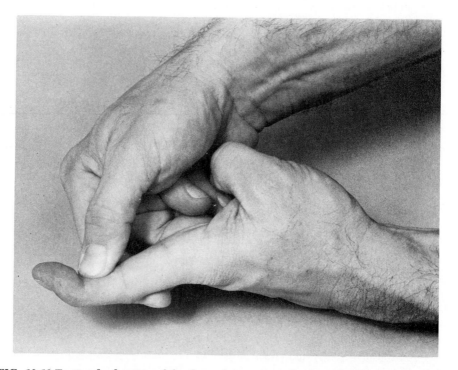

FIG. 12-13 Testing for function of the flexor digitorum profundus. The distal phalanx of the finger is forcibly flexed while the action of the superficialis tendon is blocked. Only the profundus can flex the distal phalanx.

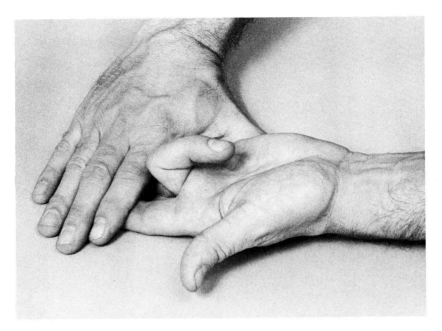

FIG. 12-14 Testing for function of the flexor digitorum superficialis. The mass action of the profundus can be blocked by holding the non-tested fingers in extension. The tested finger can only be flexed at the PIP by the superficialis tendon.

fingers so that power flexion can take place. These tendons run superficial to the deep tendons until they are split at the distal portion of the middle phalanx by the profundi. The sublimis tendons attach to the proximal portion of the middle phalanx. To test for sublimis action, the profundus group has to be blocked by the examiner. In the manner illustrated in Fig. 12-14, the examiner holds all the fingers in extension except the one being tested. The patient is then asked to fully flex his or her finger at the MP and PIP joint. If the sublimis is lacerated, the patient will be unable to flex that finger.

CIRCULATION

The circulation of the hand is extraordinarily rich and redundant (Fig. 12-15). Most people can suffer complete loss of either the radial or ulnar arteries and maintain adequate perfusion. Loss of perfusion because of damage to the vessels usually results from an extensive injury not ordinarily repaired by emergency wound-care personnel and consultation is obtained. Although pulses are always documented in any hand injury, the best indicators of perfusion are color, skin blanching with pressure, temperature, and capillary refill at the nail bed. Because arteries travel with nerves in neurovascular bundles, profuse arterial bleeding of the digit should raise the suspicion of an accompanying digital nerve injury.

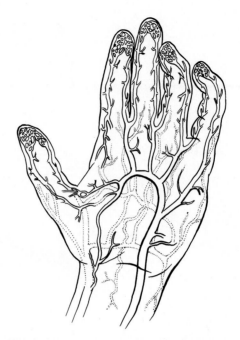

FIG. 12-15 Illustration of the profuse and redundant vascularity of the hand. It is not uncommon to be able to sacrifice either the radial or ulnar artery and still have complete perfusion of the hand. Lacerations of the digital arteries arouse suspicion of a lacerated digital nerve.

RADIOGRAPHY

Radiographs are liberally used to assist in the evaluation of the hand. For any blunt trauma associated with a laceration, underlying fractures must be ruled out. Not only do hand fractures require careful and sometimes specialized management, but a fracture with a laceration has to be considered an open fracture. Open fractures are usually managed by consultants. Foreign bodies are frequently associated with hand injuries. Radiography is particularly useful to detect metal and other debris. Contrary to popularly held opinion, almost all types of glass are easily detectable by radiographs[28] (see Chapter 15).

WOUND EXPLORATION

Ultimately, each laceration of the hand should be gently and carefully explored just prior to repair. In spite of normal functional testing, partial tendon lacerations and violation of joint capsules might remain undetected until exploration is carried out. This procedure is usually accomplished by retracting the wound with an Adson forceps or a skin hook and using a mosquito clamp to spread open the deeper tissue for a good look, preferably in a bloodless field. Chapter 8 provides further details concerning tourniquet application, wound extension, and exploration. Once again, if there is ever a doubt about an injury to an important structure of the hand, the advice of a specialist should be sought.

SELECTED HAND INJURIES AND PROBLEMS

Although there is a large variety of wounds and lacerations to the hand, those described here are those that are commonly managed and repaired by emergency wound-care personnel. Serious, complex injuries, and especially ones that cause functional deficits, are best cared for by specialists. Animal bites and burns to the hands are discussed in Chapters 14 and 16 respectively.

Uncomplicated Lacerations

The principles and techniques of wound repair discussed in Chapter 9 also apply to closing hand lacerations. Most lacerations of the dorsal and volar surfaces of the hand can be anesthetized by direct wound infiltration, which is described in Chapter 5. Large lacerations can be managed by wrist blocks. Wounds beyond the proximal phalanx are best anesthetized with digital blocks.

Debridement of the hand should to be carried out with great caution. Excessive removal of skin can lead to failure of adequate coverage, eventual wound contraction, and a resulting functional deficit. Although fat is a good substrate for bacterial growth, as much as possible is preserved on the volar surfaces of the hand, without leaving devitalized tissue behind, to maintain the padding between skin and bone. Injured fat does not regenerate. Clearly, however, truly devitalized and grossly contaminated tissues of any kind have to be sacrificed in order to prevent a serious hand infection from developing. In these cases, the opinion of a consultant is recommended.

Because of the number of important structures that lie within the small confines of the hand, deep closures with any suture material are discouraged so as to reduce the risk of tissue reaction and infection. By closing the skin alone, very little dead space will be left behind in hand injuries. In addition, natural tension across the wound is usually minimal in hand lacerations and deep closures are not needed to reduce that tension. The recommended suture material is 5-0 nonabsorbable monofilament nylon. Only as many sutures as are necessary to achieve closure are placed. Excessive numbers of superficial closures are unnecessary and possibly harmful.

Fingertip Injuries

The management of fingertip injuries is quite controversial. There are very few actual controlled studies of fingertip and fingernail problems. Therefore, the strategies and choices of repair techniques vary considerably between personnel who take care of these problems. Just the issue of whether to remove the nail following

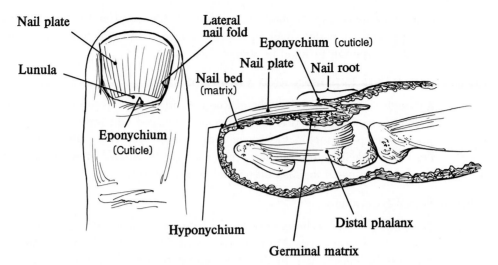

FIG. 12-16 Anatomy of the distal finger and nail components.

an injury evokes widely varying opinions. Certain principles and goals, however, are commonly held. These include: preservation of the length of the finger, preservation of proper nail growth capacity, preservation of fingertip padding and sensation, and prevention of infection.

The fingertip and fingernail apparatus comprise a complex anatomic and functional unit (Fig. 12-16). The fleshy volar pad is replete with nerve endings and capillaries. There is sufficient soft tissue to effectively pad the fingertip and distal phalanx against undue trauma. Preservation of sensation of the fingertip is crucial to all manual activities. Even with full-thickness loss of the finger pad, healing and regeneration of tissue can usually be relied upon to restore a functional pad. Numerous fibrous bands called septae anchor the skin to the underlying bony structure (Fig. 12-17). These structures prevent sliding or slipping of the skin during use of the fingers. Septae should be kept anatomically intact whenever possible.

The nail apparatus has several components. The nail itself is divided into the nail root, which is the portion that lies under the eponychium, and the nail plate, which adheres to the sterile matrix. The matrix also has two parts, the germinal matrix from which new nail is generated, and the sterile matrix, or nail bed, over which the nail passes during normal growth. The eponychium, commonly referred to as the cuticle, is the fold of skin that overlies the nail root. One of the main principles of nail management is to prevent the eponychium from adhering and scarring down onto the germinal matrix. Should this unfortunate event take place, nail regeneration can be significantly impaired. Techniques to prevent this occurrence will be discussed.

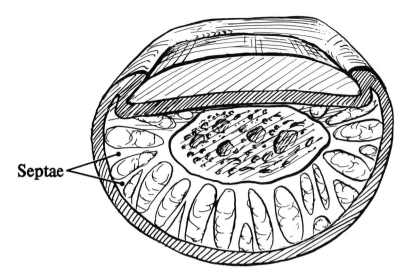

Septae

FIG. 12-17 Illustration of the fibrous septa that connect the skin to the underlying phalanges. The septa provides stability to the soft tissue of the finger.

Fingertip injuries can be divided into three groups: (1) blunt or crushing injuries, (2) sharp or shearing injuries, and (3) avulsion injuries with tissue loss. Foreign bodies lodged under a fingernail are discussed in Chapter 15.

Blunt/Crushing Injuries

The most common blunt injury is the subungual hematoma. Striking the finger with a blunt object or getting it caught in a closing door often results in a collection of blood between the matrix and the nail plate. This injury is quite painful. The blood can be drained and most of the pain can be relieved by making one or more holes through the nail plate. A common method is the use of a heated paper clip. After placing it in a hemostat, the paper clip is brought over an open flame until it is red hot. Then quickly and carefully the paper clip is passed through the nail plate, as illustrated in Fig. 12-18. There are commercially available nail drills and electric heat probes that can accomplish the same objective. Another method for drainage is to use at least an #18 gauge 1- to 1½-inch needle as a drill. A hole can be made by twirling the needle between the operator's fingers as it passes through the nail plate.

Subungual hematomas, however, signal possibly significant damage to the nail matrix. Subungual injuries that have greater than 25% of the nail bed surface covered by visible hematoma should be radiographed to rule out bony fractures. As a general rule, if the subungual collection of blood is less than 50% of the nailbed sur-

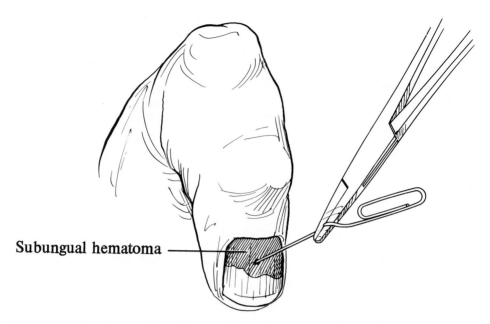

Subungual hematoma

FIG. 12-18 Heated paper clip to drain a subungual hematoma. Care is taken to avoid the nail bed after passing through the nail into the hematoma.

face, and there is no bony (usually tuft) fracture, then the simple drainage procedure is carried out and the nail is left in place.[17] If there is a fracture or the subungual hematoma is greater than 50%, nail removal is recommended to inspect the matrix. A recent study has shown that 60% of all patients with a subungual hematoma greater than 50% the area of the nail had repairable lacerations of the nail bed.[25] This figure rose to 96% if there was an accompanying fracture.

Lacerations of the matrix are probably best repaired by careful reapposition of the wound edges and suturing with 6-0 absorbable suture material. If intact, the nail that was removed earlier can be replaced for temporary splinting purposes under the eponychium, over the matrix and suture line (Fig. 12-19). Or a small piece of nonadherent dressing such as Adaptic or penrose drain can be tucked under the eponychium and the nail can be discarded (Fig. 12-20). Either nail splinting or non-adherent packing is recommended to prevent the eponychium from adhering to the germinal matrix. In this manner, the nail's capacity to regenerate is preserved. The nail, or packing, is usually left in place for 7 to 10 days to prevent adherence to the germinal matrix. The absorbable sutures are allowed to dissolve on their own.

Another common blunt injury is when the nail root avulses from under the eponychium. This injury is often seen in children. If the remainder of the nail ap-

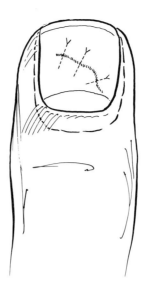

FIG. 12-19 Nail-bed injury with subungal hematoma. If the decision has been made to remove the nail, and a laceration of the bed is discovered, this laceration is repaired with 6-0 absorbable suture such as polyglycolic acid. As illustrated in this figure, the nail, if removed intact, can be replaced as a splint for 5 to 7 days. The nail will prevent adherence of the germinal matrix to the eponychium.

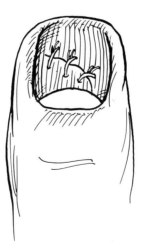

FIG. 12-20 Nail-bed injury with subungual hematoma. If the nail is in no condition to be replaced, a small stent is fashioned to separate the eponychium from the germinal matrix. This stent or packing is removed within 5 to 7 days.

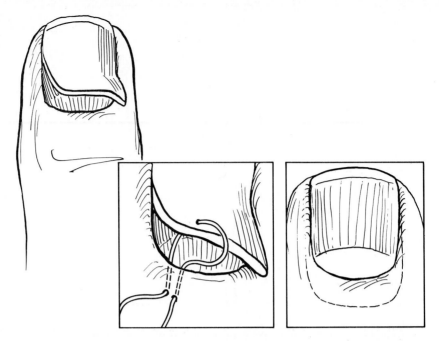

FIG. 12-21 Nail-root avulsion. Occasionally, the proximal aspect of a nail root is avulsed. The technique illustrated demonstrates how this nail root can be replaced under the cuticle. This is an injury more commonly seen in children.

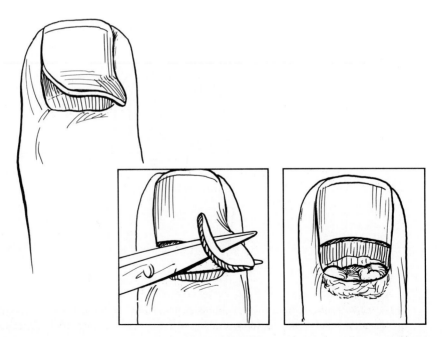

FIG. 12-22 Nail-root avulsion. If the nail root cannot be replaced as shown in Fig. 12-21, the nail root can be excised and a small penrose or adaptic packing is placed under the eponychium for 5 to 7 days. A new nail will germinate and extrude the remainder of the old portion.

pears intact and is firmly attached to the nail matrix, then the nail root can be replaced by the nail-root retrieval technique illustrated in Fig. 12-21. If this procedure is too difficult to accomplish, then the nail root is excised and the eponychium is packed with a non-adherent dressing material for 7 to 10 days (Fig. 12-22). A new nail will eventually grow out and extrude the remaining old nail.

Nail Removal Technique

When the decision is made to remove the nail, the techniques illustrated in Fig. 12-23 are suggested. A small hemostat or iris scissors is inserted under the nail plate along the nail bed. The instrument is slowly advanced as it is spread open to

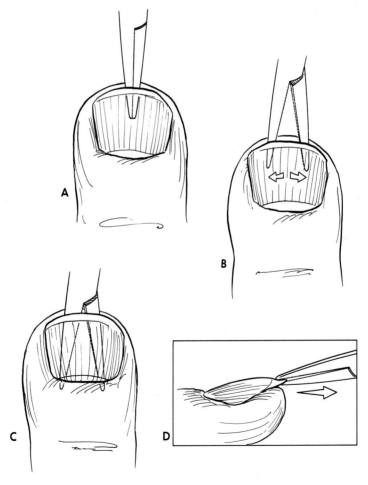

FIG. 12-23 Technique for removal of a nail. **A,** Introduce a small hemostat or iris scissors between the nail and the nail bed. **B,** Gently dissect the nail from the nail bed. **C,** Extend the dissection all the way back to the germinal matrix. **D,** Grasp the nail firmly and remove it from the nail bed.

lift the nail plate off the matrix. This process is carried back through to the nail root and germinal matrix area. Care is taken to avoid undue injury to the nail bed and germinal matrix. The eponychium is also gently pushed away from the nail plate. Once the nail plate has been loosened, a hemostat is used to grasp the nail plate firmly and pull it out from under the eponychium. The nail will not always come off easily and some measure of force must be applied.

Shearing Injuries

Lacerations of the fingertip and nail apparatus caused by sharp or shearing forces can usually be managed by simple suturing. Transverse lacerations through the nail plate and matrix can be repaired by removing the distal portion of the nail plate to

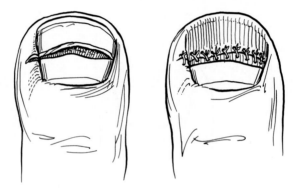

FIG. 12-24 Transverse lacerations of the nail bed can often be managed by leaving the nail root intact. The proximal portion of the nail is excised with tissue scissors proximally to the injury. The nail bed is then repaired with absorbable suture. The nail will continue to grow over the suture line well after the sutures have been absorbed.

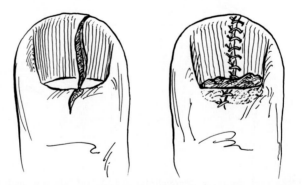

FIG. 12-25 Longitudinal lacerations of the nail bed are often best closed by removal of the nail entirely. Once the nail bed is repaired, packing of penrose drain or adaptic is used to separate the eponychium from the germinal matrix for at least 5 to 7 days.

expose the lacerated nail bed. Repair of the matrix is carried out with 6-0 absorbable suture as illustrated in Fig. 12-24. Maintaining the integrity of the nail root will prevent nail growth problems with the germinal matrix.

Longitudinal lacerations through the matrix and eponychium require careful repair of both structures. The nail bed is repaired with 6-0 absorbable suture (Fig. 12-25). The eponychium and surrounding skin is closed with nonabsorbable material like nylon. If the nail plate is removed in its entirety, then a nail replacement or packing for 7 to 10 days, as previously described, is necessary to prevent eponychial adherence to the germinal matrix. Only the nonabsorbable sutures are removed after 10 to 12 days.

Avulsion Injuries

Probably the greatest area of controversy in fingertip management concerns avulsion injuries with loss of tissue (Fig. 12-26). At issue is whether to close these avulsions by grafting or whether to leave them to heal spontaneously. Traditionally, any fingertip avulsion with less than 1 cm square area of tissue loss and no accompanying bony or nail bed injury, has been managed by allowing spontaneous healing to take place.[16] There are several studies that show that larger avulsion losses, in both pediatric and adult age groups, can be treated conservatively without grafting.[4,9,13,15,23,31] Tissue losses with dimensions of up to 1.8 × 2.6 cm have been successfully managed in this manner.[9] When bone was observed to be exposed in these studies, healing eventually took place, with successful spontaneous soft tissue cov-

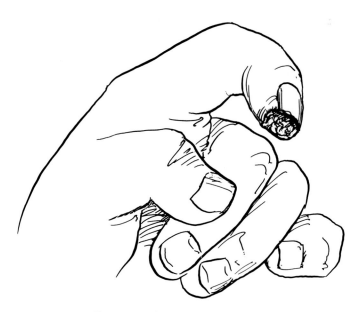

FIG. 12-26 Illustration of an avulsion injury of the fingertip.

ering of the distal phalanx.[8,31] When comparing complication rates and time lost from work, conservative management was comparable to grafting.[12] In fact, in one study the infection rate of the conservatively managed group was markedly lower than that of surgically grafted patients.[2] The one area in which conservative management appears to less optimal when compared to more meticulous surgical repair is nail bed repair and nail regeneration.[2] Unrepaired nail matrixes tended to lead more frequently to deformed nails.

Suggested recommendations for avulsion tissue loss injuries include the following:

- If the defect is less than 1 cm in diameter and no bone is exposed, then spontaneous healing is the treatment of choice.
- For losses greater than 1 cm in diameter, with an intact nail apparatus and no bone exposure, conservative management can be considered an alternative to grafting. Local practice may dictate the management of these injuries.
- For significant avulsions with uncomplicated nail apparatus involvement, repair of the matrix should be attempted if possible. The remainder of the injury, i.e., the tissue loss, can be allowed to heal spontaneously or can be grafted, depending on the clinical requirement. Consultation may be required.
- For injuries that involve exposed bone or those with complex nail apparatus involvement, consultation is recommended.
- In some patients, the avulsion is incomplete and the tissue appears intact, most commonly a partially amputated fingertip without bone involvement. Tissue can be gently re-attached by placing 6-0 nonabsorbable sutures in the skin and 6-0 absorbable sutures in the matrix. The eponychial nail folds (cuticle margins) provide good landmarks for re-apposition.

Proper dressings for fingertip avulsions include a non-adherent base like Xeroform or Adaptic, with a sponge covering and gauze wrapping as described in Chapter 17. As discussed in the later section on antibiotics for hand wounds, antibiotics are suggested for injuries with exposed bone.

Tendon Lacerations

All lacerations of flexor tendons (in the upper or lower extremity) are referred to specialists for care. An emergency wound-care setting is no place to repair flexor tendon injuries. Besides requiring a controlled surgical environment, these tendons are most effectively managed by trained surgeons using the proper instruments and magnification. Under the best of circumstances, flexor tendon injuries present considerable technical challenges, and repair can be fraught with complications. Primary closure is recommended for flexor tendons. Delayed closure up to 2-3 weeks is possible but only recommended if technical considerations prevent primary closure (e.g., excessive contamination, skin loss, unstable bony skeleton, missing tissue).

Simple, single lacerations of an extensor tendon on the dorsum of the hand, between the distal wrist and metacarpophalangeal joints, can be repaired in the emergency wound care area by an appropriately trained wound-care personnel. Extensor tendon lacerations over the forearm, wrist, and fingers are best managed by a consultant. It is recommended that training for extensor tendon repair include several supervised repairs under the guidance of a specialist. It is important to master appropriate techniques and understand proper splinting and the necessary follow-up care.

Single extensor tendons can be repaired in the emergency department under the following circumstances: (1) if the injury is between the distal wrist and the meta carpophalangeal joints; (2) if the skin and tendon wounds are sharp and not heavily macerated or contaminated; (3) if the injury is less than 8 hours old; (4) if the two ends of the tendon are easily visualized; (5) if appropriate instruments are available to minimize trauma to the tissues; and (6) if the patient is cooperative and will comply with follow-up care.

The technique for repairing an extensor tendon is shown in Fig. 12-27. A 4-0 nonabsorbable suture such as nylon or polypropylene on a straight needle is passed through the tendon in the figure-of-8 pattern until it is secure. The skin is closed with 5-0 nonabsorbable suture material. A plaster splint is placed on the palmar surfaces of the forearm-wrist-hand-digit, over the appropriate nonadherent base and the gauze sponge/wrap surface dressing. The wrist is placed at a 30-degree angle of extension and the metacarpophalangeal joints are placed at a 20-degree angle of flexion. The fingers are only slightly flexed. The splint remains in place for three weeks; however, the patient is referred much sooner to a consultant for follow-up care.

Upon careful exploration of a laceration of the hand, it is not uncommon to discover a partially lacerated extensor tendon. Successful treatment of this can be accomplished by merely closing the skin laceration and splinting.[30] As a general rule, if the tendon is more than 50% transected, it should be repaired with the technique described above. If not primarily repaired, splinting with careful follow-up and early active motion can be recommended.[30] Splinting is continued for 1 to 2 weeks post-injury after which passive motion and gently active flexion and extension is permitted for 2 to 3 weeks. After that, if the skin wound is healed and there is no excessive pain, then active motion with increasing force and stress can proceed. Again, a consultant should be involved early in the process in order to concur with decisions and to provide follow-up care.

Nerve Injuries

Lacerations associated with sensory or motor deficits of one of the major nerves of the upper extremity require immediate referral to a consultant. Injuries to the digital nerves, however, can be handled somewhat differently. There is some contro-

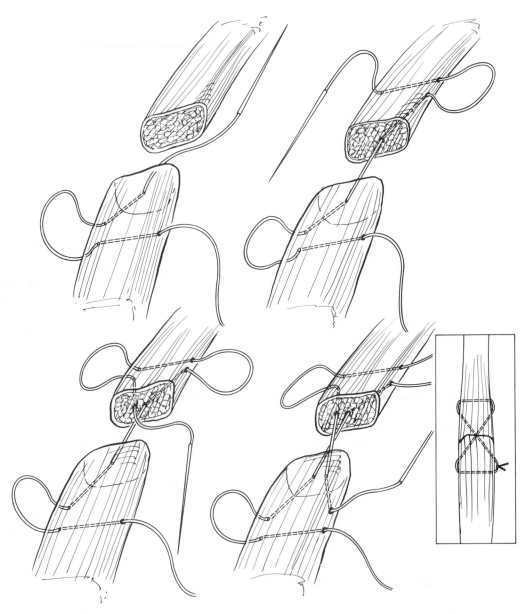

FIG. 12-27 Illustration of the figure-of-8 technique to reappose sharply divided lacerated extensor tendons. See text for further explanation.

versy over whether repair immediately post-injury is superior to repair performed up to 2 weeks later.[18] Delayed repair can have significant advantages over early repair. The repair setting and time is better controlled, the cut nerve ends are better delineated, and early skin closure is an effective barrier against infection. The delayed repair is done through a sterile field and incision. For simple lacerations in which a digital nerve sensory deficit is discovered, immediate repair is probably not necessary. With consultative support, simple skin suturing is carried out, a dressing is placed, and the patient is referred to the specialist within 1 to 2 days. Nerve repair can be carried out on an elective basis within 2 weeks.

Amputated Parts

Frequently, a patient will present to a medical facility after sustaining an injury that causes an amputation of part or all of an extremity. Although the injury is not within the realm of emergency wound-care personnel to manage, proper handling of the injured extremity and severed part is important, especially if there is a chance of reimplantation by a specialist.

The injured extremity is gently cleansed and wrapped in lightly saline-moistened gauze sponges followed by gauze wrapping. Rarely is a tourniquet needed to stop hemorrhage because natural vasospasm and platelet plugging of the severed vessels occurs rapidly after injury.

The severed part is placed in a dry sterile sponge wrapping. Saline soaking will cause unnecessary and unwanted edema and make reimplantation much more difficult. The wrapped severed part is then placed in a small plastic wrap or bag. The bag and its contents can then be put in a container with ice to cool the tissue. Great care has to be taken make sure that ice does not come into direct contact with the severed part so as not to cause necrosis from freezing. Once these steps have been taken, the patient can wait for the specialist or can be transported to an appropriate care facility.

Paronychia

The most common hand infection is a paronychia.[1] A paronychia is an infection of the eponychium and it is usually associated with a collection of pus between the eponychium and the nail root. The infection is most often localized to one side of the eponychium, the lateral nail fold. However, it can include the eponychium in the mid-line or proceed in "horseshoe" fashion to involve the entire eponychium. Pus can also invade the space under the nail plate. The most common bacteria found in a paronychia are gram-positive cocci, either *Streptococcus pyogenes* or penicillin-resistant *Staphyloccoccus aureus*.[1,5,27]

The simplest and most effective manner to drain a paronychia is to insert a #11 blade between the eponychium and the nail plate and gently sweep the blade to elevate the eponychium (Fig. 12-28). Following the drainage of pus, a small loose-fitting wick or drain fashioned from Adaptic or penrose drain rubber can be placed

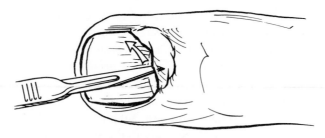

FIG. 12-28 Technique for draining simple paronychia. Note that the #11 blade is brought between the nail and the eponychium parallel to the nail plate. This simple maneuver will drain the vast majority of paronychiae.

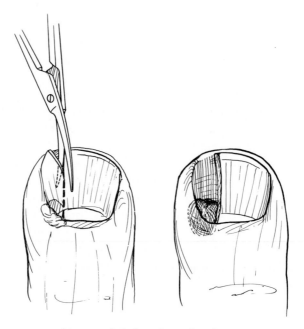

FIG. 12-29 When a paronychia extends below the nail and insinuates between the nail bed and nail plate, partial nail removal must take place. Once the nail removal is accomplished, a small packing or drain is left in place for 5 to 7 days.

under the eponychium to encourage drainage. A non-adherent dressing base is then placed and the finger is wrapped with gauze as previously described. This dressing is usually kept in place for 48 hours and the patient is brought back for reinspection at that time. Upon return to the medical care facility, the drain is removed and the patient is instructed to soak the finger 3 times a day for 20 minutes at a time to prevent resealing of the incision. This regimen will allow continued drainage to take place if necessary. Some authorities feel that neither a drain nor antibiotics are necessary for simple paronychiae and virtually all patients recover well. [19] If no drain is put in place, the patient is instructed to begin soaking immediately after the initial drainage procedure. A simple Bandaid is the dressing of choice in this case. Antibiotics can be considered optional.

Occasionally, a paronychia will extend below the nail plate between the nail and matrix. Pus can be seen through the semitranslucent nail. If pus is suspected to be in this space, partial or complete nail removal is recommended. Merely sweeping a #11 blade under the eponychium will not suffice. Fig. 12-29 demonstrates a method of partial nail removal to accomplish the drainage of both the paronychia and the pus under the nail plate. A paronychia that involves the entire eponychium and nail root area can be managed as illustrated in Fig. 12-30. An incision of the

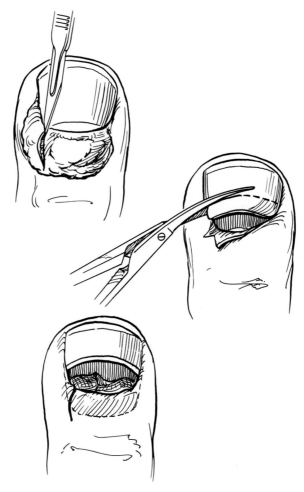

FIG. 12-30 A complex "horseshoe" paronychia usually needs to be drained both by incising the paronychia directly and removing either a portion or all the nail as illustrated. Note that a packing is left in place for 5 to 7 days to prevent adherence of the eponychium to the germinal matrix.

eponychium is made to free the nail root for removal. The eponychium is loosely packed as previously described and the patient should return for follow up in 48 hours. The eponychial packing must remain in place for 24 to 48 hours. Occasionally, the entire nail must be removed to effect complete drainage. Antibiotics are often recommended for complex paronychia. See the discussion below on antibiotics for hand wounds.

Felon

A felon is an infection with a collection of pus in the pulp space of the fingertip (Fig. 12-31). The finger pad is quite swollen and exceedingly tender. The most common bacteria found in these infections are *S. pyogenes* and penicillin-resistant *S. aureus.*[1,5,27] Several methods to drain felons have been recommended over the years. The so-called fish mouth and lateral incisions that cut through the supporting fibrous septae of the finger pad are thought to increase the occurrence of unnecessary sequelae.[14]

The simplest technique to drain a felon is to make a longitudinal incision directly through the finger pad on the volar surface of the digit into the pulp space and pus collection (Fig. 12-32).[14] The incision is kept open with a small loose-fitting wick made of a non-adherent dressing material or a small sliver of rubber such as part of a penrose drain or a rubber band. The drain is removed at follow up at 48 hours after which a soaking routine similar to the one used for paronychia is encouraged. These patients are then started on antibiotics. See the discussion on antibiotics for hand wounds later in this chapter.

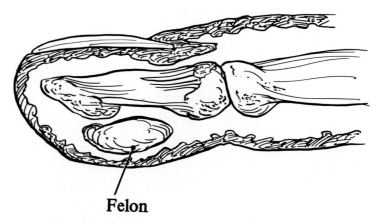

Felon

FIG. 12-31 Illustration and location of a felon in the pulp of the finger space.

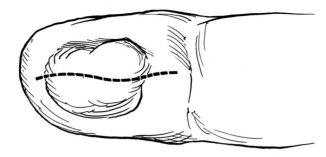

FIG. 12-32 Technique for draining a felon. Note that the incision is made directly over the area of maximal tenderness and fluctuance.

Pressure Injection Injuries

An injury to the hand that initially seems benign is caused by a high-pressure injection device such as a paint sprayer or grease gun. Through a pinhole, such a device can create a needle-thin stream that can have a pressure of up to 15,000 lbs./in^2. A variety of paints, petroleums, and other chemicals can easily pierce the skin and, under the pressure created, spread throughout the hand along natural tissue planes and tendon sheaths. Grease and paint are the two most common substances.[24]

The entry wound is often no more than a small puncture. The most common site of entry is the tip of the index finger, a result of "testing" to see if the device works. Some of the injectable chemicals, such as the petroleums, do not cause an immediate reaction or pain. The patient will often have minimal complaints. The combination of the small wound and relative lack of symptoms is deceptive. These injuries can progress over hours to marked pain, swelling, and inflammation of the entire hand. They require immediate consultation. Some authorities recommend fasciotomies of the hand before significant swelling develops in order to forestall ischemia created by an increase in tissue pressure from the intense reaction, to remove the chemical, and to debride necrotic tissue. The overall incidence of amputation has been reported to be 48%.[24]

Antibiotics for Hand Wounds

The use of antibiotics in patients with hand injuries is largely empirical because there are few definitive studies examining their use. Several studies have shown that prophylactic antibiotics are of no value in uncomplicated lacerations of the hand.[11,20,29] In more complicated injuries such as avulsions of the fingertip, antibiotics are often prescribed, but, again, there are no definitive studies to support this practice. In fact, some studies have found that antibiotics are of no value.[9,15] Only when bone is exposed under severe crushing forces has one group found a decrease in the infection rate with the use of antibiotics.[26] It is not even clear in the face of a paronychia that antibiotics improve outcome.[19] In spite of this controversy, some recommendations that rely more on traditional practice and clinical judgment can be made. Use antibiotics for:

- Wounds greater than 8 hours old
- Wounds caused by a crushing mechanism in which some tissue compromise is suspected
- Contaminated or soiled wounds in which extensive cleansing and debridement has been necessary
- Fingertip avulsions with exposed bone
- Open fractures
- Tendon or joint involvement
- Mammalian bites (see Chapter 14 for further discussion and special circumstances)
- Complex paronychia with pus under the nail
- Felons
- Immunocompromised patients or those who have diabetes

The choice of antibiotics for hand injuries also generates debate. A good first choice is dicloxacillin. It is the least expensive and combats the most important causes of infection: the gram-positive organisms. First-generation cephalosporins are effective against most of the common gram-positive and gram-negative organisms that are implicated in wound care. Another choice is amoxicillin with clavulanate, which has a similar spectrum. For penicillin-allergic patients, erythromycin is appropriate. For antibiotics to have any value, they must be administered as soon as possible in the emergency department, preferably within three hours from the time of injury.[6] For maximal effectiveness, the initial dose should be given intravenously. Intravenous preparations that are recommended include cefazolin or gentamicin (for penicillin-allergic patients). Ciprofloxacin is soon to be released in the United States as an intravenous preparation. For prophylaxis, the duration of administration is no longer than 4 to 5 days.

Dressings and Aftercare

The basic finger dressing is described in Chapter 17. Xeroform is a popular nonadherent base as is Adaptic. The latter is probably somewhat less adherent in wounds where there is more exudate and crusting. All fingertips are well padded with gauze sponges. A metal protective splint is recommended for patients who are going to return to work or resume manual activities.

Most hand wounds are best followed up within 48 hours with dressing removal for inspection. If a suture line becomes infected, suture removal and wound cleansing with thorough irrigation are carried out as soon as possible. Infections of the hand can be disastrous and often spread rapidly to important structures from a small nidus. Most sutures of the hand are removed in 8 to 10 days.

References

1. Bell M: The changing pattern of pyogenic infections of the hand, Hand 8:298-302, 1976.
2. Chow S, and Ho E: Open treatment of fingertip injuries in adults, J Hand Surg 7:470-476, 1982.
3. Custer J et al: Studies in the management of the contaminated wound, Am J Surg 121:572-575, 1971.
4. Douglas BS: Conservative management of guillotine amputation of the finger in children, Aust Ped J 8:86-89, 1972.
5. Eaton R and Butsch D: Antibiotic guidelines for hand infections, Surg Gynecol Obstet 130:119-121, 1970.
6. Edlich RF, Smith OT, and Edgerton MT: Resistance of the surgical wound to antimicrobial prophylaxis and its mechanism of development, Am J Surg 126:583-586, 1973.
7. Faddis D, Daniel D, and Boyer J: Tissue toxicity of antiseptic solutions, J Trauma 17:895-897, 1977.
8. Farrell F et al: Conservative management of fingertip amputations, J Am Coll Emerg Phys 6:243-246, 1977.
9. Fox J et al: Nonoperative management of pulp amputation by occlusive dressings, Am J Surg 133:255-256, 1977.
10. Gellis M and Pool R: Two-point discrimination distances in the normal hand and forearm, Plast Reconstr Surg 59:57-63, 1977.
11. Grossman JAI, Adams JP, and Kunec J: Prophylactic antibiotics in simple hand lacerations, JAMA 245:1055-1056, 1981.
12. Holm A and Zachariae L: Fingertip lesions: an evaluation of conservative treatment versus free skin grafting, Acta Orthop Scand 45:382-392, 1974.
13. Ipsen T, Frandsen PA, and Barfred T: Conservative treatment of fingertip injuries, Injury 18:203-205, 1987.
14. Kilgore E et al: Treatment of felons, Am J Surg 130:194-197, 1975.
15. Lamon R et al: Open treatment of fingertip amputations, Ann Emerg Med 12:358-360, 1983.
16. Louis D, Palmer A, and Burney R: Open treatment of digital tip injuries, JAMA 244:697-698, 1980.
17. Margles S: Principles of management of acute hand injuries, Surg Clin North Am 60:665-685, 1980.
18. Millesi H: Reappraisal of nerve repair, Surg Clin North Am 61:321-340, 1981.
19. Personal survey of hand specialists, 1989.
20. Roberts AHN and Teddy PJ: A prospective trial of prophylactic antibiotics in hand lacerations, Br J Surg 64:394-396, 1977.
21. Rodeheaver G et al: Bactericidal activity and toxicity of iodine-containing solutions in wounds, Arch Surg 117:181-185, 1982.
22. Rodeheaver G et al: Pluronic-F-68: a promising new skin wound cleanser, Ann Emerg Med 9:572-576, 1980.
23. Rosenthal LJ: Non-operative management of distal fingertip amputations in children, Pediatrics 64:1-5, 1979.
24. Schoo MJ, Scott FA, and Boswick JA: High-pressure injection injuries to the hand, J Trauma 20:229-238, 1980.
25. Simon RR and Wolgin M: Subungual hematoma: association with occult laceration repair, Am J Emerg Med 5:302-304, 1987.
26. Sloan JP et al: Antibiotics in open fractures of the distal phalanx, J Hand Surg 12B:123-124, 1987.
27. Stone N et al: Emperical selection of antibiotics for hand infections, J Bone Joint Surg (Am) 51(A):899-903, 1969.
28. Tanberg D: Glass in the hand and foot, JAMA 248:1872-1874, 1982.
29. Worlock P et al: The role of prophylactic antibiotics following hand injuries, Br J Clin Pract 34:290-292, 1980.
30. Wray R and Weeks P: Treatment of partial tendon lacerations, Hand 12:163-166, 1980.
31. Young WA and Andrassy RJ: Conservative management of fingertip amputations in children, Texas Medicine 79:58-60, 1983.

13 *Wound Taping and Stapling*

Wound Taping
  Indications for Taping
  Taping Technique
    Tape aftercare
Wound Stapling

Indications for Stapling
  Stapling Technique
    Staple aftercare
References

Over the last decade, the use of alternative wound closure techniques, wound taping and stapling, has increased dramatically. Although the ease of application of tapes and the speed with which staples can be inserted has focused attention on these techniques, clinical experience and scientific studies have supported the validity of their use under specified circumstances. Tapes are not only used for primary wound closure but are also an important support for lacerations after suture removal. Once thought to be limited to surgical settings for the closure of cosmetically unimportant incisions, staples have been found to compare favorably with standard suture techniques for closure of a variety of traumatically induced wounds.

WOUND TAPING

When compared to suturing, there are several advantages to wound taping. These include a reduced need for anesthesia, ease of application, even distribution of tension across the wound, no residual suture marks, application by non-physician personnel, and the elimination of need for suture removal.[10] They also have advantages in closing flap lacerations and have a greater resistance to wound infection than sutures.[1,3] On the other hand, tapes do not work well on surfaces that are oily or hair-bearing, joint surfaces, lax skin, gaping wounds under tension, or in very young or uncooperative children.

There is a bewildering variety of wound tapes currently on the market. Steri-Strips are the best known but other brands include Suture-Strip, Clearon, Nichi-Strip, and Curi-Strip. They have differing porosity, adhesion, flexibility, breaking strength, and elongation capability. An early study that compared Clearon and Steri-Strip; the latter demonstrated a better overall performance than the others.[7] In a more recent comparison study of six tapes (Curi-Strip, Steri-Strip, Nichi-Strip,

Cicagraf, Suture-Strip, and Suture-Strip Plus), an overall scoring method was devised to rank their performance under laboratory conditions.[8] The three highest ranking tapes were the Nichi-Strip, Curi-Strip, and Steri-Strip.

Indications for Taping

Wound taping can be considered under the following conditions:

- Superficial, straight lacerations under little tension. Areas suitable for taping include the forehead, chin, malar eminence, thorax, and non-joint areas of the extremities.
- Support for flaps in which sutures might compromise vascular perfusion at the wound edges.
- Lacerations with a greater-than-usual potential for infection.
- Lacerations in the elderly or steroid-dependent patient who has thin, fragile skin.
- Support for lacerations after suture removal.

Tapes do not work well on irregular wounds, those that cannot be made free of blood or secretions, intertriginous areas, scalp, and joint surfaces.

Taping Technique

Most taping of emergency wounds can be done with ¼-inch wide tape of varying lengths. For wounds that are greater than 4 to 5 centimeters in length, ½-inch width is preferable.

The following steps are carried out:

- The wound is cleansed, irrigated, and debrided if necessary. Hemostasis has to be complete and the skin surface completely dried.
- Benzoin is applied to the surrounding skin to increase adhesion. Care is taken not to spill this agent into the wound. It is left to dry until it becomes tacky.
- Tapes are cut to the length desired while they are still on the backing sheet. Usually 2 to 3 cm of overlap is allowed for each side of the wound (Fig. 13-1).
- One of the perforated end tabs is gently removed to prevent deforming of the tape ends (Fig. 13-2).
- Individual tapes are removed from the backing with forceps by pulling directly away from the backing (Fig. 13-3).
- One half of the tape is securely placed on one side of the mid-portion of the wound and held securely. The opposite wound edge is apposed with a finger of the opposite hand (Fig. 13-4). After edge apposition, the tape is completely secured (Fig. 13-5).
- Further tapes are evenly placed adjacent to the original mid-wound tape (Fig. 13-6). Repeat this process with further tapes until the wound edges are completely apposed (Fig. 13-7). Wound tapes should have a gap between them that

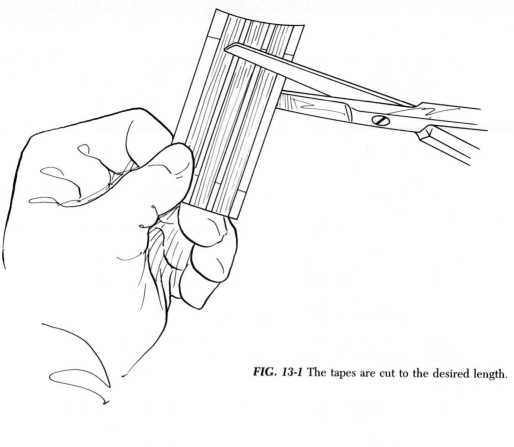

FIG. 13-1 The tapes are cut to the desired length.

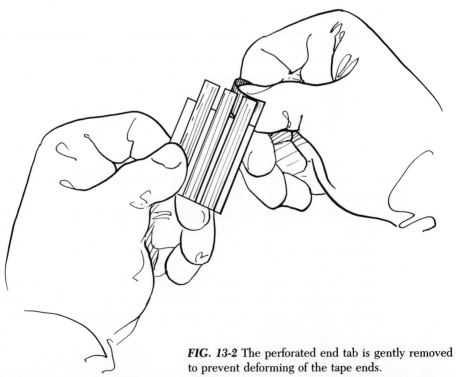

FIG. 13-2 The perforated end tab is gently removed to prevent deforming of the tape ends.

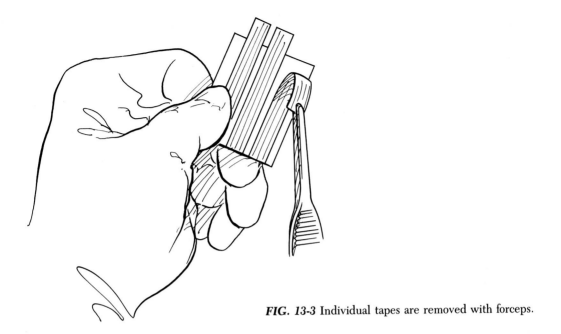

FIG. 13-3 Individual tapes are removed with forceps.

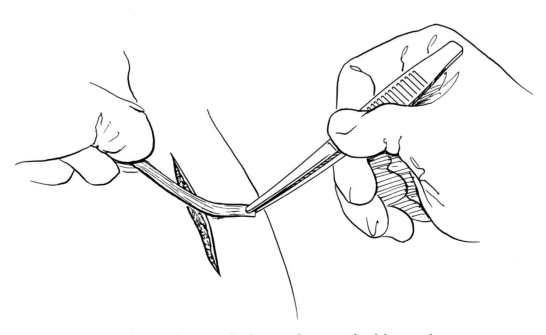

FIG. 13-4 The tape is firmly secured on one side of the wound.

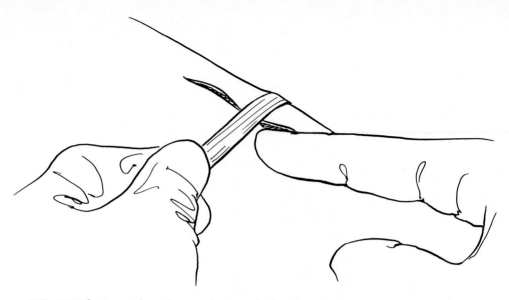

FIG. 13-5 The tape is brought over the wound after the wound is apposed with the finger of the opposite hand.

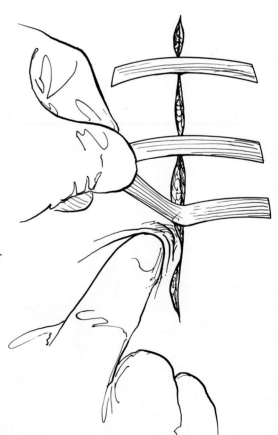

FIG. 13-6 Further tapes are placed in a similar manner.

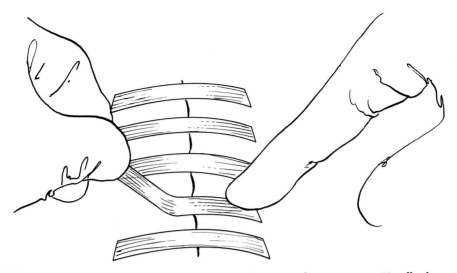

FIG. 13-7 Enough tapes are placed so that wound gapping does not occur. Usually there are 2-3 mm between tapes.

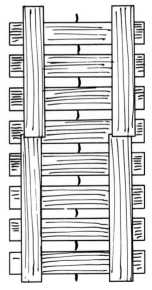

FIG. 13-8 Cross stays are placed over the tape ends to prevent skin blistering and premature removal.

is at least 2 to 3 mm wide. Complete occlusion of the wound by tapes can cause normal wound seepage to dissect under the tapes and lead to premature removal.

- The final step is to place cross stays to prevent elevation of the tape ends and minor skin blistering caused by tension of the tape ends (Fig. 13-8).

Tape Aftercare

Tapes are maintained in place for at least as long as sutures would be for the anatomic area in question. Unlike a sutured wound, a taped wound cannot be washed or moistened because premature tape removal can lead to wound dehiscence.

Note: Tapes should never be wrapped around a digit in a circumferential manner because they are not expandable and can act as a constricting band.

WOUND STAPLING

Since the introduction of automatic skin-stapling devices, there has been a reluctance to use them beyond their intended purpose of closing surgically-made incisions.* In spite of the remarkable amount of time saved by placing staples instead of sutures, early animal and clinical investigations questioned whether staples could accurately appose wound edges or promote wound tensile strength as effectively as sutures.[5] Recent studies in animals, however, have suggested that wound tensile strength is actually greater for staples when compared to sutures.[9,11] Additionally, less wound inflammatory response has been noted with staples and, most importantly, the cosmetic outcome was the same.

Clinical studies of staple use in traumatic lacerations are now beginning to demonstrate that, when compared to standard suturing methods, the ultimate cosmetic result as judged by blinded observers is no different.[2,4] In these studies, body regions that were chosen for the comparisons included the scalp, neck, arm/forearm, trunk, buttocks, and legs. Both adult and pediatric groups were studied. The time required for staple closure was approximately four to five times less than that required for suture placement. Cost has been cited as a drawback to the use of staples; however, the time saved by a busy physician and the reduced need for wound closure instruments balances that factor.[6] Patients appear to tolerate staples well while they are in place; however, there does appear to be increased discomfort upon removal when compared to sutures.[9]

Indications for Stapling

Wound stapling can be recommended under the following circumstances:

- Linear, sharp (shearing mechanism) lacerations of the scalp, trunk, and extremities. Although they have been used in hand lacerations, experience is not extensive enough to confidently recommend them for that area. Stapling is similarly avoided for facial wounds.
- Temporary, rapid closure of extensive superficial lacerations in patients requiring immediate surgery for life-threatening trauma.

---

*Staples are not optimal for body regions where computerized tomographic scan or magnetic resonance imaging is contemplated. They can create artifacts that might interfere with scan interpretation and, theoretically, they are mobile under a magnetic field.

Staples are avoided in anatomic areas to be studied by computerized tomography (CT) or magnetic resonance imaging (MRI).

Stapling Technique

Stapling devices have evolved significantly in the last several years, and there are number of products available. The Reflex One is representative of a multiple-staple device (35 staples per cartridge) with a wide staple that closes into a rectangular configuration (Fig. 13-9). This stapler is commonly used for surgical incisions or long lacerations of the trunk or extremity. The Precise Ten Shot stapler holds 10 staples that close into a smaller arcuate configuration. This device is useful for shorter, traumatically induced lacerations that might require greater precision and control. In addition to the stapler, the equipment required includes basic wound-care instruments and standard anesthetic agents.

The following steps are followed to insert staples:

- Forceps are used to evert the wound edges prior to placement of each staple (Fig. 13-10). When possible, a second operator can be very helpful in everting the edges while the primary operator uses the stapler.

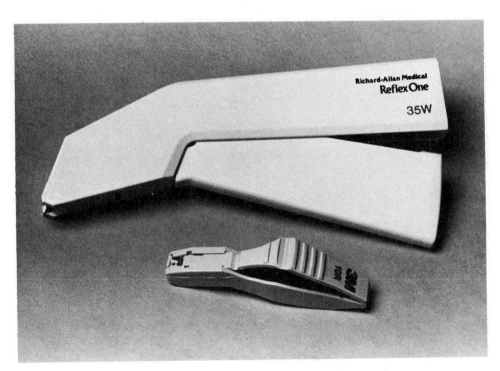

FIG. 13-9 Examples of wound stapling devices.

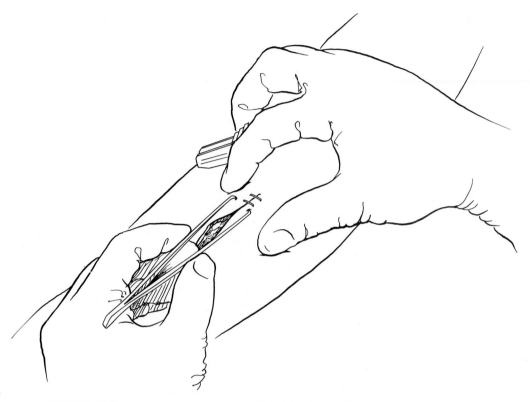

FIG. 13-10 Forceps are used to approximate and evert wound edges during stapling.

- Prior to triggering, the stapler should be placed gently on the skin over the wound without "pushing down" too hard (Fig. 13-11). A common mistake in placing staples is to go too deep.
- The trigger, or handle, is gently and evenly squeezed to advance the staple into the tissue (Fig. 13-12).
- Because of the configuration of the bending mechanism of the stapler, once the staple is seated, the stapler has to be "backed out" of the staple loop in order to disengage it.

Staple Aftercare

Staples are kept in place for the same length of time as are sutures in similar anatomic sites. Staple removal requires a special device that is provided by each manufacturer. The lower jaw is placed under the crossbar of the staple and the upper jaw is closed to open the loop of the staple as seen in Fig. 13-13, *A*, *B*, and *C*.

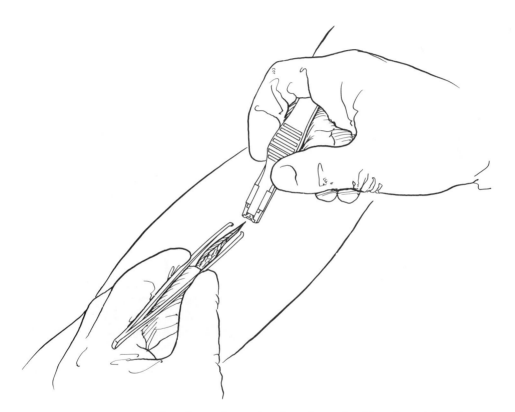

FIG. 13-11 During stapling the stapler is placed gently on the skin prior to triggering. Indenting the skin with too much pressure causes staples to be placed to deep.

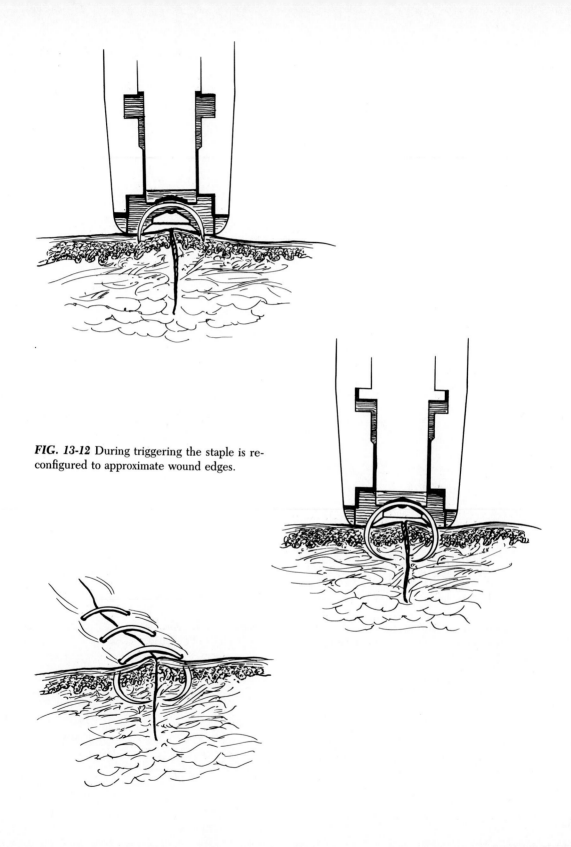

FIG. 13-12 During triggering the staple is re-configured to approximate wound edges.

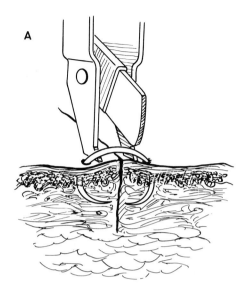

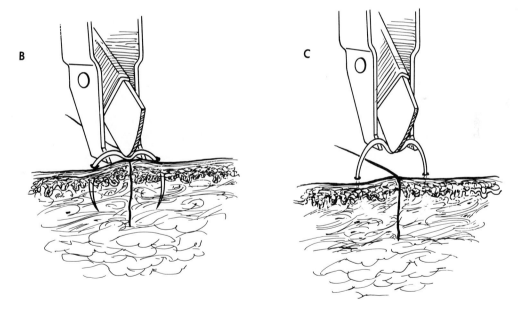

FIG. 13-13 The following procedure is used to remove staples. **A,** The lower jaws of the staple removing device are positioned under the staple cross-bar. **B,** The upper jaw is used to gently compress the staple. **C,** Once complete compression has taken place, the staple has been reconfigured for easy and gentle withdrawal.

References

1. Conolly BW et al: Clinical comparison of surgical wounds closed by suture and adhesive tapes, Am J Surg 117:318-322, 1969.
2. Dunmire SM et al: Staples versus sutures for wound closure in the peditric population (abstract), Ann Emerg Med 18:448, 1989.
3. Efron G and Ger R: Use of surgical adhesive tape (Steri-Strip) to secure skin graft on digits, Am J Surg 116:474, 1968.
4. George TK and Simpson DC: Skin wound closure with staples in the accident and emergency department, J Royal Coll Surg (Edin) 30:54-56, 1985.
5. Harrison ID, Williams DF, and Cuschieri A: The effect of metal clips on the tensile properties of healing skin wounds, Br J Surg 62:945-949, 1975.
6. Harvey CF and Hume Logan CJ: A prospective trial of skin staples and sutures in skin closure, Irish J Med Surg 155:194-196, 1986.
7. Koehn GG: A comparison of the duration of adhesion of Steri-Strips and Clearon, Cutis 26:620-621, 1980.
8. Rodeheaver GT, Spengler MD, and Edlich RF: Performance of new wound closure tapes, J Emerg Med 5:451-462, 1987.
9. Roth JH and Windle BH: Staple versus suture closure of skin incisions in a pig model, Can J Surg 31:19, 1988.
10. Trott AT: Alternative methods of wound closure: wound staples. In Roberts JR and Hedges JR, eds: Clinical procedures in emergency medicine, Philadelphia, 1985, WB Saunders Co.
11. Windle BH and Roth JH: Comparison of staple-closed and sutured skin incisions in a pig model, Surg Forum 35:546-550, 1984.

14 *Bite Wounds*

Animal and Human Bites
Microbiology of Bite Wounds
Animal Bite Risk Factors
    Location
    Type of wound
    Patient risk factors
    Biting species
Animal Bite Wound Management
    Treatment Measures for All Wounds
Specific Injuries
    Dog Bites
      Suturing
      Antibiotics
    Cat Bites
      Suturing

Antibiotics
Human Bites
    Suturing
    Antibiotics
    Indications for hospital management
Rat Bites
Fish Bites
Wound After-Care and Follow-Up
Rabies Exposure and Prophylaxis
    Animal identification
    Geographic location
    Severity of exposure
    Rabies status of attacking animal
Post-Exposure Prophylaxis
References

One of the more common problems that a medical care facility is faced with for emergency wound care is a mammalian bite. Bites can be from different sources, but the most common ones are from dogs, cats, and humans. In spite of apparently similar mechanisms of injury, each type of bite has different clinical, microbiologic, and treatment considerations that affect the management of bite-wound patients. With animal bites, there is also the possibility of secondary systemic infectious complications developing, the most important of which is rabies. It is the responsibility of any person caring for an animal bite victim to thoroughly delineate the biting circumstances and make an appropriate decision about whether or not to administer rabies prophylaxis.

ANIMAL AND HUMAN BITES

It is estimated that 500,000 to 2 million animal bites occur in the United States each year, many of which are unreported.[17] Dog bites predominate, accounting for approximately 80% of all animal bites.[9,17,40] Of reported bites 5% to 15% are caused by cats.[17,40] Other animals like rodents, monkeys, large mammals, and marine animals account for a small proportion of bite wounds. Bite injuries are more likely to occur in children, with a peak incidence between the ages of 5 and 14.[33] Dog bites are more common in males; cat bites and scratches are more often seen in females.[28,33]

Fortunately, most of the attacking animals are known to the victim and can be easily traced. Wild or possibly untraceable animals are involved in about 3% to 15% of bite incidents.[1,28] The ability to find, investigate, and quarantine animal makes the decision to administer rabies prophylaxis to a patient much easier.

MICROBIOLOGY OF BITE WOUNDS

The microbiology of bite wounds can be bewildering. Micro-organisms belonging to 30 different genera have been cultured from a dog's mouth.[3] A large variety of micro-organisms can be cultured from a normal cat mouth as well.[24] Clinical studies have shown, however, that there is little correlation between these potentially contaminating organisms and the ones that actually cause a wound infection.[7,9,23] Attempts to use a gram stain to correctly predict the presence of infecting pathogens are thwarted by the multiplicity of morphologically similar organisms that can be present merely as contaminants.[1,23]

Identification of organisms cultured from actual bite wound infections provide more useful information and predictive value with regard to prophylactic antibiotic choices than cultures of non-infected wounds. The number of species of bacteria that are implicated in true infections, although extensive, is much smaller than the total number of species that can be identified in an animal's mouth. The most frequent aerobic pathogens found in dog-bite infections are *Staphylococcus aureus*, *Staphylococcus epidermidis*, *Enterobacter* species, and other unidentifiable gram-negative rods.[7,24] Approximately 20% of cultures contain mixed flora.[7] Occasional anaerobic species are identifiable as well but with no clear predominance as to type.[24]

Another pathogen commonly identified in dog- and, especially cat-bite injuries, is *Pasteurella multocida*. Studies vary concerning the actual infection rate from this organism, ranging up to 50% in dog bites.[24,28] A recent study of dog bites, however, documents no infections with *P. multocida*.[6] An important point that can be inferred from these studies is that there is regional variation for animal-bite pathogens. Although up to 70% of cats carry this organism, the true incidence of bite wound infection is not known.[9] *P. multocida* is clinically suspected in patients who develop fulminant signs of local infection less than 24 hours after the bite. In addition to the rapidity of onset of infection, these infections are characterized by a gray, serosanguineous exudate.[17] Cat-bite infections can be caused by other organisms like *S. aureus, streptococci*, and a variety of anaerobes. Infections caused by these latter organisms usually manifest themselves later in the clinical course, between 48 to 96 hours postinjury.

The bacteriology of human bite wounds is complicated. More often than not, a culture of the bite wound will reveal the presence of multiple organisms.[9,20] Three basic patterns of bacterial species have been described in human bite wounds of the

Potential Infecting Pathogens in Bite Wounds

AEROBIC BACTERIA

Micrococcus sp.
Staphylococcus aureus
Streptococcus
Bacillus subtilis
Corynebacterium sp.
Eubacterium
Pseudomonas
Eikenella corrodens
Peptostreptococcus
Clostridium perfringens
Brucella canis
Bordetella sp.
Neisseria sp.

ANAEROBIC BACTERIA

Bacteroides sp.
Fusobacterium sp.
Peptococcus
Veillonella sp.
Propionibacterium acnes
Leptotrichia
Moraxella sp.
Acinetobacter calcoaceticus
Enterobacter sp.

Serratia marcescens
Proteus mirabilis
Aeromonas hydrophila
Pasteurella multocida
Hemophilus aprophilus
Klebsiella
CDC alphanumerics:
    IIJ
    EF-4
    DF-2

OTHER PATHOGENS (RARE)

Hepatitis virus
Yersinia pestis
Spirillum minus
Clostridium tetani
Leptospira interrogans
Simian herpes virus
Herpes virus
Rabies virus
Cat-scratch disease organism
Rio Bravo virus
Sporothrix schenckii
Streptobacillus moniliformis

(From Callaham ML: Wild and domestic animal attacks. In Auerbach and Geehr, editors: Management of wilderness and environmental emergencies, ed 2, St Louis, 1989, The CV Mosby Co.)

hand: (1) mixed gram-negative and gram-positive, organisms (i.e., *Enterobacter* species, *Klebsiella* species, a variety of *Streptococci*, *Proteus*, *Escherichia coli*, *Pseudomonas* species or others); (2) mixed gram-positive and gram-negative organisms with a predominance of coagulase-positive S. *aureus*; and (3) pure culture of S. *aureus*.[1] The recovery of S. *aureus* is usually associated with a higher incidence of and more serious suppurative complications.[20,39] In at least one study, 73% of all S. *aureus* organisms were resistant to penicillin.[26] A common and troublesome organism found in human bite wounds is *Eikenella corrodens*. It is a facultative anaerobic gram-negative rod that responds most readily to penicillin and has been reported to occur in 29% of bite wounds of the hand.[22]

ANIMAL BITE RISK FACTORS

A recent excellent review by Callaham listed the important risk factors that are possibly predictive of a higher rate of bite wound complications: These factors can influence the choice of wound management techniques (suturing) as well as the decision to use prophylactic antibiotics. Recommendations for specific biting species will be made in subsequent sections; however, all bites should be considered in the context of the Callaham risk factors (see box, p. 231).

Location

Approximately 75% of animal bites occur on the extremities.[7,28] In children, however, especially those who are under the age of 9, the predominant injury area is the face and head.[28] When examining children, the risk of skull penetration has to be considered. The anatomic location of the bite is important because there is a significant difference in the rate of infection per site. The hand appears to be at highest risk for infection, with an incidence in dog bites reported in one study to be as high as 30%.[8] The most resistant anatomic location is the face, which has an infection rate of 1.4% to 5.8%.[8,9]

All human bites to the hand are considered serious injuries. Approximately 3.6% of all bite injuries are caused by humans with 61.2% of those being inflicted on the hand and upper extremity.[34] The hand is a complex anatomic part with a high density of movable structures enclosed in limited tunnels and spaces. The hand does not tolerate infection well and can easily be devastated by even trivial injuries that introduce small inocula of bacteria.[29,36] When the hand comes into contact with the human mouth in a violent manner, it is exposed to a tremendous variety of pathogenic bacteria in high concentrations.[30]

Most human bites to the face, head, or trunk are occlusional. The hand, however, is subject to a second type of wound when it is closed into a fist to deliver a blow. This is called the clenched fist injury. Fist injuries tend to be more serious, accompanied by more suppurative complications.[30] A fist struck against the mouth can drive teeth well into the relatively unpadded surface of the dorsum of the hand at the metacarpophalangeal and distal interphalangeal joints. Tendon sheaths and joint capsules are particularly vulnerable in these locations.

Type of Wound

The mechanism of injury from an animal bite or attack plays an important role in predicting the chance of infection and, therefore, the choice of management technique. All animal bites are to be considered contaminated with potentially pathogenic bacteria. These injuries are frequently associated with crushing, tearing, and avulsion forces, and devitalized tissue. The combination of bacterial contamination with accompanying devitalized skin and fascia creates a setting ripe for the development of outright infection.

The wound that is at highest risk for becoming infected is the puncture wound where a fang has been driven deep into the tissue with only a small skin wound to show for it.[1,7,42] These wounds are difficult to adequately cleanse, irrigate, and debride and are considered at greater risk for infection. Large open wounds are less likely to develop this complication. Superficial, laceration-like wounds, without devitalized tissue, carry a low rate of infection regardless of the species.

Patient Risk Factors

Any of the conditions listed below require serious consideration for antibiotic prophylaxis.

Animal Bite Risk Factors

HIGH RISK

Location: Hand, wrist, or foot
Scalp or face in infants (high risk of cranial perforation; skull X-rays mandatory)
Over a major joint (possibility of perforation)

Type of Wound: Punctures (impossible to irrigate)
Tissue crushing that cannot be debrided (typical of herbivores such as cows, horses)

Patient: Older than 50 years
Asplenic
Chronic alcoholic
Altered immune status
Diabetic
Peripheral vascular insufficiency
Chronic corticosteroid therapy
Prosthetic or diseased cardiac valve (consider systemic prophylaxis)
Prosthetic or seriously diseased joint (consider systemic prophylaxis)

Species: Domestic cat
Large cat (deep punctures can penetrate joints, cranium)
Human (in hand wounds only)
Primates (anecdotal evidence only)
Pigs (anecdotal evidence only)

LOW RISK

Location: Face, scalp, ears, and mouth (all facial wounds should be sutured)

Type of Wound: Large clean lacerations that can be thoroughly cleansed
(the larger the laceration, the lower the infection rate)

Species: Rodents

(From Callaham ML: Wild and domestic animal attacks. In Auerbach and Geehr, editors: *Management of wilderness and environmental emergencies*, ed 2, St Louis, 1989, The CV Mosby Co.)

Biting Species

The overall infection rate of dog and cat bites varies considerably. Between 4% and 10% of dog bites become infected.[9,28,33] Sutured dog bites of the face, not treated with antibiotics, have been reported to become infected in only 1.4% of cases.[27] Up to 17% to 50% of cat bites, on the other hand, are subject to local infections.[16,28,33] Cat scratches have also been thought to carry an increased rate of infection, but a recent investigation of 14 claw injuries found no infections.[16] The rate of infection, however, is modified by several factors, including anatomic site, the patient's medical condition, and the time elapsed following the bite injury to treatment.

Practitioners have commonly concluded that human bites carry a high rate of infectious complications. Recently, one investigator estimated that the actual incidence of infection following human bites (excluding bites on the clenched fist) is 10%, with an even lower rate for bites on the face: 3%.[9] Original investigations appeared to have been biased by how much time had passed before treatment was administered.[20,30] This factor would skew the findings toward a higher infection rate. The face and ear, probably because they have a better vascularity, have a higher innate resistance to infection and tend to become infected less often.[5,41] In diabetics hand bites have to be managed with particular care because of the high morbidity associated with infection.[32]

ANIMAL BITE WOUND MANAGEMENT
Treatment Measures for All Wounds

Wound management depends on the type of wound, its severity, and its anatomic location. Simple contusions in which no obvious skin puncture, laceration, or avulsion is present are treated by thorough cleansing. In spite of the relatively minor appearance of many of these wounds, the patient still is at risk for developing rabies and this possibility has to be addressed.

For larger wounds that violate the epidermis and dermis, standard wound-care techniques are carried out:

- Povidone-iodine is the wound-cleansing solution that is recommended for wounds that are at low risk for rabies. Although it is viricidal, it has not been conclusively shown to be rabicidal.[9] When the risk of rabies is high, swabbing or scrubbing the wound with hand soap and water is recommended by the Centers for Disease Control.[38] Irrigation alone is not as effective as mechanical swabbing.*
- After thorough scrubbing of the wound periphery, copious high-pressure irriga-

---

*When there is a high risk of rabies, most authorities recommend that, whenever possible, wounds should not be sutured.[38] However, because of the extreme effectiveness of rabies prophylaxis with the immune globulin and vaccine, cosmetically important wounds should be considered for primary closure after all appropriate and meticulous wound-care steps have been taken.

tion is the next step, using a 19-gauge needle attached to a 20-cc or 35-cc syringe.

- Debridement of all devitalized tissue as well as 1 to 2 mm of dermal wound edge is essential for reducing the possibility of wound infection.
- Irrigation after debridement is recommended because dermal-edge excision provides greater exposure of the wound. Studies, both retrospective and prospective, have demonstrated that wound infection is reduced significantly after debridement.[7,8,46]
- Culture purulence or suspected infection.
- Obtain radiographs when fracture or joint penetration is suspected.
- Ensure proper tetanus immunization.
- Assess and treat for rabies exposure if necessary.

SPECIFIC INJURIES
Dog Bites
Suturing

The issue of whether to suture dog bite wounds has been controversial over the years. Recent evidence and the author's personal experience support the practice of primary suture closure of most dog-bite wounds after the above management steps have been carried out.[7,8,9] Suturing, however, is not recommended for non-facial wounds that are more than 8 to 12 hours old, deep fang wounds, hand lacerations, or those wounds that have obvious signs of infection when presented to a medical-care facility (see box on p. 231 for other high risk factors to consider). When significant risk factors are present, delayed primary closure (tertiary union) or open closure (secondary union) can be considered. Deep closures using nonabsorbable suture material are to be avoided at any time in order to avoid a foreign body nidus for infection.

Antibiotics

In spite of several studies that have researched the efficacy of prophylactic antibiotics for dog-bite wounds, the indications for prophylaxis are still somewhat controversial. Empiric use of penicillin or dicloxacillin has been felt to be of some value in preventing infection in at least one uncontrolled study.[23] Two studies, one retrospective and one double-blind controlled, have demonstrated no efficacy with prophylactic antibiotic coverage.[8,19] In another double-blind study, only hand wounds were found to have a lower infection rate when prophylactic penicillin was administered.[7] Wounds in other body areas were not similarly protected.

Based on current knowledge and risk factors, the author recommends prophylactic antibiotics to be administered in the following clinical settings: dog-bite wounds that are more than 8 to 12 hours old, wounds of the hand, deep-puncture (fang) wounds in which debridement-irrigation is difficult to carry out, and to high-risk patients like diabetics and patients who are immunosuppressed. The recommended antibiotic is a penicillinase-resistant penicillin like dicloxacillin. This drug will adequately cover most of the significant pathogens found in dog-bite wounds. Amoxicillin with clavulanate is a good alternative but more costly. For penicillin-allergic patients, erythromycin or ciprofloxacin can be used. First generation cephalosporins are often used for bite wounds, but they are less efficacious than the other drugs discussed here.

Cat Bites
Suturing

Cat-bite and scratch wounds are probably best left open and not sutured. Cat fangs can penetrate deeply into the soft tissues, and because the infection potential of these wounds is great, the most judicious course of action is to cleanse, irrigate, and debride the wound and leave it open.[44] Exceptions to this recommendation include large, easily cleansed lacerations that are not on the hand or foot. Most lacerations of the face will be protected by the good vascular supply of the face. Whenever suturing is chosen, only percutaneous nonabsorbable sutures are used. Deep closures are avoided because of the increased risk of infection.

Antibiotics

Because of the higher incidence of wound infection in cat bites, prophylactic antibiotics are recommended for all of these injuries. *Pasteurella multocida* is an organism that is frequently found in cat bites and is rapidly and particularly virulent. Protection against this organism is essential. Uncontrolled studies and observations support the practice of prophylaxis in cat bites.[43,44] A recent, small, double-blind, controlled study of cat bites indicated that prophylactic oxacillin significantly decreased the subsequent risk of infection.[18] Penicillin or dicloxacillin are the drugs of choice for cat bites and suspected *P. multocida*. Amoxicillin with clavulanate is also an effective agent. First-generation cephalosporins are less effective. The newer second- and third-generation cephalosporins, cefuroxime and ceftriaxone, are effective against all bite wound organisms, including *P. multocida*. Erythromycin is recommended for penicillin-allergic patients. Although erythromycin has shown variable activity in vitro to *P. multocida*, apparently it is effective in treating infections from which the organism could be cultured.[6,45] Ciprofloxacin can be used for penicillin-allergic patients as well.

Human Bites
Suturing

As a general rule, closure of human bite wounds has traditionally been avoided. Sutures only act as a foreign body in a clinical setting that is already high-risk. However, a recent study has cast doubt on the practice of not closing human bite wounds.[4] Sutured vs. non-sutured hand lacerations from human bites had the same outcome. Further studies, however, have not been carried out to confirm these results. The recommendation remains the same: not to close hand lacerations. Large, easily cleansed and irrigated proximal extremity or truncal wounds can be closed with a single layer of nonabsorbable material. Facial human bites can be potentially disfiguring. A fresh facial bite, less than 12 hours old, that does not show signs of infection can be safely closed with sutures.[41] Consultation is recommended when there is doubt about what management steps should be carried out.

Antibiotics

It is agreed by most authorities that all human bites of the hand, whether they are infected or not, require antibiotic coverage.[9,15,26,30] The choice is complicated because *Eikenella corrodens* is not adequately covered by dicloxacillin or the first-generation cephalosporins. Penicillin is the most effective inexpensive antibiotic for this organism. One authority recommends penicillin plus dicloxacillin to adequately cover *Eikenella corrodens* as well as *S. aureus*.[6] Others feel that amoxicillin plus clavulanate is the best choice.[25] Another appropriate drug is the second-generation cephalosporin cefuroxime. Tetracycline is the drug of choice for adults who are allergic to penicillin. Erythromycin is given to penicillin-allergic children in spite of the fact that it is less effective against *E. corrodens* than other choices.

Indications for Hospital Management

Because of the seriousness of human bites to the hand, the question of whether to admit a patient to a hospital or not often arises. It is this author's opinion that whenever there is doubt a surgical specialist should be consulted for all wounds. Patients are best served by being admitted to hospital and being administered intravenous antibiotic therapy if:

- the wound is 12 or more hours old;
- there are clear signs of infection;
- there is significant tissue loss or mutilation;
- a joint capsule or tendon has been violated, i.e., as in the clenched fist injury[43];
- a fracture is present;
- the patient is immunocompromised; or
- the patient is incompetent to care for self; that is, he or she is under the influence of drugs or alcohol.

Other human hand and non-hand wounds can be carefully considered for out-patient management with recognition that considerable judgment should be brought to bear in all cases.

Rat Bites

Most reported rat bites occur in a domestic setting. In a recent study of 50 cases, *Staphylococcus epidermidis* was the most common organism cultured from the open, fresh wound.[35] Other organisms included *Bacillus subtilis*, diphtheroids, and alpha hemolytic streptococci. Although 30% of wounds had positive cultures, only one case became infected. No patient was treated with prophylactic antibiotics. Antibiotics are recommended only if wound infection is evident. Dicloxacillin and erythromycin are effective. Rats do not carry rabies and patients do not need post-exposure prophylaxis.

Fish Bites

People who work with or own fish are susceptible to infection by the small gram-positive rod *Erysipelothrix*. This organism causes a slowly spreading cellulitis of the affected area, usually the hand. The organism responds to penicillin.

WOUND AFTER-CARE AND FOLLOW-UP

All animal-bite victims or members of their families have to be instructed about the signs of infection: pain, redness, swelling, and purulent drainage. Dressings have to be removed approximately 24 hours after the initial visit so that the wound can be inspected. A wound infection with *P. multocida* will usually be apparent by that time. If signs of infection are present, the patient should return to a medical-care facility for treatment. Otherwise, if the clinical course is benign, the patient can return for a routine wound inspection 48 to 72 hours after repair or at the appropriate time for suture removal, depending on the clinical situation. Tetanus prophylaxis is administered according to the guidelines outlined in Chapter 18.

RABIES EXPOSURE AND PROPHYLAXIS

When treating a patient with an animal bite, the issue of rabies exposure inevitably arises. In the emergency wound-care setting, the key decision is whether or not to administer rabies prophylaxis. Several factors have to be considered before that decision is made. These include the type of animal involved in the attack; the geographic location of the bite incident and whether or not rabies is carried by that species of animal in that location; the severity of exposure and whether it was sufficient to transmit the rabies virus; and finally, the status of the animal, i.e., whether or not it has been captured.

Animal Identification

Determining the type of animal that inflicted the bite is the first step in a systematic approach to a treatment decision.[31] For clarity, Figs. 14-1, 14-2, and 14-3 summarize these steps. In 1988, wild carnivores accounted for approximately 88.4% of all confirmed animals with rabies in the United States and its territories.[13] Of 4724

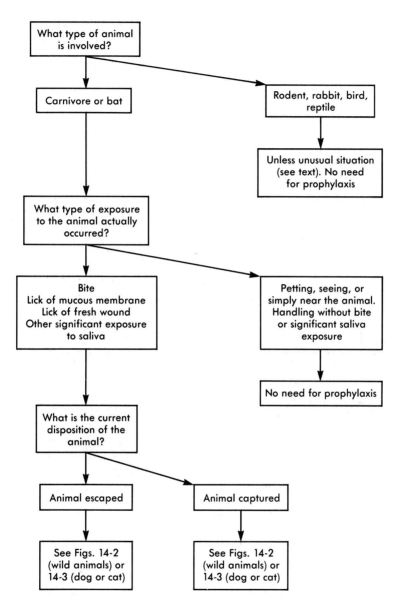

FIG. 14-1 Decision steps for post-exposure rabies prophylaxis. See Figs. 14-2 and 14-3. (Reproduced with permission from Rabies risk: systematic evaluation and management of animal bites, Comp Therapy 7:58-67, 1981.)

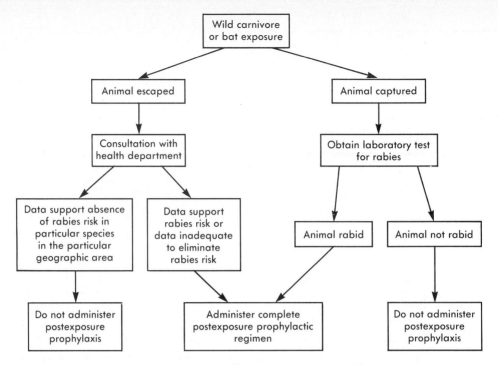

FIG. 14-2 Decision steps for post-exposure rabies prophylaxis. Wild carnivore and bat exposure. (Reproduced with permission from Rabies risk: systematic evaluation and management of animal bites, Comp Ther 7:58-67, 1981.)

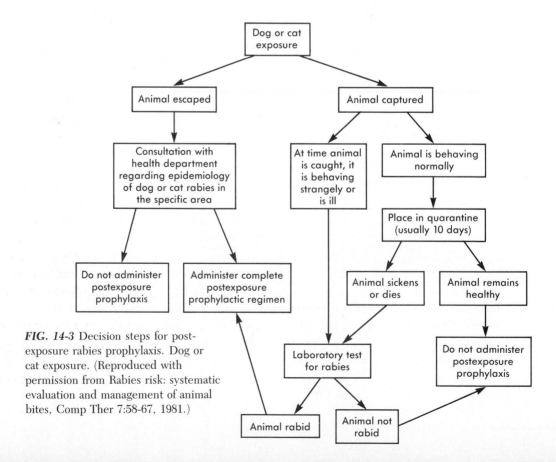

FIG. 14-3 Decision steps for post-exposure rabies prophylaxis. Dog or cat exposure. (Reproduced with permission from Rabies risk: systematic evaluation and management of animal bites, Comp Ther 7:58-67, 1981.)

confirmed cases of animal rabies reported in 1988, seven species of animals accounted for 96.6% of the cases. Skunks, at 37.9% of the total, were the most common carriers, followed by raccoons (31%), bats (13.5%), cats (4.1%), foxes (3.9%), cattle (3.6%), and dogs (2.7%). It is of epidemiologic interest that in Mexico wild dogs account for 93.5% of all animal rabies.[12] Rodents (rats and mice), rabbits, hamsters, gerbils, squirrels, and chipmunks rarely are reported to carry rabies, and bites from them are usually not considered for prophylaxis. When in doubt, consult local public health authorities. Attention has recently been focused on the ferret. It is a popular pet in certain areas of the country and, if infected with the virus, it can transmit rabies to humans.

Geographic Location

The geographic area of the bite is important because rabies is not evenly distributed in all locales. For example, although bat rabies is widely reported from all areas of the United States, only 13 states reported raccoon rabies in 1981.[10] Table 14-1 provides a state-by-state distribution of all animal types in whom animal rabies was documented in 1988.[12] From 1977 to 1986, only twenty human cases had been reported in the United States. Most of these were acquired by exposure outside the United States. Whenever there is any question about the likelihood of rabies in any bite situation, emergency wound-care personnel should not hesitate to contact their local health department for guidance.

Severity of Exposure

After determining the type of animal, some estimation is made of the severity of the bite exposure. Rabies is transmitted by animal saliva.[37] The rabies virus will not penetrate intact skin but can enter the body through mucous membranes.[31] Therefore the following clinical situations constitute a rabies exposure: (1) a bite that violates the epidermis; (2) salivary contact with a mucous membrane, i.e., a rabid dog licking a child's face or mouth; (3) salivary contact with a fresh (less than 24 hours old) abrasion or open wound. [31] Picking up or touching a dead, rabid animal but not allowing saliva to come in contact with mucous membranes or wounds does not constitute an exposure.

Rabies Status of Attacking Animal

The final step in the decision process is to determine the rabies status of the attacking animal. For wild carnivores or bats that have been captured, immediate consultation and cooperation with the local health department is necessary in order to process the animal. The animal head has to be kept refrigerated until the brain can be examined for rabies by the fluorescent antibody technique.[31] Quarantining a wild animal to observe behavior abnormalities suggestive of rabies is not appropriate. If the wild animal has escaped and cannot be apprehended, consultation with

Table 14-1 Cases of Animal Rabies, by State and Category, United States, 1988

State	Total	Total Domestic	Total Wild	Dogs	Cats	Cattle	Horses/ Mules	Sheep/ Goats	Swine	Skunks	Foxes	Bats	Raccoons	Rodents and lagomorphs*	Other Wild†	Percent Change‡
Species Total	4,724	550	4,174	128	192	171	43	9	7	1,791	183	638	1,463	25	74	-0.1
AK	34	2	32	2	0	0	0	0	0	0	32	0	0	0	0	325.0
AL	94	3	91	2	1	0	0	0	0	1	3	19	67	0	1[f]	16.1
AR	91	85	1	0	3	2	0	0	76	1	8	0	0	0	0	-26.0
AZ	45	45	0	0	0	0	0	0	10	5	30	0	0	0	0	-46.4
CA	402	8	394	3	1	2	2	0	0	256	8	129	1	0	0	1.8
CO	28	0	28	0	0	0	0	0	0	1	0	27	0	0	0	-15.2
CT	8	0	8	0	0	0	0	0	0	0	0	8	0	0	0	166.7
DC	13	2	11	1	1	0	0	0	0	0	0	0	11	0	0	-71.1
DE	61	2	59	0	2	0	0	0	0	7	4	8	36	4[a]	0	577.8
FL	184	14	170	0	14	0	0	0	0	1	8	32	127	0	2[g]	65.8
GA	292	13	279	7	6	0	0	0	0	24	9	6	237	0	3[h]	39.7
HI	0	0	0	0	0	0	0	0	0	0	0	0	0	0	0	0.0
IA	175	74	101	15	16	36	5	1	1	96	0	5	0	0	0	-35.7
ID	11	0	11	0	0	0	0	0	0	0	0	11	0	0	0	10.0
IL	32	4	28	2	0	1	1	0	0	16	0	11	0	0	1[i]	-30.4
IN	36	0	36	0	0	0	0	0	0	26	2	8	0	0	0	80.0
KS	41	3	38	1	1	1	0	0	0	35	0	3	0	0	0	-2.4
KY	106	23	83	15	1	5	2	0	0	78	2	2	1	0	0	-22.6
LA	13	1	12	0	1	0	0	0	0	8	0	4	0	0	0	0.0
MA	3	0	3	0	0	0	0	0	0	0	0	3	0	0	0	-40.0
MD	338	16	322	0	13	2	0	1	0	19	21	21	255	5[b]	1[j]	-24.9
ME	1	1	0	0	1	0	0	0	0	0	0	0	0	0	0	-66.7
MI	35	4	31	2	2	0	0	0	0	8	2	21	0	0	0	25.0
MN	142	42	100	7	6	27	2	0	0	92	1	7	0	0	0	-44.3
MO	36	6	30	3	2	1	0	0	0	18	0	12	0	0	0	-39.0
MS	9	0	9	0	0	0	0	0	0	0	0	9	0	0	0	0.0
MT	214	16	198	1	4	8	3	0	0	182	1	16	0	0	0	14.4
NC	8	0	8	0	0	0	0	0	0	4	1	3	0	0	0	0.0
ND	105	24	81	4	6	11	3	0	0	78	0	1	2	0	0	-18.6
NE	21	5	16	1	1	3	0	0	0	12	0	4	0	0	0	23.5

	Total													Other wild†	% Chg‡
NH	4	1	3	0	0	0	0	0	0	0	0	0	3	0	0.0
NJ	15	0	15	0	0	0	0	0	0	0	0	0	15	0	−16.7
NM	15	4	11	0	2	0	2	0	0	6	1	4	4	0	400.0
NV	20	0	20	0	0	0	0	0	0	0	0	0	20	0	33.3
NY	40	1	39	0	1	1	0	0	0	0	0	0	38	0	−29.8
OH	6	0	6	0	0	0	0	0	0	0	0	0	6	0	−60.0
OK	38	6	32	2	3	3	2	0	0	31	0	0	0	0	8.6
OR	6	0	6	0	0	0	0	0	0	0	0	0	6	0	20.0
PA	543	48	495	3	16	8	0	0	0	73	18	11	380	12ᶜ	1ʲ	67.6
PR	73	21	52	9	3	3	9	0	0	0	0	0	0	0	52ᵏ	4.3
RI	0	0	0	0	0	0	0	0	0	0	0	0	0	0	−100.0
SC	127	26	101	5	20	0	0	1	1	10	11	9	67	2ᵈ	2ˡ	115.3
SD	137	40	97	5	10	22	1	1	1	92	1	3	0	0	1ᵐ	−39.9
TN	111	9	102	8	0	1	1	0	0	87	5	10	0	0	14.4
TX	434	78	356	21	30	14	9	4	0	266	20	57	4	0	9ⁿ	0.5
UT	10	0	10	0	0	0	0	0	0	0	0	0	10	0	42.9
VA	366	19	347	1	13	2	1	0	2	89	24	11	220	2ᵉ	1ᶠ	1.1
VT	0	0	0	0	0	0	0	0	0	0	0	0	0	0	00.0
WA	4	0	4	0	0	0	0	0	0	0	0	4	0	0	−60.0
WI	55	14	41	4	3	6	1	0	0	38	3	3	0	0	14.6
WV	103	8	95	1	2	1	0	4	0	31	3	7	54	0	30.4
WY	39	6	33	1	3	2	0	0	0	20	13	13	0	0	−45.8
Percent§	100	11.6	88.4	2.7	4.1	3.6	0.9	0.2	0.2	37.9	3.9	13.5	31.0	0.5	1.6
Total 1987‖	4,729¶	559	4,169	170	166	174	39	8	2	2,033	119	629	1,311	12	65
% Chg§	−0.1	−1.6	+0.1	−24.7	+15.7	−1.7	+10.3	+12.5	+250.0	−11.9	+53.8	+1.4	+11.6	+108.3	+13.9

*Rodents and lagomorphs include: (a) 4 groundhogs; (b) 5 groundhogs; (c) 11 groundhogs, 1 rabbit; (d) 1 squirrel, 1 rat; (e) 2 groundhogs.
†Other wild includes: (f) 1 bobcat; (g) 2 otter, 1 bobcat; (h) 3 bobcats; (i) 1 coyote; (j) 1 deer; (k) 52 mongooses; (l) 2 bobcats; (m) 1 badger; (n) 6 coyotes, 1 deer, 1 ringtail, 1 bobcat.
‡Percent change from 1987.
§Percentage of all rabid animals in 1988.
‖1987 total by species.
¶Total includes one human case.
From CDC Surveillance Summary, vol 38, no 55-1; 1989.

the local health department to determine the likelihood of rabies being present in that animal species in that region is necessary. If the animal is wild and has escaped, the decision to give prophylaxis is made in conjunction with the local public health authorities. Table 14-1 can be used to estimate the probability of rabies in the attacking species for a given state.

For domestic dogs and cats, a somewhat different approach is taken.[31] If the animal is captured, an immediate examination by a qualified veterinarian or animal control officer is undertaken to determine if there are signs or symptoms of animal rabies. If there is a suspicion that rabies is present, then the animal is sacrificed and its brain is examined for rabies. For a normal-appearing animal without signs of being rabid, quarantining is indicated for a 10-day period. Should the animal sicken and die, rabies testing of brain tissue is carried out and rabies prophylaxis is administered as necessary. An animal that remains healthy for that period is assurance enough that rabies is not present. On the average, animals with rabies die within 3 to 4 days from the onset of illness.

If the dog or cat has escaped, every attempt is made to capture the animal. Local authorities such as police and animal control officers can assist in this effort. Should this effort be futile, consultation with the local health department is initiated to help determine the risk of exposure given the particular geographic region and epidemiology of rabies in that area.

One crucial question that often comes up during the process of investigating a possible rabies exposure is how long after the incident prophylaxis can be administered in order for it to be effective. The incubation period of rabies has been reported to be as short as 5 days and as long as 2 years, with an average of 30 to 90 days.[21,37] Once the virus has traveled from the bite site to the central nervous system, entering the "neural" phase, post-exposure prophylaxis is believed to be ineffective. In practical terms, delays of up to 7 to 10 days for bites that are not considered high risk are acceptable but not optimal.[31] Early administration of prophylaxis, however, is preferable for high-risk bites (skunk, raccoon, fox, or bat), bites of the head, neck or hands, and in patients taking corticosteroids or other immunosuppressive agents.[21,31] If the patient does not present until after 7 days from exposure, consultation with the local health department is recommended, but prophylaxis is often administered anyway if the bite circumstances are high risk.

POST-EXPOSURE PROPHYLAXIS

The current recommendations for post-exposure prophylaxis by the Immunization Practices Advisory Committee (ACIP) for the Centers for Disease Control require that rabies immune globulin and human diploid cell vaccine (HDCV) be administered.[11] The combined use of these drugs is necessary to prevent prophylaxis failure that might occur if either one is omitted. Table 14-2 summarizes the current guidelines for administration of these agents. Rabies immune globulin is adminis-

Table 14-2 *A Guide to Rabies Post-Exposure Prophylaxis*

	Animal Species	Condition of Animal at Time of Attack	Treatment of Exposed Person*
Domestic	Dog or cat	Healthy and available for 10 days of observation	None, unless animal develops rabies[1]
		Rabid or suspected rabid	RIG[2] and HDCV
		Unknown (escaped)	Consult public health officials if treatment is indicated, give RIG[2] and HDCV
Wild	Skunk, bat, fox, coyote, racoon, bobcat, and other carnivores	Regard as rabid unless proven negative by laboratory tests[3]	RIG[2] and HDCV
Other	Livestock, rodents, and lagomorphs (rabbits and hares)	Consider individually. Local and state public health officials should be consulted on questions about the need for rabies prophylaxis. Bites of squirrels, hamsters, guinea pigs, gerbils, chipmunks, rats, mice, other rodents, rabbits, and hares almost never call for antirabies prophylaxis.	

*All bites and wounds should immediately be cleansed thoroughly with soap and water. If antirabies treatment is indicated both rabies immune globulin (RIG) and human diploid cell rabies vaccine (HDCV) should be given as soon as possible, regardless of the interval from exposure. Local reactions to vaccines are common but do not contraindicate continuing treatment. Discontinue vaccine treatment if fluorescent-antibody tests of the animal are negative for rabies.

[1]During the usual holding period of 10 days, begin treatment with RIG and vaccine (preferably with HDCV) at the first sign of rabies in a dog or cat that has bitten someone. The symptomatic animal should be killed immediately and tested.

[2]If RIG is not available, use antirabies serum, equine; do not use more than the recommended dosage.

[3]The animal should be killed and tested as soon as possible. Holding for observation is not recommended.

From ACIP, Rabies Prevention—U.S., 1984. MMWR 33:393-402, 407-408, 1984.

tered in a total does of 20 IU/kg. One-half of that dose is given subcutaneously around the bite wound and the other half is injected intramuscularly in the gluteal site. When the bite area is too small, such as the fingertip, the bulk of the rabies immune globulin is given intramuscularly in order to accommodate local injection. Complications following administration of rabies immune globulin are unusual. The most common ones are pain at the injection site and an occasional temporary rise in body temperature.

The vaccine (HDCV) is administered according to a fixed schedule (see Table 14-3). The first dose is given at the first visit to a medical facility. The vaccine is deliv-

Table 14-3 *Post-Exposure Rabies Prophylaxis Immune Globulin and Vaccine Dosing Schedule*

All post-exposure treatment should begin with immediate thorough cleansing of all wounds with soap and water.

A. Persons not previously immunized — RIG, 20 IU/kg body weight, one half infiltrated at bite site (if possible), remainder IM; 5 doses of HDCV, 1.0 mL (i.e., deltoid area), one each on days 0, 3, 7, 14, and 28.

B. Persons previously immunized* — Two doses of HDCV, 1.0 mL, IM (i.e., deltoid area), one each on days 0 and 3. RIG should not be administered.

*Pre-exposure immunized with HDCV, prior post-exposure prophylaxis with HDCV; or persons previously immunized with any other type of rabies vaccine *and* also had a history of positive antibody response to the prior vaccination.
From ACIP. Rabies Prevention—U.S., 1984. MMWR 33:393-402, 407-408, 1984.

ered intramuscularly at a site away from the injection of the rabies immune globulin. The deltoid muscle is preferred because of reported vaccine failures when given in the gluteal region.[21] The patient is then required to return according to the scheduled protocol. The ACIP recommends 5 doses, with the last one being given on the twenty-eighth day following the initial visit. Early in the clinical use of the vaccine, measuring antibody titers in patients was believed to be necessary to ensure adequacy of immunization following the prophylaxis course. Because of the documented effectiveness of the vaccine in virtually all patients, this practice is no longer thought to be necessary.[2] Local reaction at the injection sites occur more frequently with the vaccine than the rabies immune globulin. Swelling, erythema, and induration have been noted.[14] Systemic reactions to the vaccine are infrequent, but mild headache, malaise, myalgia, and abdominal pain have been reported.[14] Allergic and neurologic reactions, more frequently associated with the older duck embryo vaccine, are exceedingly rare with the use of the human vaccine.[14]

References

1. Aghababian R and Conte J: Mammalian bite wounds, Ann Emerg Med 9:79-83, 1980.
2. Anderson L, Sikes R, and Langkop C: Post-exposure trial of a human diploid cell strain rabies vaccine, J Infect Dis 142:133-138, 1980.
3. Bailie W, Stove E, and Schmitt A: Aerobic bacterial flora of oral and nasal fluids of canines with reference to bacteria associated with bites, J Clin Microbiol 7:223-231, 1978.
4. Bite U: Human bites of the hand, Can J Surg 27:616-618, 1984.

5. Brandt F: Human bites of the ear, Plast Reconstr Surg 43:130-134, 1969.

6. Callaham ML: Controversies in antibiotic choices for bite wounds, Ann Emerg Med 17:1321-1330, 1988.

7. Callaham ML: Prophylactic antibiotics in common dog bite wounds: a controlled study, Ann Emerg Med 9:410-414, 1980.

8. Callaham ML: Treatment of common dog bites: infection risk factors, J Am Coll Emerg Phys 7:83-87, 1978.

9. Callaham ML: Wild and domestic animal attacks. In Auerbach PS and Geehr EC, eds: Management of wilderness and environmental emergencies, ed 2, St Louis, 1989, The CV Mosby Co.

10. Centers for Disease Control: Rabies in the United States 1981, Morbid Mortal Weekly Rep 23(suppl):33-37, 1983.

11. Centers for Disease Control, Rabies Prevention United States 1984, Morbid Mortal Weekly Rep 33:393-402, 1984.

12. Centers for Disease Control: Rabies Surveillance United States 1986, Morbid Mortal Weekly Rep 36(suppl):1-27, 1986.

13. Centers for Disease Control: Rabies surveillance United States 1988, Morbid Mortal Weekly Rep 38(ss-1);1-21, 1989.

14. Centers for Disease Control: Recommendations of the Immunization Practices Advisory Committee (ACIP): Rabies prevention, Morbid Mortal Weekly Rep 29:265-280, 1980.

15. Chuinard R and D'Ambrosia R: Human bite infections of the hand, J Bone Joint Surg 59 A:416-418, 1977.

16. Dice DJ: Cat bite wounds: risk factors for infection (abstract), Ann Emerg Med 18:471, 1989.

17. Doan L: Animal bites and rabies. In Rosen P et al, eds: Emergency medicine: concepts and clinical practice, St Louis, 1983, The CV Mosby Co.

18. Elenbaas R, McNabney W, and Robinson W: Evaluation of prophylactic oxacillin in cat bite wounds, Ann Emerg Med 13:155-157, 1984.

19. Elenbaas R, McNabney W, and Robinson W: Prophylactic oxacillin in dog bite wounds, Ann Emerg Med 11:248-251, 1982.

20. Farmer C and Mann R: Human bite infections of the hand, South Med J 59:515-518, 1966.

21. Fishbein DB and Arcangeli LS: Rabies prevention in primary care, Postgrad Med 82:83-95, 1987.

22. Goldstein EJC, Barones MF, and Miller TA: *Eikenella corrodens* in hand infections, J Hand Surg 8:563-566, 1983.

23. Goldstein EJC, Citron D, and Finegold S: Dog bite wounds and infection: a prospective clinical study, Ann Emerg Med 9:508-512, 1980.

24. Goldstein E, Citron D, and Wield B: Bacteriology of human and animal bite wounds, J Clin Microbiol 8:667-672, 1978.

25. Goldstein EJC et al: A comparative study of augmentin versus penicillin ± dicloxacillin: a special report, Postgrad Med 56:105-110, 1984.

26. Guba A, Mulliken J, and Hoopes J: The selection of antibiotics for human bites of the hand, Plast Reconstr Surg 56:538-541, 1975.

27. Guy RJ and Zook EG: Successful treatment of acute head and neck dog bite wounds without antibiotics, Ann Plast Surg 17:45-48, 1986.

28. Kizer K: Epidemiologic and clinical aspects of animal bite injuries, J Am Coll Emerg Phys 8:134-141, 1979.

29. Koch S: Acute rapidly spreading infections following trivial injuries to the hand, Surg Gynecol Obstet 59:277-308, 1934.

30. Malinowski R et al: The management of human bite injuries to the hand, J Trauma 19:655-658, 1979.

31. Mann J: Systemic decision-making in rabies prophylaxis, Ped Infect Dis 2:162-167, 1983.

32. Mann R and Peacock J: Hand infections in patients with diabetes mellitus, J Trauma 17:376-380, 1977.

33. Marcy S: Infections due to dog and cat bites, Ped Infect Dis 1:351-356, 1982.

34. Marr J, Beck A, and Lugo J: An epidemiologic study of the human bite, Public Health Rep 94:514-521, 1979.

35. Ordog GJ, Balasubramaniam S, and Wasserberger J: Rat bites: fifty cases, Ann Emerg Med 14:126-130, 1985.

36. Peeples E, Boswick J, and Scott F: Wounds of the hand contaminated by human or animal saliva, J Trauma 19:655-658, 1979.

37. Plotkin S and Clark H: Prevention of rabies in man, J Infect Dis 123:227-240, 1971.

38. *Report of the Committee on Infectious Diseases*, Twenty First Edition, American Academy of Pediatrics, 1988.

39. Shields C et al: Hand infections secondary to human bites, J Trauma 15:235-236, 1975.

40. Strassburg M et al: Animal bites: patterns of treatment, Ann Emerg Med 10:193-197, 1981.

41. Thomasetti B, Walker L, and Bormby M: Human bites of the face, J Oral Surg 37:565-568, 1979.

42. Thomson H and Svitek V: Small animal bites: the role of primary closure, J Trauma 13:20-23, 1973.

43. Tindall J and Harrison C: *Pasteurella multocida* infections following animal injuries, especially cat bites, Arch Dermatol 105:412-416, 1972.

44. Vietch J and Omer G: Case report: treatment of cat bite injuries of the hand, J Trauma 19:201-202, 1979.

45. Weber DJ et al: *Pasteurella multocida* infections: report of 34 cases and review of the literature, Medicine 63:133-154, 1984.

46. Zook E et al: Successful treatment protocol for canine fang injuries, J Trauma 20:243-246, 1980.

15 *Foreign Bodies, Puncture Wounds, and Abrasions*

Foreign Bodies
    Techniques for removal
Puncture Wounds
    Treatment of puncture wounds

Fishhooks
Abrasions
References

There are many problems that lend themselves to emergency wound-care techniques. These include retained foreign bodies and fishhooks, puncture wounds, and abrasions. Although these may seem trivial, each one of these problems presents special concerns and, occasionally, requires sophisticated diagnostic and management procedures. In addition, certain anatomic areas of the body, particularly the structures of the hand and face, are fraught with difficulties that can be successfully managed by a thorough understanding and application of proper technique.

FOREIGN BODIES

Any material can potentially become a foreign body should it penetrate the skin and lodge in the soft tissue. In a clinical study of foreign bodies retained in the hand, the most common objects, in order of frequency, were wood splinters, glass fragments, various metallic objects, and needles.[1] Included in the list were pencil leads, thorns, nails, and plastic objects. Each one of these foreign substances can cause a variety of problems unless they are removed.

Inert materials like metal, even if they are bacteria-free upon penetration, can cause chronic pain and discomfort, especially in weight-bearing areas or near joints. Only metallic fragments that are lodged in non-crucial areas can be left permanently within the tissue. The clinical decision to remove an inert object has to be weighed against the potential damage that could be created during a search for the object. If left alone, noncritical inert foreign bodies will encapsulate within soft tissue and cause no further problem. It is preferable to remove glass whenever possi-

247

ble, but small insignificant fragments can be left behind as described above for unimportant metallic objects.

Objects that are not inert, particularly wood and other organic materials like thorns, must be removed in their entirety. These materials can cause a variety of bacterial and fungal infections.[3,21] Synovitis from joint penetration, periosteal reactions, foreign body granulomas, draining fistulas, and pseudotumors of the soft tissue have all been reported with non-inert foreign objects.[1,4,15] Retained wood objects have been reported to cause chronic inflammation, drainage, and pain for up to 7 years following penetration.[4] Therefore, a missed diagnosis or failure to remove all fragments of a non-inert object can lead to prolonged disability and patient discomfort.

The discovery of a foreign object depends on the material, size, and body area location. Very often patients can accurately report the presence of a foreign body sensation. It behooves emergency wound-care personnel to heed these complaints even if the object is not readily visible, palpable, or apparent on x-ray. Metallic objects are the easiest ones to find and localize because they are radiodense to radiographic examination. Glass is also easy to find on radiographs in spite of a common misconception that it needs to be leaded to become radiodense.[22] Studies have shown that glass is visible by radiograph in 88% to 100% of the cases, even glass that is .5 mm in size.[1,7] Xeroradiography has been reported to increase the yield in finding foreign objects like glass, plastic, and thorns.[23] Wood, on the other hand, is elusive to both standard radiographs and xeroradiographs. In a plain radiograph study of foreign objects retained in the hand, wood splinters could be detected no more than 17% of the time.[1] A promising but not thoroughly studied technique to find wood and other non-radio-opaque objects is computerized axial tomography.[20] Another method that has shown variable results is ultrasonography.[16]

Techniques for Removal

Once the diagnosis is made, localizing the foreign body and retrieval is carried out. These steps are often frustrating and attended by unanticipated difficulties. It seems a simple matter to make a small incision and retrieve an object that appears to be close to the surface of the skin. However, simple retrieval is not always possible. For objects that are located below the surface and out of direct sight, careful localization is necessary before proceeding with exploration. Radiodense objects can be localized by a variety of techniques using markers and radiographs. A simple technique recommended by this author is to bend a paper clip to form a flat plane with an extended arm. The extended arm is placed over the skin entry point of the foreign object and the paper clip is secured with a small piece of tape (Fig. 15-1). Two radiographs are taken *exactly* at an angle of 90° to each other (antero-posterior and lateral views) using the plane of the clip as a geometric point of reference (Figs. 15-2 and 15-3). In this manner, both the location and depth of the object relative to

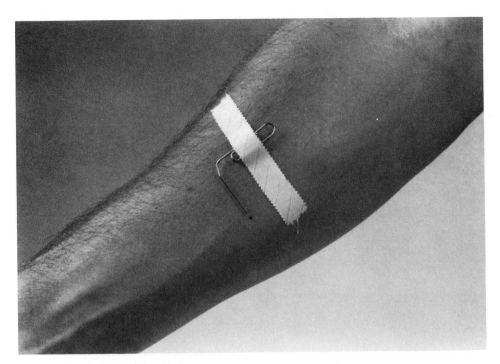

FIG. 15-1 Technique for placing a reconfigured paper clip with the extended arm directly over the entry point of a foreign-body penetration.

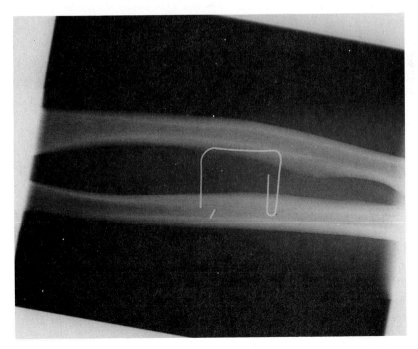

FIG. 15-2 Direct anteroposterior view of the paper clip and foreign body.

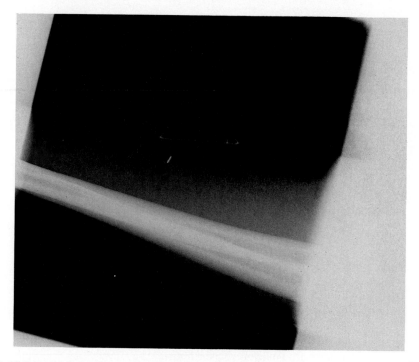

FIG. *15-3* Direct lateral view of the paper clip and foreign body. Note that these two radiographs can be used to locate accurately the position of the foreign body relative to the extended arm by the anteroposterior view and its depth by the lateral view.

the extended arm of the paper clip can be determined. After appropriate cleansing and the administering of an anesthetic, a small incision is made and exploration is carried out until the object can be removed. NOTE: Do not remove the paper clip until just prior to wound preparation and exploration.

Non-radiodense objects are best served by more generous incisions and thorough exploration by direct visualization. Incisions permit debridement and removal of tissue that is embedded with foreign material. Copious irrigation under pressure as described in Chapter 5 will aid in exposing and removing nonradiodense objects.

For objects that are partially protruding from the skin, the temptation to "grab and yank" has to be resisted. If a wood splinter is pulled injudiciously, small fragments can be stripped off the splinter and left behind to cause future difficulty. The technique illustrated in the knuckle area of the finger shown in Fig. 15-4 demonstrates how a small incision is made parallel to the course and angle of the object. By creating a small incision, the splinter can be removed without leaving behind smaller splinters. In addition, the wound can be copiously irrigated to decrease the level of bacterial contamination. It is important to note that these small incisions must not be closed with sutures. They should be left open to drain if necessary and

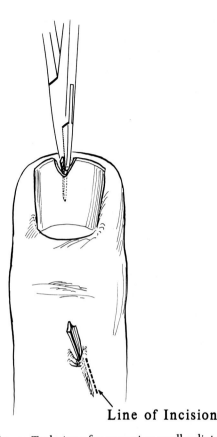

Line of Incision

FIG. 15-4 Top half of figure: Technique for removing small splinter from between the nail plate and nail bed. Note that a small wedge of nail has been removed in order to gain exposure of the protruding of the splinter. A small hemostat is then used to gently extract the splinter. Bottom half of figure: Technique for removing a penetrating foreign body, a splinter, that is protruding from the skin. Note that a small incision is made directly away from the entry point, parallel to the shaft of the foreign body. The splinter can be removed in its entirety without leaving smaller splinters.

prevent the accumulation of purulence that might lead to the formation of an abscess.

A common problem is a splinter or other object that is lodged under a nail plate. If the object can be grasped by a hemostat, then it can be carefully pulled out from under the nail. Again, care has to be taken not to strip fragments off a wooden object. For a splinter that cannot be grasped, removal of a small part of the nail plate in a wedge-shape fashion can be carried out in order to expose the splinter, as shown in the top half of Fig. 15-4. A simple technique for removing small splinters lodged under the nail plate is to bend the tip of a 25- or 27-gauge needle so that a small barb equal in size to the diameter of the needle is created.[5] The shaft of the needle is then introduced adjacent and parallel to the splinter and carried back to the most proximal portion of the object. Then the barb is raked along the splinter and both the needle and the foreign object are pulled out from under the nail. Removing objects from under nails is best carried out when the patient is anesthetized. The anesthetic is usually delivered via a digital block as described in Chapter 5.

Particularly troublesome are cactus spines that can accidentally become embedded in skin in large numbers, usually in children. In a controlled rabbit experiment, Elmer's Glue-All was applied under a single layer of gauze and was allowed to dry. Gentle peeling successfully removed 95% of all spines.[17] The next most effective method was manual removal with tweezers, with a 76% rate of spine removal. Although the glue method has not been reported as having been tested in humans, it is a novel and promising idea.

Occasionally, a foreign body cannot be successfully retrieved by attempts at localization and exploration in a minor wound-care setting. A good rule of thumb is that if exploration with unsuccessful removal exceeds 30 minutes, then the procedure should be discontinued. The most common situation in which this eventuality arises is deep foreign objects of the foot. These foreign bodies are best removed in radiology department suites where image intensifiers and stereotaxic localization can be applied while a consultant explores the affected area.[18,24]

PUNCTURE WOUNDS

Puncture wounds are a very common problem for facilities that treat emergency wound-care problems. The vast majority of these wounds are to the soles of the feet and are caused by stepping on nails.[9,12] Although puncture wounds often appear simple and benign, they are accompanied by a significant incidence of complications. In two large series, the rate of infection and of cellulitis was reported to range from 11% to 15%.[9,12] In a group of pediatric cases, osteomyelitis occurred in 2% of the patients.[9] In this same group, 3.5% of the patients had retained foreign bodies like small pieces of tennis shoe, sock, dirt, grass, etc. Although *Staphylococcus aureus* and *Streptococcus pyogenes* have been implicated in puncture wound infections, *Pseudomonas aeruginosa* has been found to have a particular predilection for this wound environment and is an important cause of puncture wound osteomyelitis.[8,13,14] In a recent study, the anatomic site most likely to become infected is the plantar portion of the foot that extends from the metatarsal necks to the toe creases.[19] There was also a strong correlation with *P. aeruginosa* infection and the use of tennis shoes.[19]

Treatment of Puncture Wounds

Because of the significant incidence of infection and retained foreign bodies, management of puncture wounds has to be thorough. Merely soaking the foot in a soapy solution and applying a dressing will not suffice. Each wound should be carefully inspected for foreign material and early signs of infection. For a better look at the deep tissues, the epidermal edges of the wound can be trimmed back using iris scissors (Fig. 15-5). Using the same scissors, the wound edges are gently spread to explore the subdermal area for foreign material. Following exploration, high-pressure irrigation as described in Chapter 6 is carried out until all debris is removed. A simple Band Aid can then be applied as a dressing.

Prophylactic antibiotics are not recommended for puncture wounds. In the studies previously mentioned, no benefit could be documented when prophylaxis was instituted. In fact, in all cases where osteomyelitis developed, antibiotics had been administered prior to the development of this problem. Patients are instructed to return if any signs of infection develop. If the patient returns with excessive redness, drainage, pain, or swelling, antibiotics, such as dicloxacillin or a first-generation cephalosporin, can be begun at this time. Erythromycin can be started in pen-

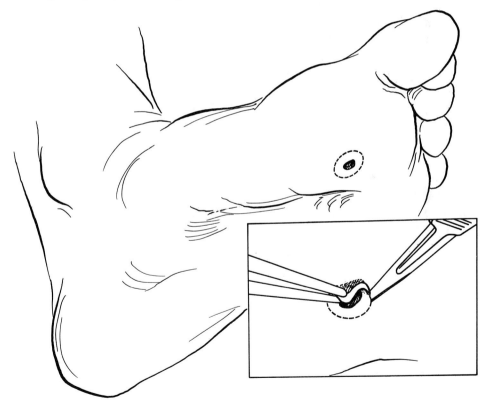

FIG. 15-5 Technique for incising small edge of tissue from puncture wound site to gain better exposure to the puncture wound. In addition, this excision acts as a form of debridement of a small portion of devitalized tissue. (Adapted from Zukin D and Simon R: Emergency wound care: principles and practice, Rockville, Md, 1987, Aspen Publishers Inc, p 116.)

icillin-allergic patients. Ciprofloxacin is useful for penicillin-allergic patients as well and provides coverage against *P. aeruginosa.* Because of the problem of *P. aeruginosa,* all infected wounds are cultured. Antibiotic failure will require hospitalization, further wound care, and consideration for institution of anti-pseudomonal therapy. Because deep puncture wounds of the foot are moderately tetanus-prone, every effort is made to ensure that the patient is current in his tetanus immunization. Proper administration of tetanus toxoid and tetanus immune globulin is described in Chapter 18.

FISHHOOKS

Hooks with small barbs or hooks that are only very superficially embedded can often be backed out through the original site of penetration. Experienced fishermen will make a small incision in the dermis at the entry site and pull the hook out with a needle-nose pliers. Dermis is the most likely layer to resist removal of the hook and barb because of its naturally tough consistency. This extraction procedure can easily be duplicated in an emergency wound-care facility. After basic cleansing with

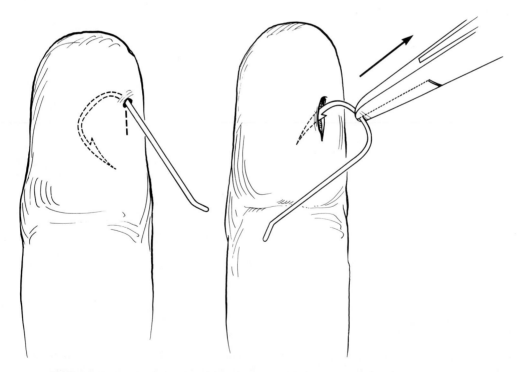

FIG. 15-6 Technique for removing fish hook with small barb. Note that a small incision is made in line with the concavity of the curve of the hook. The needle is then gently backed out through this incision.

an appropriate solution like povidone-iodine, a small amount of anesthetic is injected adjacent to the penetrating shaft. With a #11 or #15 blade, a small incision is made in line with the barb, inside the concave portion of the hook (Fig. 15-6). The portion of the shaft closest to the barb is grasped with a hemostat and the hook is removed with a sharp, rapid pulling motion. The pulling motion is in direct line with that portion of the shaft closest to the barb of the hook.

Another method for removing a hook with small barbs requires the use of some string with good tensile strength like umbilical tape or 0-silk suture (Fig. 15-7). The string is looped around the curved portion of the shaft of the hook and is gently drawn parallel to and in the opposite direction of the straight portion of the shaft. The straight shaft and eyelet portions are depressed against the skin to slightly rotate the barb from its point of attachment in the skin. The string is given a sharp pull to release the hook. Caution is suggested as bystanders might find themselves in the pathway of the hook. This method of hook removal does not require the administration of an anesthetic.

Another removal method is carried out with the use of an 18- or 16-gauge needle. As illustrated in Fig. 15-8 the needle is introduced into the skin through the original wound entry site. It is passed adjacent to the shaft until the hollow portion of the needle point can be placed over the barb. While both are held firmly together, the needle and hook are brought back out through the wound site. The needle effectively sheaths the barb and prevents it from snagging on tissue during removal.

For deeply embedded hooks or those with large barbs, the push-through method is recommended. Trying to back out a deeply penetrated or large barbed hook can

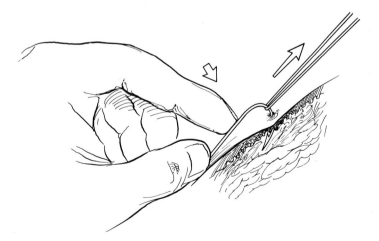

FIG. 15-7 Technique for removing fish hook with small barb by using traction with 0 silk or umbilical tape. Note that pressure is applied to the shaft of the hook towards the skin as a swift "yank" of the cord is applied in the direction opposite the barb. Care is taken to warn bystanders that the fish hook could fly across the room. Place a small piece of adhesive tape around the hook and string might help avoid this hazard.

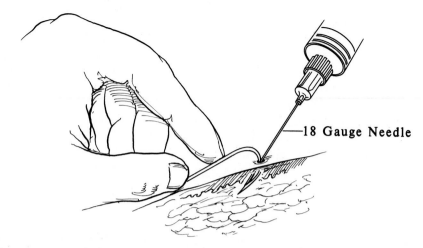

FIG. 15-8 Technique for removing fish hook by placing an 18-gauge needle on the barb of the hook and backing it out through the puncture wound.

cause excessive tissue damage. Basic skin preparation is carried out, and a small amount of local anesthetic is injected at the site through which the hook point is to be extruded. Using a hemostat as a grasping instrument, the hook shaft is manipulated in such a manner so as to push the hook point out through the dermis (Fig. 15-9). The hook is then clipped off with wire cutters and the shaft is backed out of the wound. Occasionally, the string method will work on deeply embedded hooks with small barbs.

Certain anatomic sites deserve separate mention. Hooks embedded in cartilage, most commonly the ear or nose, cannot be successfully backed out. The push-through method is recommended in this setting. Hooks that penetrate into joint capsules are also best removed by the push-through method because barbs can break off in the joint space when backed out. Violation of a joint space can lead to serious complications, therefore consultation is encouraged. Occasionally, fishhooks penetrate the cornea or other part of the globe. This complication constitutes an emergency. No attempt is made to remove the hook in an emergency wound-care area. Ophthalmologic consultation is mandatory. If the patient has to be transferred to another facility for hook removal, he or she should be placed in a semi-recumbent position to decrease eye pressure. Light padding or a metal eyeshield is taped gently over the eye, avoiding any undue contact or pressure on the hook. Pressure-patching with gauze sponges is totally contraindicated in order to avoid extrusion of intra-occular contents through the eye wound.

ABRASIONS

Abrasions are skin wounds caused by tangential trauma to the epidermis and dermis. The skin is forced against a resistant surface in a rubbing or scraping fashion. The resultant injury is roughly analogous to a burn. Varying thicknesses of epider-

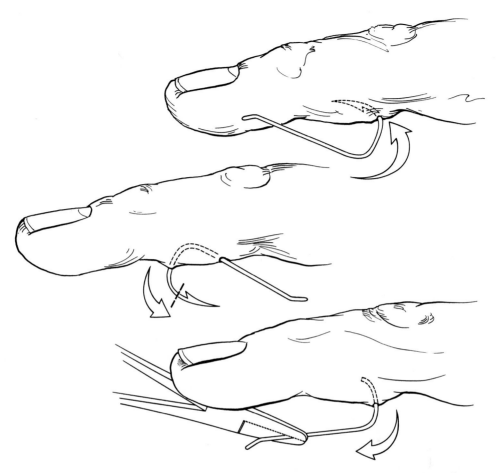

FIG. 15-9 The push-through technique for removing hooks with large barbs or those that are lodged in cartilage or joint spaces. The anesthesic is infiltrated in the area of the hook and the projected exit site. Once the exit has been accomplished, the barb is removed and the shaft is backed out through the original puncture site.

mis and dermis can be lost, including tissue as deep as the superficial fascia and even bone. Abrasions can be very small or can cover large body surface areas. Frequently these injuries are impregnated with dirt, debris, and road tar. The principles for management of these include prevention of infection, promotion of rapid healing, and prevention of "tattooing" from the retained foreign material. This latter problem is of special cosmetic importance because, once the healing process traps unsightly debris in the epidermis and dermis, it cannot easily be removed by later surgical manipulations.

Most abrasions are small and relatively clean. Like burns, however, they are extremely sensitive and painful to touch. Cleansing has to be gentle yet thorough. An appropriate wound-cleansing solution will suffice to remove surface contaminants and to prepare the wound for dressing. Because wound-cleansing solutions like povidone-iodine scrub solution and chlorhexidine contain ionic detergents, excessive pain can be caused during their use. Povidone-iodine solution, without detergent, or Polaxamer 188, as described in Chapter 6, are preferable for cleaning abrasions.

Cleansing of contaminated and debris-laden abrasions can be tedious and difficult. If the abrasion is small, a local anesthetic can be injected around the area in a "field" or circumferential pattern. Once the pain is eliminated, scrubbing with a sponge or soft surgical brush can take place, using an appropriate cleansing solution. If necessary, meticulous removal of all particulate debris can be aided by using a needle, a #11 surgical blade, or a small-jaw tissue forceps.

Large abrasions that are heavily contaminated are difficult to manage in an emergency wound-care area because the volume of local anesthetic necessary to achieve anesthesia would exceed toxic limits. In these cases, parenteral sedation is recommended, and in extreme cases, the patient might be better served in an operating suite.

One of the most common foreign contaminants of abrasions is road tar or asphalt. If permanently impregnated in skin, tar is a cosmetic disaster because of its dark color. All tar or asphalt particles must be removed during initial wound-cleansing and debridement. A cleansing adjunct that is very useful for tar removal is polyoxyethylene sorbitan, a monionic surface-active agent with both hydrophilic and lyophilic properties.[2] It is an emulsifying agent that is virtually nontoxic to tissue. This substance is most commonly available as a component of Neosporin G antibacterial cream. Plain Neosporin or Polysporin ointments, with a petrolatum base, are also helpful in dissolving tar and can be substituted for the cream when it is not available.[6] However, the ointment is not as effective and is not water soluble like the cream. The water-solubility of the cream makes it easy to wash off after it has been applied to the tar-laden abrasion. Another effective commercial tar removal agent is Medi-Sol, a high-purity hydrocarbon that contains limonenes, lanolin, and aloe vera. It is also an adhesive remover.

Once an abrasion is initially cleansed and debrided, follow-up management is usually the patient's responsibility. The abrasion must be kept clean to prevent secondary infection. The abrasion must not be allowed to desiccate, particularly if it is deep or in a cosmetically important area. Wound desiccation has been demonstrated experimentally in humans to retard wound healing and impede epithelial cell covering of the injured surface.[11] For wounds that can be easily covered with a dressing, any non-adherent dressing can be applied over a thin coating of an ointment like Neosporin or Polysporin. There is a bewildering variety of dressing materials available. Adaptic, Telfa, and vaseline gauze are the least expensive. Other options include products such as membrane (Tegaderm), foam (Epilock), and hydrocolloid (Duoderm) dressings. The dressing can be removed every two or three days for gentle cleansing and redressing. Experimentally, topical antibiotic ointments alone have been demonstrated to increase the rate of wound re-epithelialization.[10] Therefore it is recommended that wounds that cannot be easily dressed be kept moist with a thin coating of an antibiotic ointment like Neosporin or Polysporin. The ointment is usually applied three or four times a day to maintain the moist wound environment.

References

1. Anderson M, Newmeyer W, and Kilgore E: Diagnosis and treatment of retained foreign bodies in the hand, Am J Surg 144:63-565, 1982.
2. Bose B and Tredget T: Treatment of hot tar burns, Can Med Assoc J 127:21-22, 1982.
3. Byron T: Foreign bodies found in the foot, J Am Pod Assoc 71:30-35, 1981.
4. Cracchiolo A: Wooden foreign bodies in the foot, Am J Surg 140:585-587, 1980.
5. Davis L: Removal of subungual foreign bodies (letter), J Fam Pract 11:714, 1980.
6. Demling R, Buerstatte W, and Perea A: Management of hot tar burns, J Trauma 20:242, 1980.
7. Feldman AH and Fisher MS: The radiographic detection of glass in soft tissue, Radiology 92:1529-1531, 1969.
8. Fischer MC, Goldsmith JF, and Gilligan PH: Sneakers as a source of *Pseudomonas aeruginosa* in children with osteomyelitis following puncture wounds, J Ped 106:607-614, 1985.
9. Fitzgerald R and Cowan J: Puncture wounds of the foot, Orthop Clin North Am 6:965-972, 1975.
10. Geronemus R, Mertz P, and Eaglestein W: Wound healing: the effects of topical antimicrobial agents, Arch Derm 115:1311-1314, 1979.
11. Hinman C and Maibach H: Effect of air exposure and occlusion on experimental human skin wounds, Nature 200:377-378, 1963.
12. Houston A et al: Tetanus prophylaxis in the treatment of puncture wounds of patients in the deep South, J Trauma 2:439-450, 1962.
13. Jacobs RF, Adelman L, and Sack CM: Management of *Pseudomonas* osteochondritis complicating puncture wounds of the foot, Pediatrics 69:432-435, 1982.
14. Joseph WF and LeFrock JL: Infections complicating puncture wounds of the foot, J Foot Surg 26:S30-S33, 1987.
15. Kahn B: Foreign body (palm thorn) in knee joint, Clin Orthop 135:104-106, 1978.
16. Lammers RL: Soft tissue foreign bodies, Ann Emerg Med 17:1336-1347, 1988.
17. Martinez TT et al: Removal of cactus spines from the skin: a comparative evaluation of several methods, Am J Dis Child 141:1291-1292, 1987.
18. McFadden J: Stereotaxic pinpointing of foreign bodies in the limbs, Ann Surg 175:81-85, 1972.
19. Patzakis MJ et al: Wound site as predictor of complications following deep nail punctures of the foot, West J Med 150:545-547, 1989.
20. Rhoades C et al: Detection of a wooden foreign body in the hand using computed tomography—case report, J Hand Surg 7:306-307, 1982.
21. Rudner E and Mehregan A: Implantation dermatosis, J Cutan Pathol 7:330-331, 1980.
22. Tanberg D: Glass in the hand and foot, JAMA 248:1872-1874, 1982.
23. Tountas C, MacDonald C, and Artman R: Detection of foreign bodies in the hand utilizing xeroradiography, Minn Med 61:296-297, 1978.
24. Wayne R and Carnazzo A: Needle in the foot, Am J Surg 129:599, 1975.

16 *Minor Burns*

Initial Management and General Patient
    Assessment
Burn Assessment
    Cause of the Burn
    Body Location
    Depth of the Burn
    Extent of the Burn
Guidelines for Hospital vs. Non-hospital
    Management of Burn Victims
Treatment of Minor Burns
    Epidermal Burns

Partial-Thickness Burns
    Cleansing
    Debridement
    Burn dressing
    Home management and follow up
Full-Thickness Burns
Chemical Burns
Frostbite
Tetanus and Antibiotic Prophylaxis
References

The treatment of burns is a common activity for facilities and personnel who care for emergency wounds and injuries. A thorough understanding of burns is necessary to properly select those that can be managed appropriately on an outpatient basis and those that need referral for specialized care. The depth, type, and extent of the burn, body location, and underlying patient condition are all important factors in making that decision. Although individual aspects of treatment of minor burns remain somewhat controversial, basic management principles do not vary greatly. The three main principles for treating the patient with burns are: relief of pain, prevention of infection and additional trauma, and minimization of scarring and contracture.[2]

INITIAL MANAGEMENT AND GENERAL PATIENT ASSESSMENT

No matter how small or trivial a burn appears, the patient must be assessed for more severe associated problems and injuries. If the patient sustained the burn at the scene of a fire or explosion, immediate evaluation for inhalation injury, carbon monoxide exposure, and other trauma is mandatory. Inhalation injury is the most common cause of mortality in fire victims.[24] Clinical signs of inhalation injury include burned nasal hairs, soot on the face, hoarseness, cough, shortness of breath, and wheezing. Even if these signs are not present at the outset, inhalation injury must be suspected in patients who were trapped in an enclosed, smoke-filled space. Respiratory tract injury is often delayed and observation of the patient for 24 hours is indicated.[1] Carbon monoxide exposure is suspected in any patient who is alert and has a headache or in a patient with confusion or other alteration of mental status.

Once the patient is initially stabilized, vital signs have been taken, and unnecessary articles of clothing removed from the burned area, attention can be turned to the burn itself. The most salient clinical symptom of minor burns is pain. Epidermal (first-degree) and superficial partial-thickness (superficial second-degree) burns are often extremely painful and require immediate pain relief. The simplest and most rapid manner in which to abolish burn pain is by placing moist, cool towels over the burned area. There is clinical and experimental evidence demonstrating that cooling of burned surfaces can decrease the eventual damage to burned tissues.[4,7,16] The water should not be very cold because excessive cold itself can compound the burn injury. A water temperature of 20° to 25° C appears to be optimal to obtain both pain relief and some measure of protection for burned tissue.[7] Care must be taken to ensure that large burn areas are not covered with cool, moist towels for excessive periods of time because hypothermia can set in. In addition to cool towels and sponges, parenteral pain medicine such as morphine sulfate or meperidine can be used, especially for patients who have a significant component of anxiety associated with their burns.

While the patient is being stabilized and pain relief is being administered, a thorough history is taken. Items of importance in the history include the age of the patient, any associated conditions and illnesses, psychosocial considerations, and drug allergies. Patients under the age of 2 have thin dermises and poorly developed immune systems.[9] These children are rarely treated on an outpatient basis. Likewise, patients over 65 tolerate burns poorly and often need inpatient care. Patients with underlying diseases such as diabetes, pulmonary disease, severe cardiac problems, and disorders requiring chronic immunosuppressive therapy are at higher risk with burns and require special consideration for hospital management.

Frequently, burn victims have significant psychosocial problems. Like automobile trauma victims, burn victims often have alcohol- or drug-related disorders. Although these impairments may have nothing to do with the treatment of the burn itself, a severe alcohol or drug dependency may preclude outpatient management, even for minor burns. The worst psychosocial problem associated with burns is child abuse. Experienced burn-care personnel see this catastrophe all too frequently and tend to think of all children with burns as potential victims of child abuse, until proven otherwise. Finally, during the history, a thorough detailing of allergies is necessary because a large number of drugs can be administered or applied to a burn victim during the course of his or her management.

BURN ASSESSMENT
Cause of the Burn

Knowing the cause of a burn can make a difference in predicting its depth and extent. Brief scalding burns, which occur with the spilling or splashing of hot water, usually result in epidermal or superficial partial-thickness burns. Burns caused by immersion into a hot liquid and flame contact more frequently cause deep partial-thickness or full-thickness burns. These burns can be complicated and serious, especially when important anatomic parts like the hands or face are involved. Electrical burns almost always cause full-thickness injuries at the burn site. In addition, electrical injuries can be associated with muscle necrosis, fractures, and cardiac arrhythmias.[18]

Body Location

The anatomic location of a burn is an important factor in determining management. Because of the complexity and crucial function of the hands, extensive partial-thickness or full-thickness burns on the hands are best managed, at least at the outset, in a controlled setting. Not only do hand burns require careful cleansing, debridement, and dressing, but there is also a danger of joint stiffening secondary to the immobility caused by pain and edema. Patients must observe strict elevation of the burned extremity in addition to early motion exercises to prevent "freezing" of the hand. This complication more frequently occurs in patients over the age of 50. Partial-thickness burns of the face not only raise the possibility of airway obstruction and inhalation injury, but they can be very difficult to manage surgically.

Burns of the perineum are technically difficult to manage and are extremely uncomfortable for the patient. It is beyond the capabilities of most patients or families to care for these problems at home. Among the most frustrating burns to manage on an outpatient basis are those of the foot. The dependent nature of this anatomic part and its weight-bearing function cause frequent failure of outpatient management. It is very difficult for patients to voluntarily maintain the necessary strict elevation of his or her leg, a failure that can lead to edema, pain, and tissue breakdown at the burn site.

Depth of the Burn

Burns are traditionally divided into three depths of tissue injury: epidermal (first-degree burns); partial-thickness (second-degree burns); and full-thickness (third-degree burns). Partial-thickness or second-degree burns are further subdivided into superficial and deep partial-thickness burns.

Epidermal or first-degree burns are the most common type of burns. Heat induces dermal vasodilation, giving the epidermis its characteristic red color. Blistering does not occur and these burns heal without treatment. The superficial epidermis will slough or peel about 5 to 7 days after the burn was sustained and the vasodilation will gradually disappear. Sunburn is the most common example of an epidermal burn. Occasionally, what appears to be an epidermal burn will blister and become a superficial partial-thickness burn 12 to 24 hours after heat exposure if this exposure was especially intense or prolonged.

Partial-thickness or second-degree burns are so designated because the epidermis and part of the dermis are destroyed. However, dermal appendages like pilosebaceous units and eccrine sweat glands survive, giving the skin a chance to regenerate epidermis from these preserved dermal foci. These remaining appendages are crucial to eventual healing and recovery.

Clinically, it is important to distinguish between superficial and deep partial-thickness burns. There are important differences in the time they require to heal and in eventual cosmetic appearance. Superficial partial-thickness burns classically blister and are extremely painful. When the necrotic epidermis is removed, the injured dermis is homogeneously pink and moist in appearance. It is extremely sensitive to touch, but will heal without scarring in a 2- to 3-week period. Deep partial-thickness burns are not as painful to touch and they appear drier and whiter when debrided. Sometimes the surface of these burns is interspersed with reddish spots, indicating underlying dermal plexi. However, there still is some awareness of pinprick and some of the dermal appendages are preserved. These burns take longer than 3 weeks to heal.

With full-thickness or third-degree burns the dermis as well as the dermal appendages have been totally destroyed. A dry, taut, leatherlike surface that is insensitive to examination or pinprick characterizes the appearance of these burn injuries. The color of these burned areas can vary from white to brown to outright black. There is frequent difficulty in distinguishing between deep partial-thickness and full-thickness burns upon initial presentation of a patient to a wound-care facility. Often these two types of burns are treated in the same manner and require grafting for final coverage of the damaged area.

Extent of the Burn

Proper estimation of the extent of body surface area affected is crucial to burn management. Only partial-thickness (second-degree) and full-thickness (third-degree) injuries are considered in the calculation. Epidermal (first-degree) burns are not included. The "rule of nines" is still the most efficacious way to estimate burn size in adults (Fig. 16-1). Surface anatomy can be divided into areas that represent 9% or multiples of 9% of the body surface. The head and each arm constitute a 9% surface area apiece, while one leg is 18%. The entire surface area of the thorax and abdomen combined, anterior and posterior, is 36%.

Greater precision in estimating burn size can be obtained by using standard, more detailed charts that subdivide the anatomic parts. These diagrams also take into account the variations in surface area that occur with age (Fig. 16-2). In young children the surface area of the head constitutes a much greater area relative to the rest of the body than in adults. As an individual grows, the lower extremities get proportionately larger, while the trunk and arms stay relatively the same throughout life. Final surface area proportions are not reached until after the age of 15.

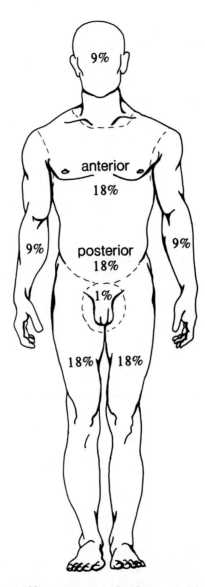

FIG. 16-1 Rapid estimation of burn extent can be determined by the "rule of nines." This rule is illustrated above. Only partial-thickness (second-degree) and full-thickness (third-degree) burns are considered for percentage area determination.

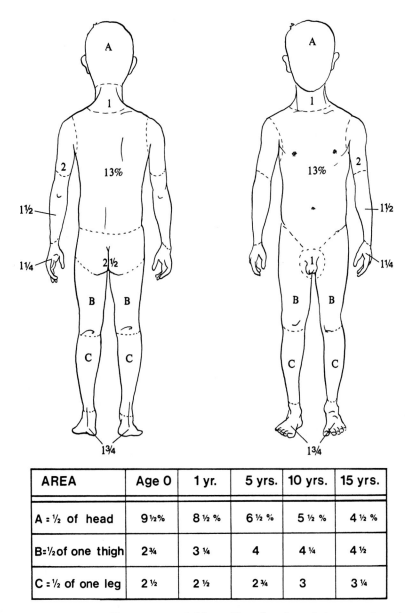

AREA	Age 0	1 yr.	5 yrs.	10 yrs.	15 yrs.
A = ½ of head	9½%	8½ %	6½ %	5 ½ %	4 ½ %
B=½of one thigh	2¾	3 ¼	4	4 ¼	4 ½
C = ½ of one leg	2 ½	2 ½	2 ¾	3	3 ¼

FIG. 16-2 Estimation of burn size in children. Note that the relative area sizes change significantly with age.

GUIDELINES FOR HOSPITAL VS. NON-HOSPITAL MANAGEMENT OF BURN VICTIMS

Table 16-1 lists suggested criteria for hospital management of burns. Patients not meeting these criteria can be considered to be "minor" burn victims and can be treated as outpatients. Different authorities vary on what an appropriate burn size is that can be treated without having to admit the patient to hospital. The total extent of burn limit for outpatient management varies between 10% to 15% of the area that has sustained a superficial-thickness burn.[4,9] The author who advocates 10% burn-surface area as the cut-off point feels that pain relief, initial cleansing, debridement, and patient education are best accomplished in a controlled patient setting. Highly motivated, responsible adults with good family support systems probably can do well on an outpatient basis with burns approaching the 15% range.

Children are best managed on an inpatient basis with any partial-thickness burn that is greater than 10%. Again, pain relief, wound cleansing, debridement, and dressings are easier to manage in the hands of experienced personnel. After the traumatized parents are brought under control, they can be properly educated in the care of the burn before the child is discharged. Except for the most trivial burn, children under 2 years of age should all be managed in-house. On the other end of the age scale, it is recommended that patients over the age of 65 be considered for similar treatment.

As previously discussed, burns in crucial anatomic locations such as the hands, feet, face, and perineum are best managed in an inpatient setting. Full-thickness burns of greater than 3% of the body surface area will require surgical management and grafting. Even smaller full-thickness burns, if initially treated out of hospital, need to be referred to a specialist for continued management and possible later skin grafting.

If there is any suspicion of inhalation or airway injury, no matter how small or superficial the burn, the patient must be admitted for observation. Inhalation injury can be insidious, and overt signs and symptoms often will not appear for several

---

Table 16-1 *Guidelines for Hospital Admission of Burn Victims*

Partial-thickness burns >15% surface area (>10% surface area of child)
Full-thickness burns >3% surface area
Suspected inhalation injury
Age <2 or >65
Partial- or full-thickness burns of hands, face, perineum, or feet
Electrical burns
Severe underlying systemic disease
Acute alcohol or drug abuse
Suspected child abuse

hours post-exposure.[1] Finally, the decision to treat patients in the hospital is often determined by the extent of underlying disease, alcohol or drug abuse, and suspicion of potential child abuse.

TREATMENT OF MINOR BURNS

The large majority of burns that is treated on an outpatient basis are epidermal or superficial partial-thickness burns. Because these burns tend to have an overwhelmingly favorable outcome irrespective of treatment, some of the controversies over management are not crucial. However, for the sake of completeness, these controversies will be mentioned in context with each management step.

Epidermal Burns

Epidermal or first-degree burns usually are called to the attention of medical care personnel only if the burns are extensive or very painful. A gentle cleansing with a non-irritating soap such as Ivory Flakes or Dreft soap mixed in a solution of cool saline (20° to 25° C) is recommended. Diluted (with 2 to 4 parts cool saline) chlorhexidine (Hibiclens) can also be used.[2] For home symptom relief, the patient can apply any number of commercial preparations containing at least 60% of aloe vera. Not only does this compound have some antimicrobial activity, but it affords local pain relief as well.[9] Analgesia can be supplemented with aspirin, ibuprofen, acetaminophen, or codeine for up to 48 to 72 hours, after which the acute pain eventually subsides.

These burns usually heal within 5 to 7 days after going through epidermal desquamation. Occasionally, epidermal burns convert to superficial-thickness injuries with blistering 12 to 24 hours after heat exposure. Should this occur, returning to a medical-care facility or contacting the primary-care physician is recommended.

Partial-Thickness Burns
Cleansing

Partial-thickness burns are also best managed by an initial cleansing with a nonirritating soap or with chlorhexidine (Hibiclens) diluted in 2 to 4 parts of cool saline. Ice chips can be mixed into the solution to provide a cooling effect. Hair can be clipped but should not be shaved with a razor in the burn site in order to prevent any further damage to the remaining dermal appendages from which new epidermis will arise. In order to effectively clean and debride a partial-thickness burn, which is extremely sensitive to touch or manipulation, a parenteral narcotic is often recommended for the patient.

Debridement

Once cleansing has taken place, the next step is debridement. Obviously necrotic and partially sloughed epidermis and dermis is removed by using forceps and tissue scissors. This skin is dead and insensitive. Therefore local anesthetics are not required. A major controversy in burn management is whether to remove intact blisters. Proponents for blister removal point to the ideal culture media that blister fluid represents with a concomitant risk of burn infection.[9] There is clinical and experimental evidence, however, that leaving blisters intact has several beneficial effects on burn wounds.[13,14,26] Intact blisters tend to prevent capillary stasis and retard necrosis within burn injury sites as well as decrease desiccation of the burn wound. It is also believed that retention of blisters aids in the control of pain, a benefit that is especially important over joint surfaces where pain can limit active movement, thereby leading to potential joint stiffness.[22] As a general rule, large confluent blisters are likely to break easily and should be removed. Small intact blisters on the hands, feet, and over joints should be left intact. It can be argued that blisters on noncompliant patients should be removed to prevent infection from neglect or improper home care.

Burn Dressing

Preferences for burn dressings vary widely among practitioners who care for minor burns. Topical agents recommended range from no agent at all to a variety of topical antibiotics as well as several newer synthetic wound coverings.[2,6,9,20] Because the eventual outcome of limited-area superficial partial-thickness burns is uniformly good, no clear preference for one agent or dressing can be made over another. Another controversial choice that practitioners have to make is whether to keep burns completely open, without an occlusive dressing or to keep the wound occluded until healing takes place.[26] Additionally, there is some divergence of opinion as to whether dressings should be changed at least daily or left in place for several days at a time before removal.[13-15]

It is this author's opinion that superficial partial-thickness wounds do well with a topical antimicrobial agent and the application of an occlusive dressing. The Burn Treatment Center at the University of Cincinnati recommends that the ointment be reapplied twice a day after gentle cleaning by the patient and a new gauze occlusive wrap be applied after each cleaning over a layer of a topical antimicrobial agent. Silvadene is currently the agent of choice in most burn centers.[4] Bacitracin and Neosporin are good alternatives and are preferred by the Burn Treatment Center. In an experimental comparison with other petrolatum-based topical agents, wound healing was faster and bacterial colonization was more effectively retarded by Neosporin.[10] Petrolatum ointments are easier to apply and avoid exposing potentially allergic patients to sulfa.

Specifically, once the burn wound is cleaned and debrided, the ointment is applied directly to the affected area in a thin layer (2 to 4 mm thick for Silvadene) by using either a sterile tongue depressor or a gloved finger. The topical agent is then covered with a non-adherent mesh like Adaptic (Fig. 16-3). Gauze sponges made into fluffs followed by gauze wrapping complete the dressing.

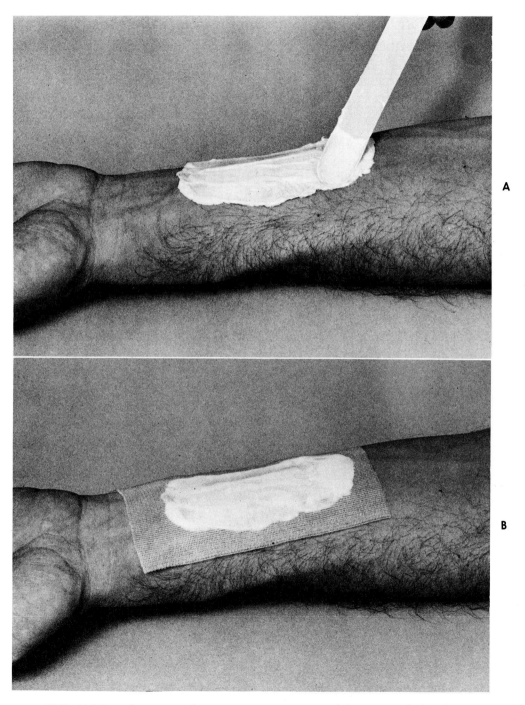

FIG. 16-3 Burn dressing application. **A,** Burn ointment of choice is applied with a sterile blade. **B,** A non-adherent dressing material is placed directly over the cream.

Continued.

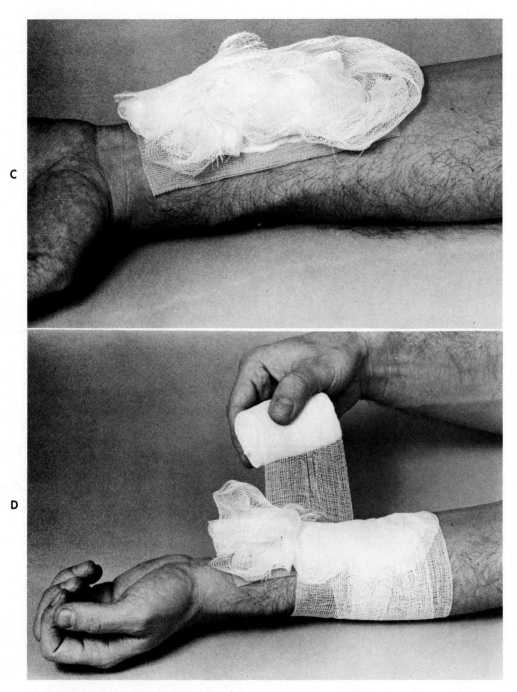

FIG. 16-3, cont'd **C,** Gauze sponges or gauze "fluffs" are placed over the non-adherent base. **D,** Gauze wrapping completes the dressing.

In the interest of thoroughness, other topical agents and dressing alternatives are mentioned here. Simple petrolatum-impregnated gauze has been widely used, but some authors believe that it macerates wounds.[15] Mafenide (Sulfamylon) is no longer recommended for minor burns because it is painful and causes excessive drying. There is hesitation to use gentamicin ointment for fear of causing the emergence of gentamicin-resistant *Pseudomonas* species organisms.[17] Other agents used to varying degrees are furacin, povidone-iodine, and scarlet red. Experience in minor human burns with newer wound coverings like Tegaderm, Hydron gel, and Vigilon wound coverings is less extensive than with older methods. The chief advantage of Hydron gel is that it affords good pain relief; however, it was found in two studies to be time-consuming and difficult to apply and the Hydron dressing peeled and cracked inappropriately as it dried over the wound.[6,25]

The only recommended open or nonocclusive treatment is for minor facial burns. The face is difficult to dress appropriately and heals well without wound coverings. Twice-a-day cleansing is recommended, as with other burns, followed by an application of petrolatum-based antibacterial ointment like Bacitracin or Neosporin. The consistency of silver sulfadiazine and the necessity to apply it in a layer that is several millimeters thick makes it difficult to use on the face. The patient is encouraged to sleep with his or her head elevated at night to decrease unwanted edema at the burn site.

Home Management and Follow Up

Burn supplies, including gauze sponges, gauze wrap, antibacterial soap, and a sterile tongue depressor are dispensed or prescribed along with written and verbal instructions on how to use them. A small jar or tube of topical agent is also dispensed or prescribed. The patient is instructed to remove the first dressing the morning after his or her first wound-care visit. The burned area is gently washed with the soap and two or three of the sterile sponges provided. A topical agent is spread over the wound and gauze wrapping is applied. This process is repeated once or twice daily. Some authorities believe that the first dressing can remain in place for 2 or 3 days. At the University of Cincinnati it is believed that once- or twice-a-day changes prevent the exudate build-up and crusting that can disrupt epitheliazation when infrequent dressing changes are made. Again, there is no clear evidence to support any specific dressing change interval for minor burns.

All minor burn victims are seen in follow up 48 hours after initial treatment. From that time on, individualized treatment regimens are prescribed. Strict elevation of the burned part is essential to proper healing. The use of slings for upper-extremity and hand burns can accomplish this goal while the patient is in an upright position. Gentle but frequent motion of joints within the burn-injured anatomic parts is also mandatory. Pain will often deter a patient from this activity, so appropriate oral medication like aspirin, ibuprofen, acetaminophen, or codeine may be required early during convalescence. Usually, however, if the patient thoroughly understands the need for joint motion, cooperation with burn-care personnel quickly follows in spite of some wound discomfort.

Full-Thickness Burns

Full-thickness burns that cover less than 3% of the body surface area and that are in a noncritical site (hand or face) can be treated in the manner described above for partial-thickness burns. However, before proceeding it is best to discuss the case with a consultant. These patients require close follow-up care and initial treatment decisions are best made in concert with a consultant.

Chemical Burns

There are approximately 25,000 chemicals that are capable of causing burns.[5] The most common classes of chemicals are the corrosives (acids and alkalis). Sulfuric acid and sodium hydroxide are, by far, the most common offenders.[12] Another common alkali is powdered concrete that contains either lime (calcium oxide) or cement (various metal oxides). The pathophysiology of chemical injury to the skin is capillary dilatation, inflammation, blistering, or tissue loss. Chemical burns can be classified like thermal burns in terms of depth and extent. An important difference from thermal burns is that chemical burns (usually caused by alkalis) can continue to cause damage up to 36 hours after exposure.[2,21] This fact has implications in treatment and follow-up.

There is no question that the most important treatment for chemical burns is copious irrigation immediately after exposure. Delay in irrigation, by as little as three minutes, can significantly worsen the burn.[8] Therefore, first-aid measures in the workplace or home are the most important therapeutic measures. In the emergency department, copious saline irrigation (at least 1 to 2 liters) is continued or instituted for all chemical exposures. Special care is taken to thoroughly irrigate alkali burns and, occasionally irrigation with several liters of saline in conjunction with wound cleansing is necessary. Chlorhexidine or povidone-iodine can be used as cleansing agents. There are exceptions to immediate irrigation. Elemental (metal) lithium and sodium can cause a reaction when exposed to water and should be covered with mineral oil before cleansing. Phenol can be inadvertently spread with water and should be covered with glycerol before cleansing is started.

After irrigation of a chemical burn, the patient is treated according to the guidelines and recommendations for thermal burns. Admission criteria to the hospital are similar to those for thermal burns, as are guidelines for local wound care and dressings. The most important difference is that all except the most trivial chemical burns should be reassessed within 24 hours. The delayed effect of alkalis, in particular, has to be monitored and treated appropriately.

A chemical that deserves special mention is hydrofluoric acid. This chemical is a strong acid that causes extreme local pain. If the skin is not obviously affected (no erythema, blistering, tissue loss) copious irrigation is followed by placing a bulky dressing that is soaked in the antidote calcium gluconate or calcium chloride. These chemicals inactivate the acid by forming calcium fluoride. If there is skin involvement and severe local pain, 0.5 mL of calcium gluconate (10% solution) per square centimeter of skin involved is injected into the subcutaneous layer. In areas like the fingertips, injection might not be feasible, so the calcium gluconate can be mixed with lubricant jelly and applied to the affected fingers. Hydrofluoric-acid burns are best managed with the cooperation of a consultant, particularly for follow-up care.

Frostbite

Frostbite is the result of the exposure of unprotected skin to temperatures that are below freezing. Extracellular tissue ice-crystal formation can lead to cellular membrane destruction and cell death.[11] Microthrombosis has been observed as well. Frostnip is a skin response that precedes actual tissue damage. The patient complains of cold and pain in the affected area. The skin is blanched and numb. Immediate rewarming with water at 38° to 41° C for at least twenty minutes can prevent progression to actual frostbite.

Frostbite is recognized by the continued pale, cool, gray, and bloodless appearance of the affected skin in spite of rewarming. In 24 to 48 hours blisters can appear. Other than rewarming the affected part, little can be done to fully assess or treat frostbite in the initial visit to the emergency department. Blisters, if present, are left intact. The skin is gently cleaned with diluted chlorhexidine. Aggressive emergency-department debridement is not carried out because true demarcation of necrotic and viable tissue may not be evident for 30 to 90 days. Dressings and slings are fashioned to gently cradle affected extremities rather than to occlude tissue. Digits are separated with gauze. Only open, obviously nonviable and nonprotective blister skin is removed and covered with an occlusive non-adherent dressing material (Adaptic) and an ointment such as Neosporin. The remainder of the injured area is left open. At home, strict elevation of the affected area is observed. A consultant is involved early in the care of the patient.

Tetanus and Antibiotic Prophylaxis

Finally, there are the considerations of tetanus prophylaxis and the possibility of wound infection. Tetanus toxoid and tetanus immune globulin should be given to all burn wounds in accordance with the recommendations in Chapter 18. Currently, there are no studies that support the use of prophylactic oral or parenteral antibiotics in the minor superficial burn setting.[3,14,23] Control- and antibiotic-treated groups consistently yield the same infection rate of approximately 3% to 4%. Should a burn-wound infection develop, it is best managed with local wound care and appropriate antibiotics at that time.

References

1. Achauer B et al: Pulmonary complications of burns, Ann Surg 177:311-319, 1973.
2. Baxter CR and Waeckerle JF: Emergency treatment of burn injury, Ann Emerg Med 17:1305-1315, 1988.
3. Boss WK et al: Effectiveness of prophylactic antibiotics in the outpatient treatment of burns, J Trauma 25:224-227, 1985.
4. Cone JB: Minor burns: standards for outpatient treatment, Consultant 27:37-42, 1987.
5. Cupreal WR et al: Treatment of chemical burns: specialized diagnostic, therapeutic and prognostic implications, J Trauma 10:634-638, 1970.
6. Curreri W et al: Safety and efficacy of a new synthetic burn dressing, Arch Surg 115:925-927, 1980.
7. Davies J: Prompt cooling of burned areas: a review of benefits and the effector mechanisms, Burns 9:1-6, 1983.
8. Gruber RP, Laub DR, and Vistness LM: The effect of hydrotherapy on the clinical course and pH of experimental cutaneous chemical burns, Plast Reconstr Surg 55:200-203, 1975.
9. Heimbach D, Engrav L, and Marvin J: Minor burns, Postgrad Med 69:22-32, 1981.
10. Leyden JJ et al: Comparison of antibiotic ointments, a wound protectant, and antiseptics for the treatment of human blister wounds contaminated with *Staphylococcus aureus*, J Fam Pract 24:601-604, 1987.
11. McCauley RL et al: Frostbite injuries: a rational approach based on histopathology, J Trauma 23:143-147, 1983.
12. Moran KD, O'Reilly T, and Munster AM: Chemical burns: a ten-year experience, Am Surg 53:652-653, 1987.
13. Moserova J, Runtova M, and Broz L: The possible role of blisters in dermal burns, Acta Chirurgiae Plast 25:51-53, 1983.
14. Moylan J: Outpatient treatment of burns, Postgrad Med 73:235-242, 1983.
15. Ollstein R: Burn injury, Qual Rev Bull 5:9-11, 1979.
16. Pushkar N and Sandorminsky B: Cold treatment of burns, Burns 9:101-110, 1983.
17. Richards R and Mahlangu G: Therapy for burn wound infection, J Clin Hosp Pharm 6:223-243, 1981.
18. Sances A et al: Electrical injuries, Surg Gynecol Obstet 149:97-108, 1979.
19. Saranto J, Rubayi S, and Zawacki B: Blisters, cooling, antithromboxanes, and healing in experimental zone-of-stasis burns, J Trauma 23:927-933, 1983.
20. Shuck J: Outpatient management of the burned patient, Surg Clin North Am 58:108-117, 1978.
21. Steele RH and Wilhelm DL: The inflammatory reaction in induced superficial injury. III. Leukocytosis and other histologic changes, Br J Pathol 51:265-266, 1970.
22. Swain AH et al: Management of blisters in burns, Br Med J 295:181, 1987.
23. Timmons M: Are systemic prophylactic antibiotics necessary for burns? Ann Royal Coll Surgeons (Engl) 65:80-81, 1983.
24. Trunkey D: Inhalation injury, Surg Clin North Am 58:1133-1140, 1978.
25. Warren R and Snelling C: Clinical evaluation of the Hydron gel burn dressing, Plast Reconstr Surg 66:361-368, 1980.
26. Zawacki B: Reversal of capillary stasis and prevention of necrosis in burns, Ann Surg 180:98-102, 1974.

17 *Wound Dressing and Bandaging Techniques*

Wound Dressing Principles
    Tidiness
    Non-adherent, porous base
    Moist environment
    Protection
    Partial immobilization
Basic Wound Dressing
    Dressing Application
Home Care and Dressing Change Intervals
Body Area Dressings
    Scalp Dressings

Face Dressings
Ear or Mastoid Dressings
Neck Dressings
Shoulder Dressings
Truncal Dressings
Groin, Hip, and Upper Thigh Dressings
Hand and Finger Dressings
Elbow and Knee Dressings
Ankle, Heel, and Foot Dressings
References

The choice of a dressing for emergency wounds is very much subject to the preference of the person who applies it. There are no hard and fast rules that can be followed when selecting a dressing. What follows is a discussion of the general principles of wound dressing and some recommendations for dressing and bandaging depending on the type of wound, body location, and other factors. A discussion of specialized dressings for burns is found in Chapter 16.

WOUND DRESSING PRINCIPLES

The first decision to be made after repairing a wound is whether to apply a dressing at all. Uncomplicated lacerations of the face and scalp are often left open. The head and face are very vascular, and wounds in these areas are very resistant to infection. If the patient is careful and keeps the wound clean, a sutured laceration will heal without trouble. These wounds merely need the regular application of a petrolatum based antibacterial ointment to maintain a moist environment and help prevent crusting that can interfere with suture removal.[12] Neosporin and Silvadene have been shown experimentally to be agents that effectively encourage epithelialization when compared to other ointments such as Furacin and Pharmadine, which contains povidone-iodine.[3] Neosporin is easier to apply to the face than Silvadene, which needs to be laid down in a relatively thick layer.

The generally accepted practice for wounds and lacerations that are not on the head and face is to apply a wound covering, although there is little evidence that a dressing improves the eventual outcome of sutured lacerations. One study of un-covered wounds that were sutured post-operatively could not document an increase in the rate of infection when compared to dressed incisions.[5] When the decision is made to apply a dressing, the following principles should be observed.

Tidiness

A dressing must be neat and uncomplicated. Sloppy or poorly applied dressings and bandages do not convince a patient that good wound care has been delivered. A great number of small wounds will be best served by a simple Band-Aid or two. This dressing remains one of the most versatile and appropriate wound coverings yet devised.

Non-adherent, Porous Base

The base of a dressing, which is the portion that comes into direct contact with the wound surface, cannot be adherent.[7] Plain, fine-mesh gauze is an example of a dressing that sticks to wounds by becoming incorporated in the coagulum. When it is removed, it can disrupt healing by disturbing the delicate epithelial covering. A good wound covering also has to allow for the passage of exudate so that excessive accumulation does not occur.

Moist Environment

At the same time, the wound has to remain moist. Experimental studies convinc-ingly show that desiccation by exposure can significantly delay epithelial layer for-mation.[4,7] Fig. 17-1 illustrates the pathways for epidermal healing in moist and dry environments. In a non-occluded wound, epithelial cells are forced to find a path-way beneath dry coagulum/exudate and dermal remnants.

In practice, synthetic dressings like Adaptic, Xeroform, and Telfa are traditional non-adherent, porous coverings that allow for the drainage of exudate, but do not permit excessive desiccation.

A point of controversy that has yet to be resolved is whether the application of antibacterial creams or ointments under dressings has any value.[6] Claims against the use of these agents include excessive maceration of tissue and the emergence of resistant bacteria.[1,10] Suppression of infection and improved wound-edge healing, particularly for flaps, are reasons given in support of the use of topicals.[3,8] Cur-rently, these agents are recommended for facial wounds (lacerations, abrasions, burns) or any other wound that will be treated without dressing and bandaging. These agents can be considered optional for wounds that will be dressed.

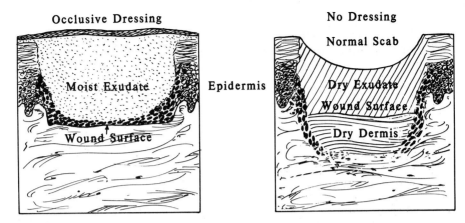

FIG. 17-1 Note the different pathways necessary for epithelial cells to migrate in order to provide an epithelial cell covering of an open wound. The moist environment experimentally appears to provide for more rapid healing than a dry environment as seen in open, uncovered wounds.

Protection

Protection from contamination is best accomplished by ensuring that in addition to the non-adherent base, the wound is also well covered with gauze sponge material and an appropriate gauze wrap. Gauze sponges help meet this requirement of wound dressing. Most minor wounds and lacerations produce very little exudate; therefore, a simple 2 × 2 or 4 × 4 gauze sponge or even a Band-Aid will suffice for this purpose. Complicated or contaminated wounds with a potential for infection are likely to exude freely and copiously. In addition to several layers of gauze sponges, frequent dressing changes are often necessary.

Partial Immobilization

Finally, dressings should protect the healing wound as well as provide partial immobilization of the injured part. Any number of forces can disrupt a suture line, ranging from clothing contact to accidental minor trauma to the wound. Gauze sponges in combination with gauze wrapping will suffice for the purpose of protection. Occasionally, rigid splinting, particularly for lacerations over joints, is necessary. In general, however, excessive wrapping should be avoided to prevent complete immobilization of a moving anatomic part, particularly the hand. Although rest for the injury is necessary, some movement is encouraged within the bandage. The goal is to prevent the stiffening of joints that can occur, especially in elderly patients.

Young children present a particularly difficult challenge in wound dressing. Fortunately, their wounds heal rapidly and, in practice, seem to be quite resistant to infection. Again, the principle of simplicity is important. A Band-Aid, when it can be appropriately used, is the dressing of choice for small wounds. If the Band-Aid is removed by the child, it can easily be replaced by a parent. Children are more likely to leave band-aids in place because this dressing is recognized as a "badge" for other children to appreciate. When more complicated dressings have to be used, as on the hand, a "mittenlike" bandage that encompasses the entire hand is often recommended. If the laceration or wound is serious, most older children seem to have an instinctive understanding that prevents them from removing dressings.

BASIC WOUND DRESSING

The basic wound covering consists of four materials: a non-adherent base, absorbant gauze sponges, gauze wrapping if needed, and tape to secure the dressing. Standard non-adherent bases include Adaptic (a porous synthetic mesh), Telfa, and Xeroform (a treated fine-mesh gauze).

Recent developments in the manufacture of dressings have produced several semi-permeable, occlusive, non-adherent wound dressings that have been applied to lacerations, burns, and abrasions.[9] In a study of a modified polyurethane foam on those three types of wounds, it was found that wounds tended to heal faster, were less painful, and were easier to care for when compared to standard dressing controls.[13] Although this was potentially encouraging, the investigators terminated their comparison after only 20 days of observation. Final healing outcome may have been no different. Other parameters that remain to be fully explored before these new dressings can be routinely recommended for general use include bacterial growth potential at the wound site and effect on wound tensile strength.[2,7] There are conflicting data concerning possible adverse effects in these two areas. Some of these dressing materials are also considerably more expensive than older, standard materials.[13]

Dressing Application

After repair, an antibacterial ointment can be thinly and gently spread over the wound. Based on the preceding discussion, application of a topical agent for sutured lacerations can be considered optional. If one is chosen, Neosporin is recommended. For patients sensitive to Neosporin, Silvadene or Polysporin can be substituted. Although sensitivity to neomycin (a component of Neosporin) is a concern, an actual allergic response to patch testing is very low. Of a total of 3,333 patients reported in a review of topical agents, only 14 or .3% were found to be sensitive to neomycin.[8] Patients allergic to sulfa cannot be given Silvadene.

In a sterile fashion, the non-adherent base is cut to conform with the general wound area as shown in Fig. 17-2, A through D. Depending on the potential for wound drainage and exudation, one or more gauze sponges are placed over the

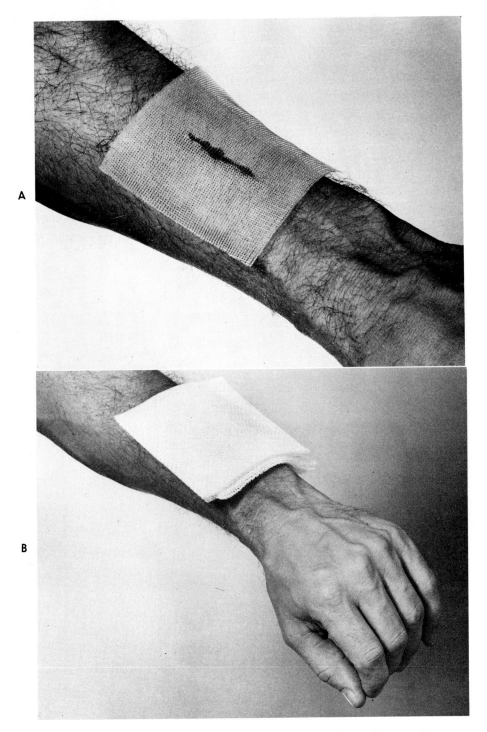

FIG. 17-2 Basic components of a wound dressing. **A,** A nonadherent base. **B,** Gauze sponge covering.

Continued.

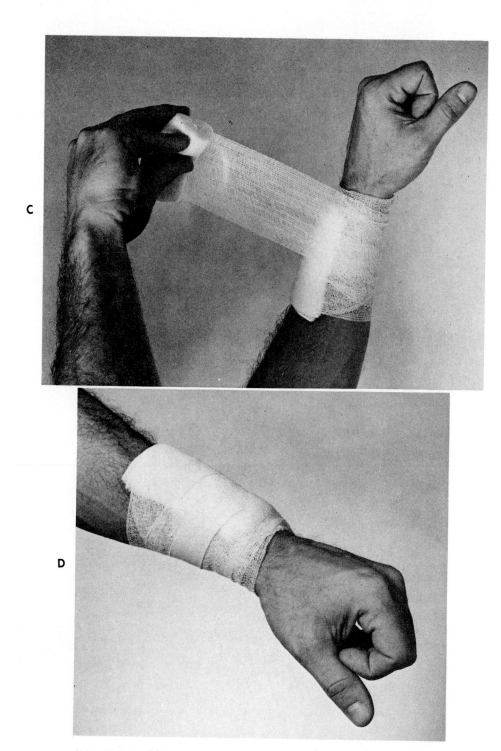

FIG. 17-2, cont'd **C**, Gauze wrap. **D**, Tape application to secure dressing.

base. On an extremity, a gauze wrap is applied, followed by tape. On flat surfaces where gauze wrapping is not appropriate, the tape is placed directly over the gauze sponges.

A common tape adhesive adjunct is tincture of benzoin. This substance is very effective in keeping tape adherent to the skin for the duration of the dressing. Precautions have to be taken, however, not to spill benzoin directly into the wound. Under experimental conditions, this compound has been shown to increase the potential for wound infection when it comes into direct contact with the raw wound surface.[11]

One of the most important precautions in dressing and bandaging is never to wrap tape circumferentially around an extremity or digit (Fig. 17-3). Tape, if brought around the finger or wrist to adhere to itself, becomes a non-expanding band that causes a tourniquet effect upon the vascular blood supply to the distal regions of a hand or finger. Pressure builds up as congestion and edema develop. In fact, this pressure can cause complete cessation of blood flow with attendant ischemic necrosis of the anatomic part. This is one of the worst potential complications of wound care.

HOME CARE AND DRESSING CHANGE INTERVALS

Recommendations are discussed in detail in Chapter 18.

BODY AREA DRESSINGS
Scalp Dressings

Most simple sutured lacerations of the scalp can be left open to the air. A small amount of blood coagulum will quickly develop along the suture line and act as a wound covering. Because the scalp is very vascular, however, and tends to bleed profusely when injured, occasionally there is a need to apply a bulkier dressing to the area after repair. Fig. 17-4, *A* through *F*, demonstrate the basic bandage and the method to continue that wrapping as a recurrent dressing for wounds closer to the crown. An important point to remember is that the initial gauze wrap should include the greatest diameter of the skull in order to prevent inadvertent slippage. The forehead just above the brow and the external occipital protuberance are the landmarks that are the center points for the wrap. Otherwise, the dressing will slip over the crown and fall off.

This dressing can often be supplemented by gently applied elastic wrap for 24 hours. The elastic wrap is then removed, leaving the basic bandage intact. Great care must be taken when applying a scalp dressing, particularly with an elastic support, not to cause excessive pressure on the ears. Whenever possible, the ears should be brought out from underneath the bandage to prevent the complication of an ischemic necrosis of the skin of the ear or of the cartilage skeleton.

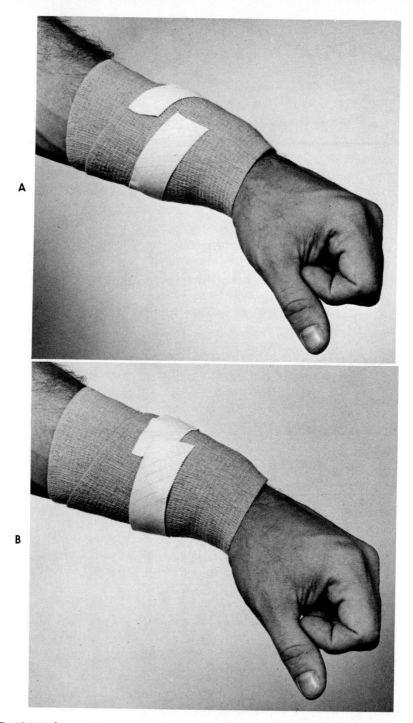

FIG. *17-3* Technique for correct taping of a bandage. **A,** Correct: tape does not overlap if it surrounds a extremity. **B,** Incorrect: overlapping tape can cause unwanted constriction and distal edema.

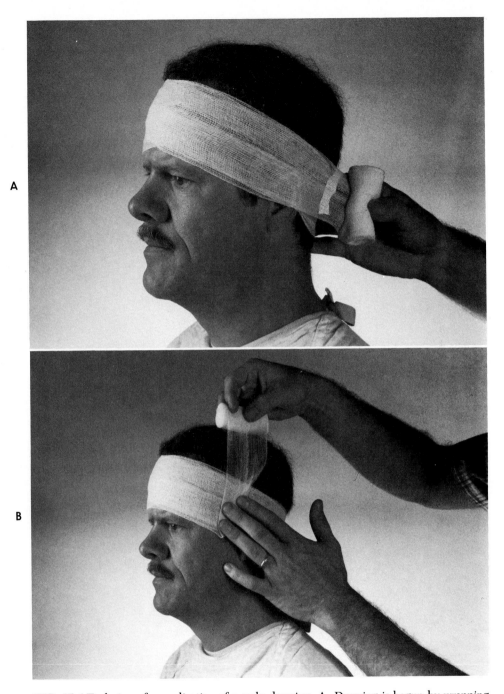

FIG. 17-4 Technique for application of a scalp dressing. **A,** Dressing is begun by wrapping gauze around the mid-forehead and directly over the occipital protuberance. This beginning allows for stabilization of the scalp dressing. Attempts to wrap the dressing higher on the scalp will lead to inevitable loosening of the dressing. **B,** If a recurrent portion of the dressing is necessary in order to cover lacerations or wounds on the top of the head, or vertex, the recurrent portion is begun as illustrated.

Continued.

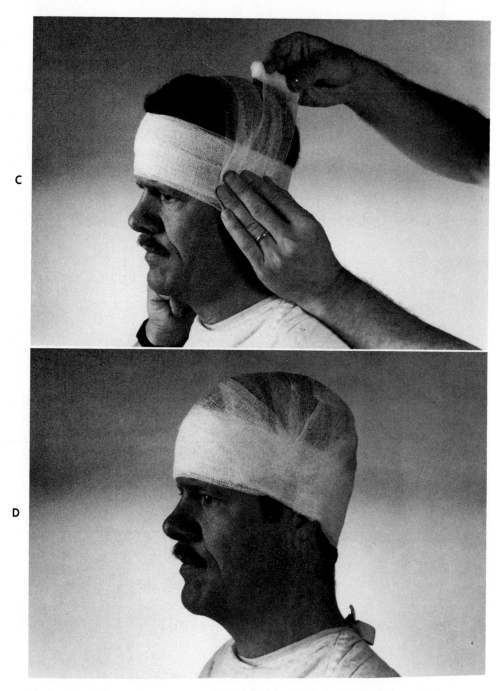

FIG. 17-4, *cont'd* C, The recurrent portion is brought back and forth over the area of concern. **D,** The recurrent portion is then anchored by continued circumferential wrapping of the gauze around the forehead and external occipital protuberance.

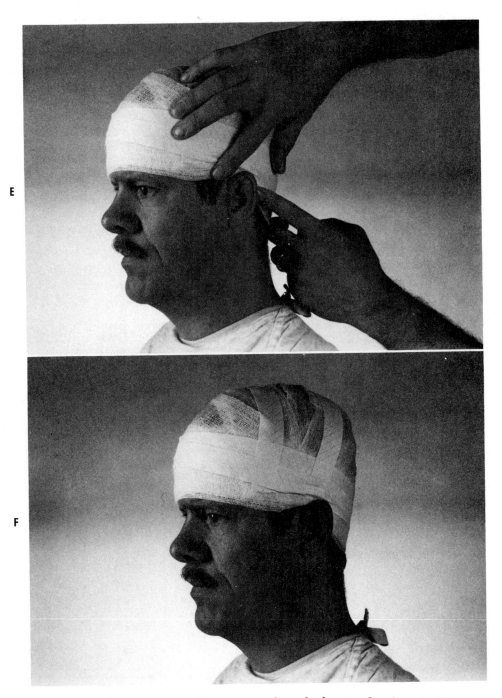

FIG. 17-4, cont'd E, Tape is applied to secure the scalp dressing. It is important to remove the ears from underneath the circumferential portion of the dressing in order to avoid ischemia of the ear skeleton. **F,** View of a completed recurrent scalp dressing.

Face Dressings

As mentioned previously, facial lacerations can be left uncovered following repair. Small, uncomplicated lacerations of the ear, eyelid, nose, and lip are included in this recommendation. A very thin film of an antibacterial ointment like Neosporin can be applied daily by the patient. The antibiotic nature of this ointment is of questionable value at best, but the ointment base is useful in preventing the crusting of coagulum around the wound. By preventing crusting, sutures are much more easily removed with minimal wound disruption. When a facial wound needs covering to protect it from the environment, Band-Aids are recommended. Bulky bandages of the face are poorly tolerated by patients and tend to come off quickly.

Ear or Mastoid Dressings

Complicated ear injuries that are at risk for forming perichondral hematomas require a more involved dressing that applies pressure evenly over all of the contours of the ear. One or two 4 × 4 gauze sponges are cut in the contoured fashion shown in steps A through G of Fig. 17-5. They are placed around and behind the ear to

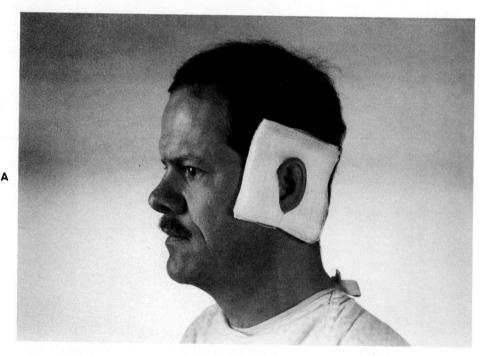

A

FIG. 17-5 Technique for application of a mastoid dressing. **A,** With bandage scissors, cut a center portion out of two or three 4 × 4 gauze sponges so that they fit behind the cartilaginous skeleton of the ear. It is important that the cartilaginous skeleton is well supported and not "crushed" against the scalp.

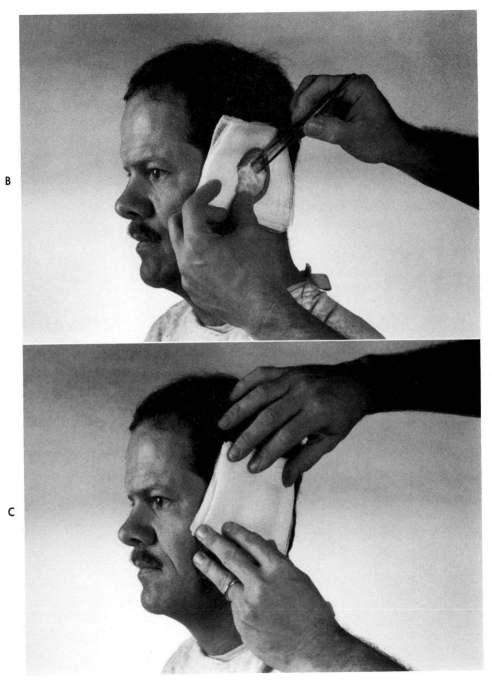

B

C

***FIG. 17-5, cont'd* B,** Petrolatum gauze packing is placed and molded within the cartilaginous skeleton. **C,** Fresh sponges are placed over the molded petrolatum gauze.
Continued.

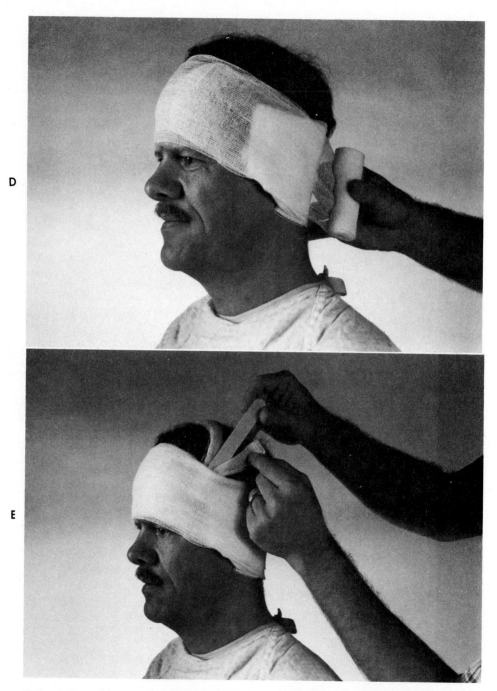

FIG. 17-5, *cont'd* **D,** Circumferential gauze wrapping is placed from the mid forehead directly over the external occipital protuberance. This portion is then secured with tape. **E,** A gauze tie is inserted anterior to the affected ear using a tongue blade.

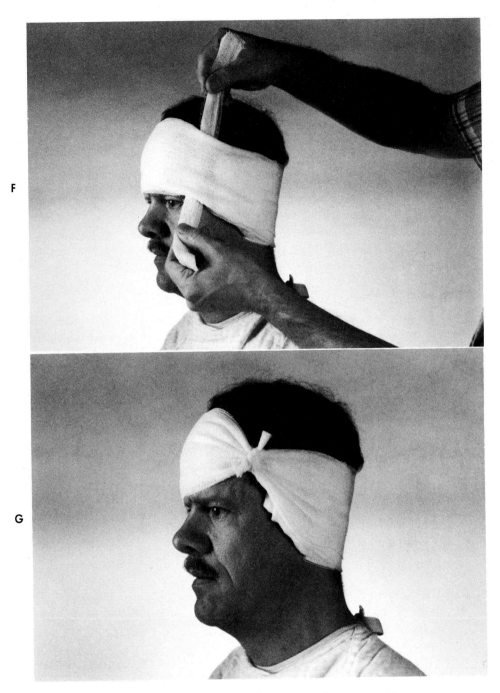

FIG. 17-5, *cont'd* **F,** This gauze is firmly tied in a square knot to provide even pressure over the ear. **G,** The final appearance of a mastoid dressing.

provide support and a "bed" for the cartilaginous skeleton. The area within the helix is filled with petrolatum gauze and "molded" over the antihelix, antitragus, and external canal. Two more intact sponges are placed over the entire ear and 3- or 4-inch gauze bandage is brought around the head and over the ear several times. After the bandage is taped, it is tightened by placing a gauze tie just anterior to the ear. The net effect is to provide even pressure over the ear without compromising its blood supply.

Neck Dressings

The neck is an uncommon site for lacerations and other wounds. Dressings need to be effectively secured without compromising the airway or venous return through the jugular system. Simple wrapping with a gauze bandage over the dressing base will suffice in most cases. For wounds of the posterior neck in the region of the occiput, the gauze bandage can be wrapped around both the head and the neck to provide for adequate coverage and security, as seen in Fig. 17-6, *A* and *B*.

Shoulder Dressings

The shoulder can be a difficult area to dress, especially if the wound is large, is in the axilla, or is directly over the articular surfaces. The dressing illustrated in *A*, *B*, and *C* of Fig. 17-7 takes advantage of the trunk to anchor the shoulder portion. The wrap is brought alternately around the trunk and shoulder/upper arm until it is complete. This dressing configuration is also useful for the upper arm, an area in which bandages tend to slip down with arm motion and gravity. For clarity, a schematic of the shoulder dressing is illustrated in Fig. 17-8.

Truncal Dressings

Most wounds on the trunk can be covered with the standard base described above and taped over benzoin. Larger wounds, such as burns, need larger bandages. The dressing described above to cover the shoulder can be extended downward over the trunk and will not slip toward the abdomen. Another method to dress the trunk is illustrated in Fig. 17-9.

Groin, Hip, and Upper Thigh Dressings

The groin, hip, and thigh are also difficult regions to properly cover. The technique illustrated in Fig. 17-10 is an all-purpose one that will protect most large wounds in those areas. Like the shoulder, the gauze wrap is brought alternately around the trunk and thigh until it is complete.

Hand and Finger Dressings

Fingers can be bandaged in one of two ways: gauze wrapping or tube gauze application. After applying ointment and a non-adherent base, 2 × 2 sponges are placed

Text continued on p. 296.

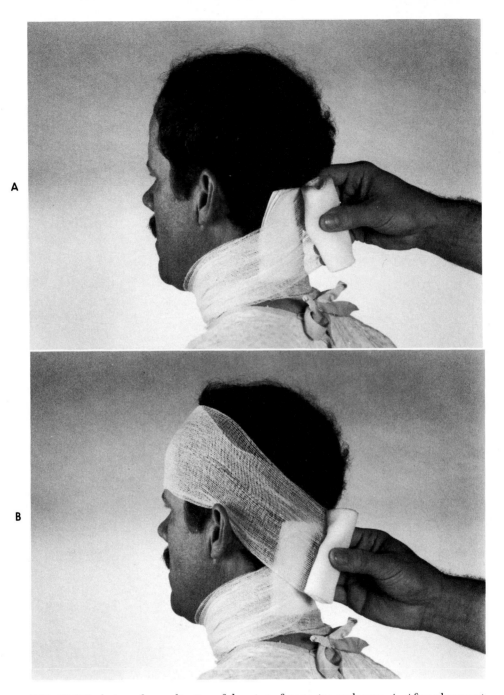

FIG. 17-6 Technique for application of dressing of posterior neck area. **A,** After placement of 4 × 4 sponges, gauze wrapping is gently brought around the neck to secure the gauze. **B,** In a recurrent manner, the dressing is then continued around the frontal area and neck in a figure-of-8 fashion to secure the dressing completely. Note that the ear is clear of the dressing.

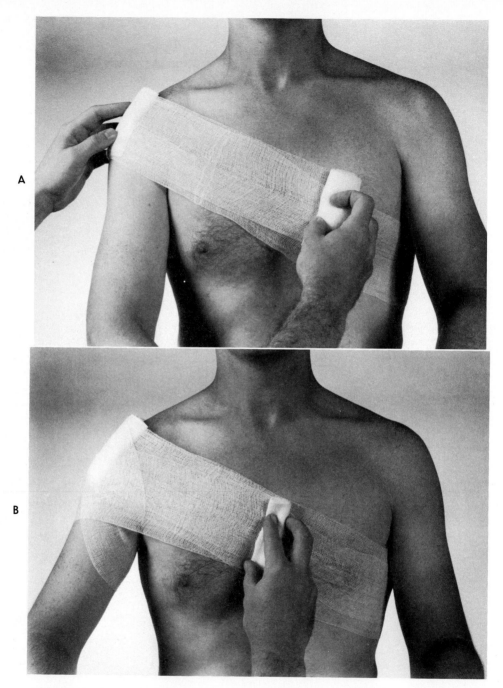

FIG. 17-7 Technique for application of shoulder and upper arm dressing. **A,** Note that the gauze base is placed in the area of injury and the gauze wrapping is begun by circumferentially placing it around the trunk and shoulder area. **B,** The gauze is then continued around the upper arm and the chest in an alternating manner.

C

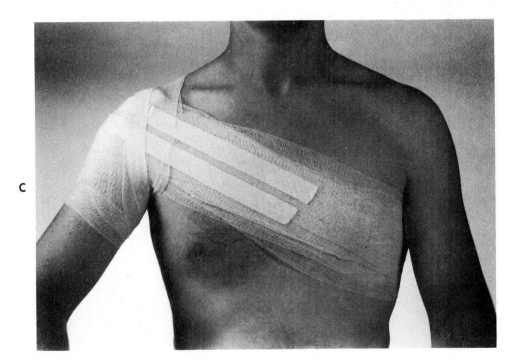

FIG. 17-7, cont'd C, The final appearance of a shoulder dressing.

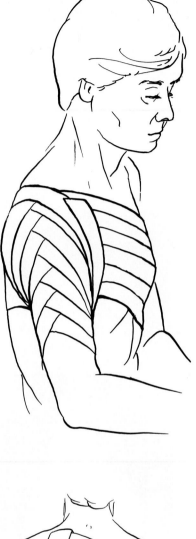

FIG. 17-8 A schematic of the shoulder dressing is presented for clarification.

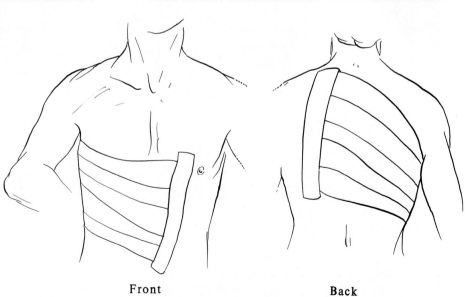

Front   Back

FIG. 17-9 Technique for application of truncal dressing. Note that gauze wrapping is brought around the hemithorax and secured with benzoin and tape.

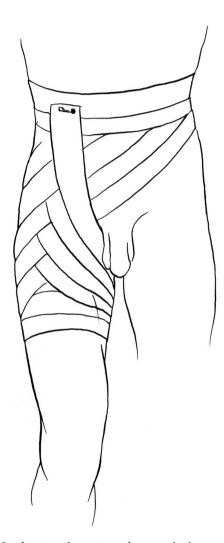

FIG. 17-10 Technique for dressing the groin and upper thigh area. Note that, like the shoulder dressing, the gauze is brought in an alternating manner first around the trunk and then the thigh.

over the actual wound. One or two layers of 2-inch gauze bandage are then placed over the finger in the manner illustrated in *A* through *G* of Fig. 17-11. The bandage is then turned in order to circumferentially wrap the entire finger from finger base to tip and back to the base again. In order to complete the bandaging, the gauze is carried in a figure-of-8 pattern down around the palm and is finally anchored at the wrist. Gauze bandaging of the finger alone tends to be inadequate and the dressing can come off prematurely. The basic technique of tube gauze bandages is illustrated in Fig. 17-12.

Injuries of the hand itself are bandaged as illustrated in Fig. 17-13, *A* and *B*. Depending on the size of the hand, 2- or 3-inch gauze wrapping is placed over the non-adherent base and sponge covering. The gauze wrap includes the wrist to ensure proper anchoring. When two or more fingers are incorporated in a hand dressing, they have to be separated by gauze or sponge strips to prevent skin to skin contact and subsequent maceration (Fig. 17-14).

Text continued on p. 302.

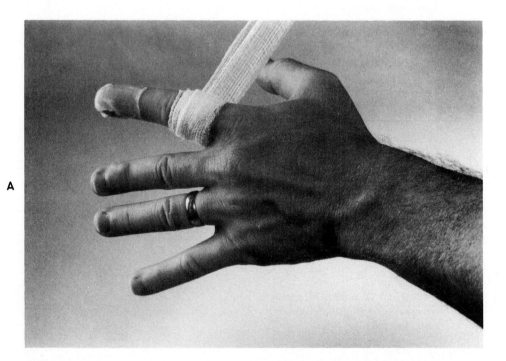

A

FIG. 17-11 Technique for dressing a finger and finger tip. **A,** Note that the non-adherent base is placed over the finger tip. This base can be supplemented by 2 × 2 sponges. The gauze is begun around the base of the finger to initially secure the bandage.

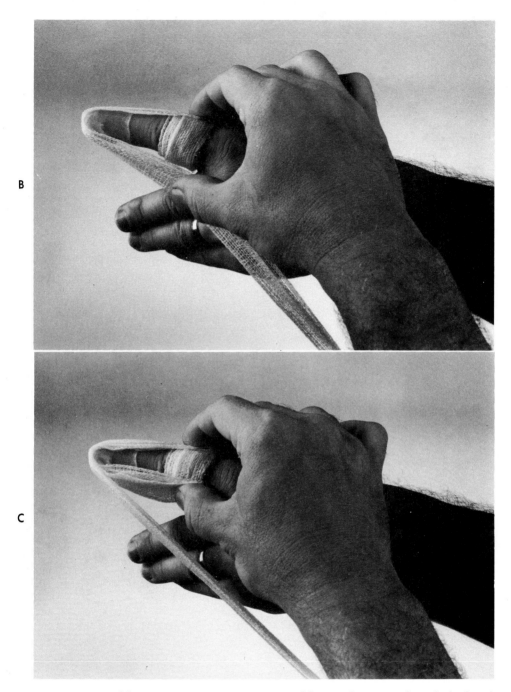

B

C

FIG. 17-11, cont'd **B,** In a recurrent manner, several layers of gauze are brought back and forth over the tip of the finger to ensure coverage of the distal portion of the digit. **C,** These layers are continued until deemed sufficient.

Continued.

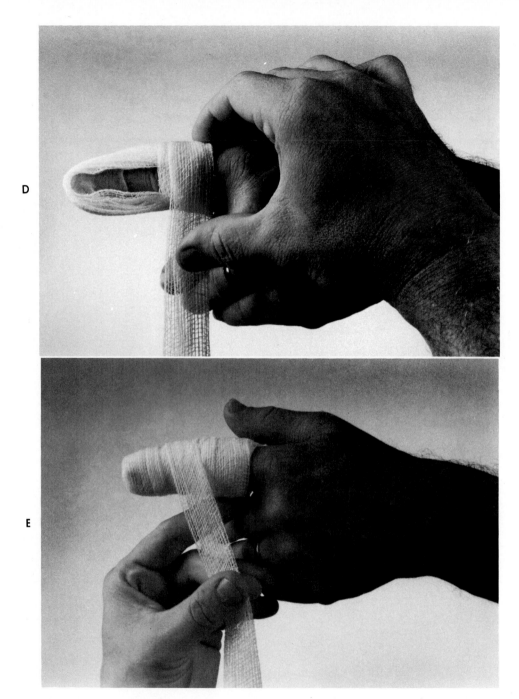

FIG. 17-11, cont'd **D,** The gauze wrap is then brought back around the finger at its proximal point. **E,** The wrapping is continued to cover the entire digit.

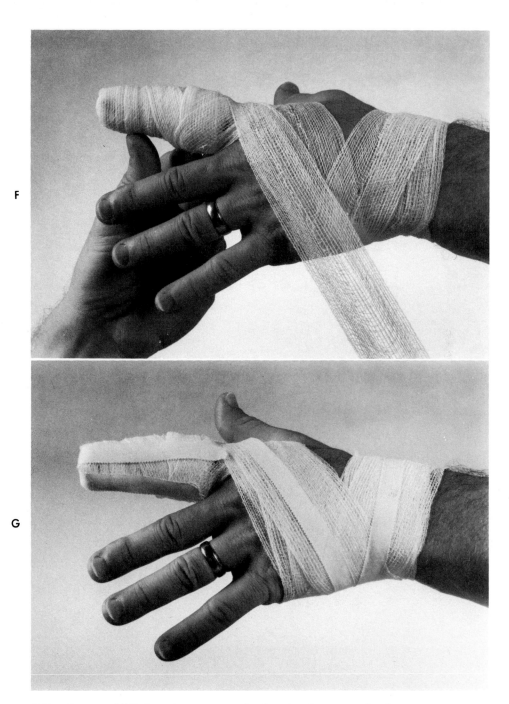

FIG. 17-11, cont'd F, In order to secure the digit bandage properly, the gauze is continued around the palm and the wrist to secure the bandage firmly. **G,** Final appearance of a proper finger bandage. Note that tape has been applied to secure all elements of the gauze. Also note that none of the tape is wrapped in a circumferential manner.

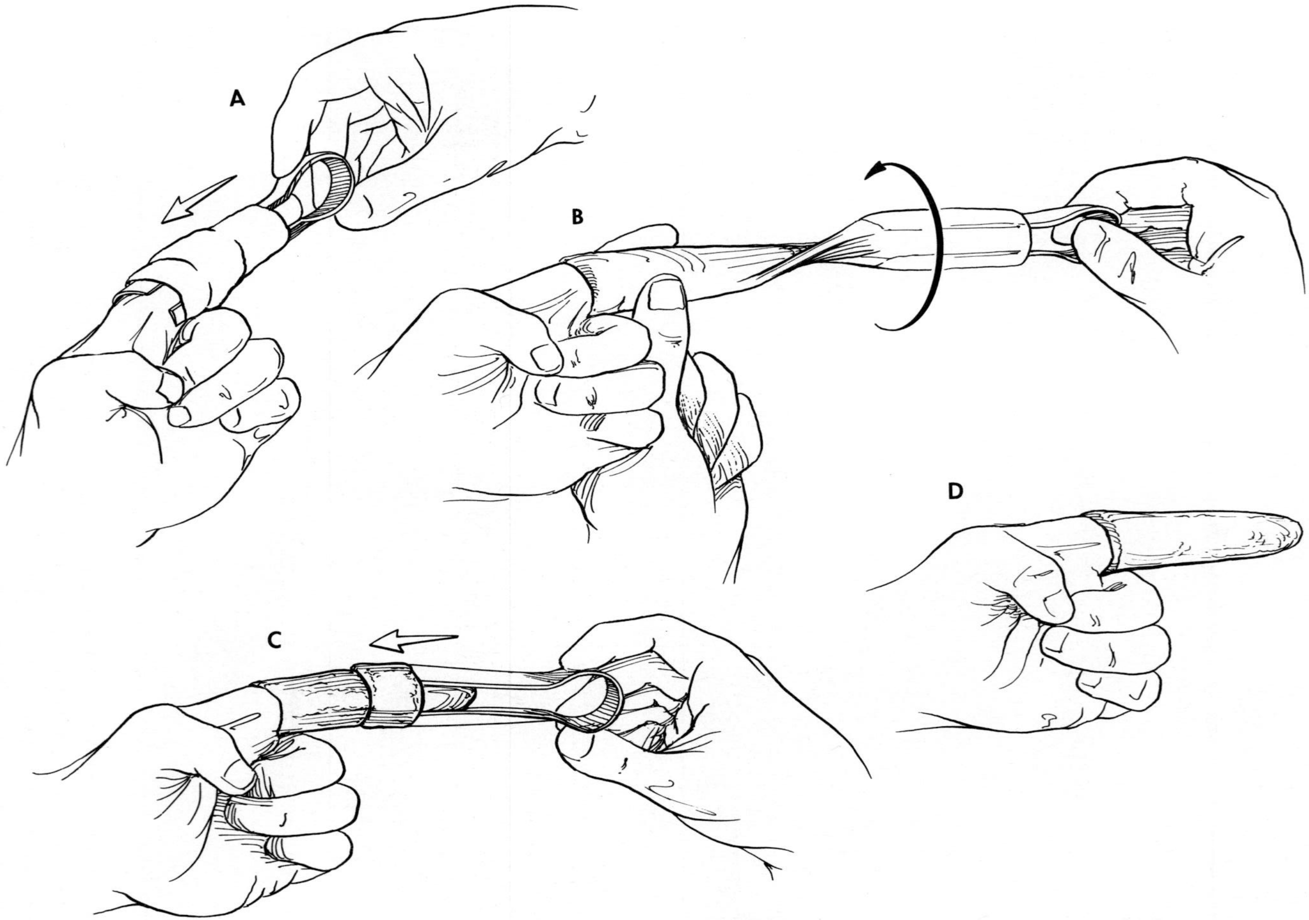

FIG. 17-12 Technique for placement of a tube gauze finger bandage. **A,** Note that sufficient tube gauze is slid onto the applicator and then brought over the finger. **B,** The first layer of tube gauze is secured as the applicator is brought distally from the finger and rotated 180 degrees. **C,** The next layer of tube gauze is placed by the applicator over the digit. **D,** This process is repeated until an adequate number of layers of tube gauze has been applied.

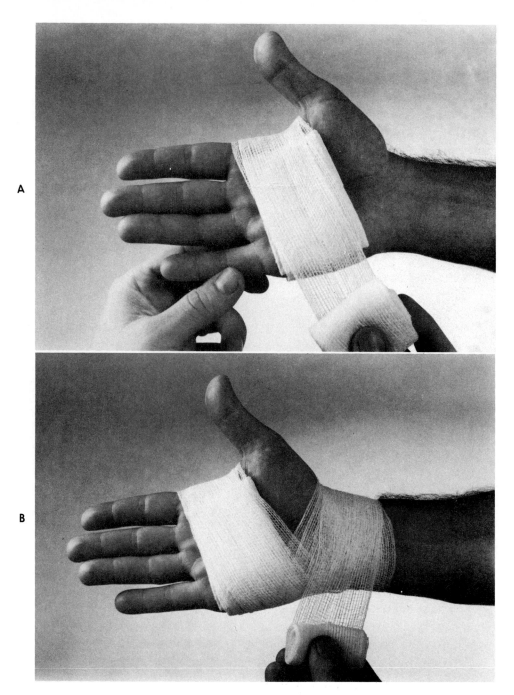

FIG. 17-13 Technique for placing a dressing on the palmar or dorsal surface of the hand. **A,** The non-adherent base and 4 × 4s are placed on the palm or dorsum of the hand. The gauze wrapping is begun by securing this dressing base. **B,** The dressing is completed by alternate wrapping of both the palm and the wrist with the gauze wrap. Tape is applied in a noncircumferential manner to complete the dressing.

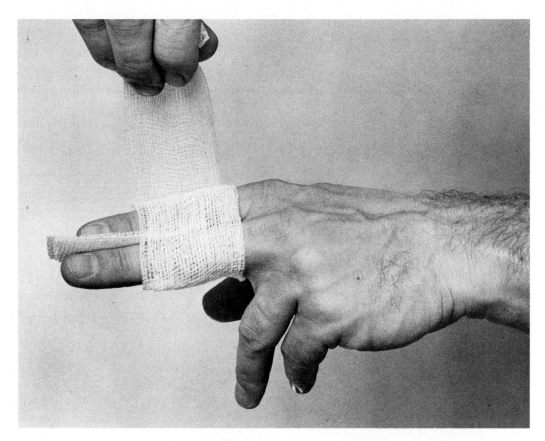

FIG. 17-14 Always place gauze between skin-to-skin contact areas to prevent maceration.

Elbow and Knee Dressings

The elbow and knee can be wrapped circumferentially with 4-inch gauze. Although the dressing will be adequate, it will limit motion of the joint. The figure-of-8 technique illustrated in *A* through *D* of Fig. 17-15 when placed with the joint in some flexion allows for more freedom of movement. 4 × 8-inch gauze sponges are placed over the extensor surfaces and incorporated into the bandaging. These large sponges allow for "travel" as the joint is flexed and extended.

Ankle, Heel, and Foot Dressings

Ankle and foot dressings are straightforward. The gauze bandage wrapping is in the same figure-of-eight style as for the knee and elbow. When bandaging the foot, always include the ankle as the anchoring point. The difficult area to cover is the heel. As illustrated in Fig. 17-16, the wrapping starts around the heel and anterior

Text continued on p. 308.

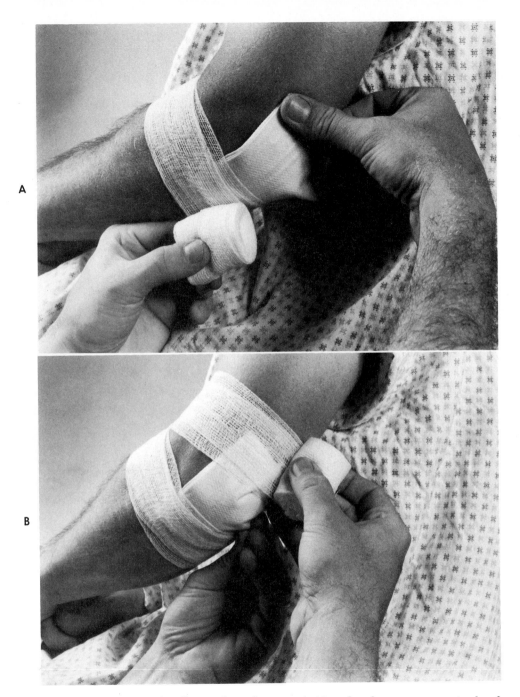

FIG. 17-15 Technique for elbow or knee dressing. **A,** Note that the gauze sponge is placed over the extensor surface of the knee or elbow and secured with the beginnings of a gauze wrap. **B,** The gauze wrap is then brought over to the opposite side of the gauze dressing base.

Continued.

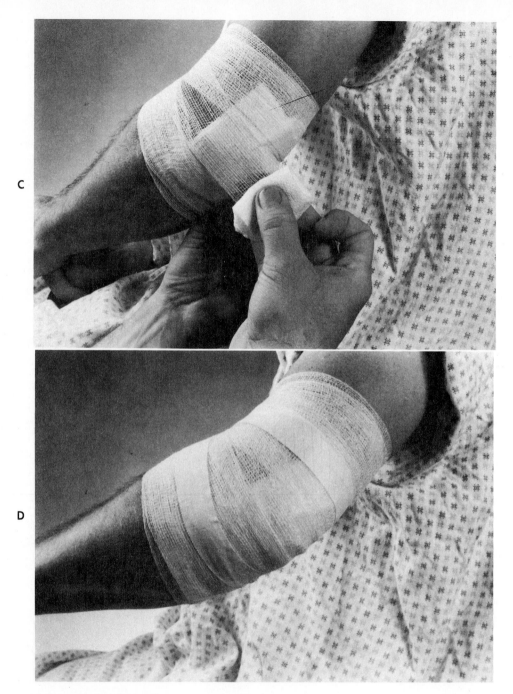

FIG. 17-15, cont'd **C**, The gauze wrapping is then continued over the center portion of the dressing base. **D**, An example of a completed dressing. Most elbow and knee dressings are fashioned with the knee or elbow in a slightly flexed position to provide for better patient mobility.

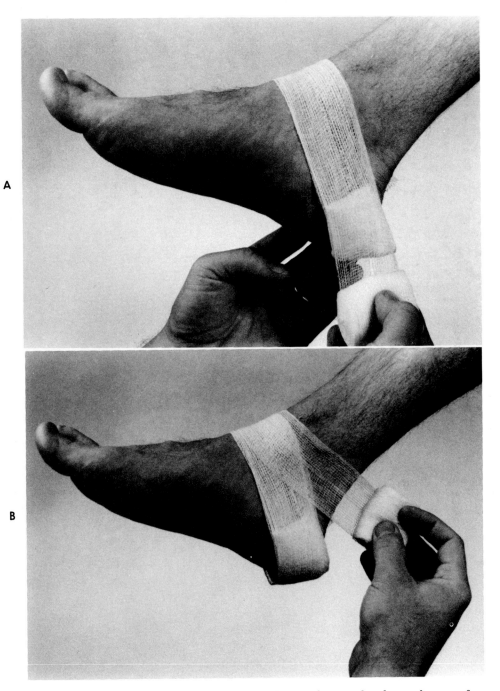

A

B

FIG. 17-16 Technique for heel dressing. **A,** The dressing base is placed over the area of concern of the heel and the initial gauze wrap secures that base. **B,** The gauze wrap is continued around the ankle.

Continued.

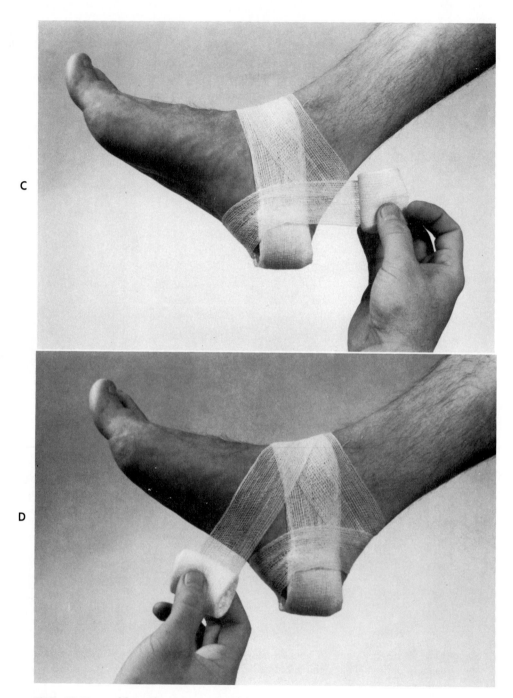

FIG. 17-16, cont'd C, The gauze wrap is then brought directly across and around the heel. **D,** Once it has crossed the heel it is brought over the ankle and then around the foot.

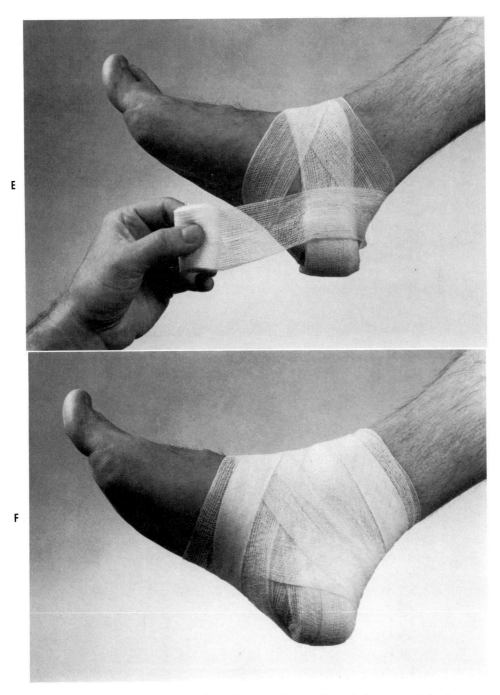

***FIG. 17-16, cont'd* E,** After being brought around the ankle and then around the foot, it is brought back in the reverse manner over the heel. **F,** Completed example of heel dressing.

portion of the ankle. After three or four wraps, the bandage is brought around the heel alone, then around the foot. This process is continued until the foot, heel, and ankle are all part of the dressing.

References

1. Ayliffe GA et al: Antibiotic-resistant *Staphylococcus aureus* in dermatology in burn wounds, J Clin Pharmacol 30-32, 1977.
2. Bothwell JW and Rovee DT: The effects of dressings on the repair of cutaneous wounds in humans. In Harkiss KJ, ed: Surgical dressings and wound healing, London, 1971, Bradford Univ Press.
3. Eaglestein WH and Mertz PM: Effect of topical medicaments on the rate of repair of superficial wounds. In Dineen P, ed: The surgical wound, Philadelphia, 1981, Lea & Febiger.
4. Hinman C and Maibach H: Effect of air exposure and occlusion on experimental human skin wounds, Nature 200:377-378, 1963.
5. Howells C and Young H: A study of completely undressed surgical wounds, Br J Surg 53:436-439, 1966.
6. Lammers RL: Principles of wound management. In Roberts JR and Hedges JR, eds: Clinical procedures in emergency medicine, Philadelphia, 1985, WB Saunders Co.
7. Lawrence J: What materials for dressings? Injury 13:500-512, 1981-82.
8. Leyden JJ and Sulzberger MB: Topical antibiotics and minor skin trauma, Am Fam Physic 23:121-125, 1981.
9. Millikan LE: Wound healing and dermatologic dressings, Clin Dermatol 5:31-36, 1987.
10. Norton LW: Trauma. In Hill GJ, ed: Outpatient surgery, Philadelphia, 1980, WB Saunders Co.
11. Panek P et al: Potentiation of wound infection by adhesive adjuncts, Am Surg 38:343-345, 1972.
12. Stuzin J, Engrav LH, and Buehler PK: Emergency treatment of facial lacerations, Post Grad Med 71:81-83, 1982.
13. Wayne MA: Clinical evaluation of Epi-Lock—a semiocclusive dressing, Ann Emerg Med 14:20-24, 1985.

18 *Patient Discharge and Follow-up Care*

Tetanus Prophylaxis
   Immunization Schedules
   Complications of Tetanus Toxoid
Suture Removal
   Technique for Removal
Prophylactic Antibiotics for Emergency
   Wounds
Analgesia
Instructions to the Patient

Wound area protection
Dressing change and follow-up
   intervals
Wound cleansing
Signs of wound infection
Written instructions
Advising Patients about Wound Healing
References

Wound aftercare includes tetanus prophylaxis, instructions to the patient, and proper follow-up care. If they are carefully and fully informed, most patients take good care of their wounds and dressings. Merely handing patients a written list of instructions in a hurried manner does not mean that the responsibility of the person repairing the wound has ended. Written instructions are best followed when they are reinforced with unhurried verbal explanations. Because each wound and each patient is different, information about dressing care, activity, bathing, and suture removal has to be individualized.

TETANUS PROPHYLAXIS

For virtually every patient with an emergency wound or laceration, a decision has to be made about whether or not to administer tetanus prophylaxis. Although contaminated wounds with extensive devitalized tissue are considered more tetanus-prone than clean minor wounds, up to one third of documented cases of tetanus have originated from seemingly trivial injuries.[1,10,15] A common portal of entry for tetanus is a puncture wound to the foot.[10] Tetanus occurs almost exclusively in patients who have never been immunized or who never completed a proper immunization program.[7] Probably for this reason, most cases are reported in patients who are over the age of 50.[7] A high proportion of older adults, when tested for serum tetanus antibody, have been shown to have inadequate levels of protection.[6] Young adults and children are more likely to have appropriate levels of protection because of widespread immunization programs that have been put into place in recent years. In any event, a careful immunization history is taken for every patient with a minor wound. This history should establish whether initial immunization has been properly completed and the date of the last tetanus toxoid dose.

Immunization Schedules

The guidelines in Table 18-1 for the administration of tetanus prophylaxis are those recommended by the Immunization Practice Advisory Committee (ACIP) of the Centers for Disease Control.[8] The currently recommended preparation of tetanus toxoid includes the diphtheria toxoid and is designated Td. The risk of contracting diphtheria in adulthood is of sufficient magnitude that, as a public measure, prophylaxis against this disease is recommended.[15] The trivalent diphtheria, tetanus, and pertussis (DTP) is administered to children under 7 who have not been fully immunized. It is important to be aware that there is a DT preparation with a higher concentration of diphtheria toxoid. This preparation is not recommended for patients over 7 and is only occasionally administered to patients under 7 who cannot tolerate the pertussis (P) component of DTP.

For adolescent and adult patients who have never been immunized and who received their first dose of Td at the time of their wound repair, follow-up care should include subsequent visits to a medical care facility to complete immunization. Table 18-2 summarizes the time guidelines for administration of the second, third, and booster doses of Td.

Table 18-1 *Summary Guide to Tetanus Prophylaxis in Routine Wound Management—United States, 1985**

History of Adsorbed Tetanus Toxoid (Doses)	Clean, Minor Wounds		All Other Wounds†	
	Td‡	TIG	Td‡	TIG
Unknown or < three	Yes	No	Yes	Yes
≥ three§	No‖	No	No¶	No

*Important details are in the text.

†Such as, but not limited to, wounds contaminated with dirt, feces, soil, saliva, etc.; puncture wounds; avulsions; and wounds resulting from missiles, crushing, burns, and frostbite.

‡For children under 7 years old; DTP (DT, if pertussis vaccine is contraindicated) is preferred to tetanus toxoid alone. For persons 7 years old and older, Td is preferred to tetanus toxoid alone.

§If only three doses of *fluid* toxoid have been received, a fourth dose of toxoid, preferably an adsorbed toxoid, should be given.

‖Yes, if more than 10 years since last dose.

¶Yes, if more than 5 years since last dose. (More frequent boosters are not needed and can accentuate side effects.)

From ACIP guidelines: Diphtheria, tetanus and pertussis. Guidelines for vaccine prophylaxis and other preventive measures—US 1985. MMWR 34:405-414, 419-426, 1985.

Table 18-2 *Routine Diphtheria and Tetanus Immunization Schedule Summary for Persons 7 Years Old and Older—United States, 1985**

Dose	Age/Interval	Product
Primary 1	First dose	Td
Primary 2	4-8 weeks after first dose†	Td
Primary 3	6-12 months after second dose†	Td
Boosters	Every 10 years after last dose	Td

*Important details are in the text.
†Prolonging the interval does not require restarting series.
From ACIP guidelines: Diphtheria, tetanus, and pertussis. Guidelines for vaccine prophylaxis and other preventive measures—US 1985 MMWR 34:405-414, 419-426, 1985.

Complications of Tetanus Toxoid

Occasionally, a patient will report an allergic reaction to a prior tetanus shot. In a study of 740 patients who claimed to be allergic to tetanus shots, the true incidence of allergy, upon skin challenge testing, was very low.[16] Of the 740 patients 7 developed local reactions that were self limited. One patient became syncopal and one developed a fever that lasted for 4 days. Only 1 of 740 patients had a true urticarial response but still tolerated a full immunizing dose. In spite of these reassuring figures, the possibility of a serious reaction still must be considered.[16] For patients considered at high risk for a reaction, tetanus immune globulin (TIG; 250-500 units) is given in the emergency department. TIG will confer immunity in that event but not for future exposures. This preparation consists only of anti-tetanus antibody and does not cross-react with the toxoid. Referral to an allergist for skin testing, and subsequent immunization with toxoid, is recommended as prudent follow-up.

Local and systemic reactions to Td are not common but do occur in up to 7% to 9% of pediatric patients.[4] Pain, swelling, and erythema can occur at the injection sight but are usually self-limited. Preparations containing the pertussis vaccine (DTP), on the other hand, are associated with a much higher rate of adverse reactions. Fever can occur in up to 50% of infants receiving DTP.[7] It can last for 24 to 48 hours and can be accompanied by somnolence, nausea, vomiting, and irritability. Other rare reactions that have been reported include arthus-type hypersensitivity, urticaria, anaphylaxis, and neurologic complications.

SUTURE REMOVAL

The recommended intervals between wound repair and suture removal are detailed in Table 18-3. In the face area, where cosmetic appearance is paramount, sutures are removed as early as possible. This is done, however, with the knowledge that a

Table 18-3 *Recommended Intervals for Removal of Percutaneous Sutures*

Region	Days Until Removal	
	Adults	Children
Scalp	6-8	5-7
Eyelid	3-5	3-5
Ear	4-5	3-5
Nose	3-5	3-5
Lip	4-5	3-5
Forehead/Other Face	3-5	3-5
Chest/Abdomen	8-10	6-8
Back	12-14	10-12
Arm	8-10	6-8
Hand	8-10	6-8
Fingertip	10-12	8-10
Joint—Extensor Surface	10-14	8-10
Joint—Flexor Surface	8-10	6-8
Lower Extremity	8-12	6-10
Foot	10-12	8-10
Penis	7-10	6-8

wound has barely begun to gain tensile strength. Minimal accidental force can cause disruption and open the laceration. Therefore, the application of wound tapes over healing lacerations for a minimum of 7 days is recommended. A return visit for tape removal is not necessary. If wound tapes are the primary method of wound closure, they can be left in place for up to 10 days without causing complications. At the least, they should remain over a wound for the time recommended for sutures for any given body area.

It is important to understand that suture punctures are small wounds. Epithelial cells invade these small wounds and keratinized epithelial "plugs" can be caught in the wound during healing. This phenomenon produces unnecessary visible marks, which can be avoided if sutures are removed in less than seven days.[5] The use of skin tapes as either the sole wound closure method or for wound support after early suture removal is an alternative technique to avoid suture tracking. The pull-out dermal closure described in Chapter 10 is another "trackless" closure option.

In other areas of the body, where cosmesis is not as important and wound healing is not quite as rapid as in the highly vascular face, sutures are left in for longer periods. Extensor surfaces of joints require somewhat longer times before removal because of the mechanical forces brought to bear on the healing wound. Because of the dependency of the lower extremities and their relatively slower rate of healing, sutures are also left in place for longer in those sites.

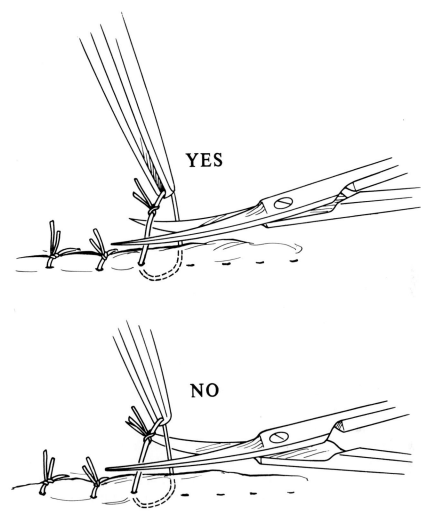

YES

NO

FIG. 18-1 Technique for correct removal of a suture. Note that the scissors cut between the knot and skin. The lower figure indicates the incorrect technique to remove sutures. (Adapted from Zukin D and Simon R: Emergency wound care: principles and practice, Rockville, Md, 1987, Aspen Publishers Inc, p 130.)

Technique for Removal

The technique for suture removal is illustrated in Fig. 18-1. The basic reason for cutting the suture under the knot, close to the skin surface, is so that when it is pulled from the wound the previously exposed, possibly contaminated portion of the suture does not travel back through the wound. Although standard scissors can be used for most suture removal tasks, iris scissors or a #11 scalpel blade are recommended to cut very fine sutures, usually 6-0 on the face. Bandage or commercial suture-removal scissors have tips that are often too blunt to cut small closely-spaced sutures easily. Before removal, all dried coagulum is gently removed from the suture line with cotton swabs and hydrogen peroxide. Cleaning away the coagulum makes locating small sutures and knots much easier. In addition, it prevents the unnecessary tugging and pulling that often accompanies suture removal when sutures are excessively crusted.

PROPHYLACTIC ANTIBIOTICS FOR EMERGENCY WOUNDS

For small, uncomplicated minor wounds and lacerations, there is no good clinical evidence that systemic antibiotics provide protection against the development of wound infection.[12-14,17] In a study in which intramuscular penicillin was administered to alternate patients with lacerations treated in an emergency department, there was no difference in the rate of infection between the study and control groups.[14] A randomized, controlled study using oral cephalexin for prophylaxis also demonstrated no efficacy of the antibiotic for minor lacerations.[17] In two randomized, controlled studies using oral or parenteral cephalosporins for minor hand lacerations, there was no increase in the infection rate of non-antibiotic treated patients when compared to those treated with antibiotics.[12,13]

Although not all authorities agree, nor is there strong scientific evidence underlying any specific set of recommendations for wound antibiotic prophylaxis, clinical and empirical experience suggests that there are wound characteristics and circumstances that warrant antibiotic intervention.[2,3,9] If the decision to initiate antibiotic therapy is made, there is evidence that the initial dose has to be administered as soon as possible. In an experimental study, a variety of antibiotics lost their protective effect if administered 3 hours after injury and bacterial contamination.[2] In Chapter 8, guidelines are given for clinical settings in which immediate intravenous antibiotic therapy is recommended. The following are guidelines for which oral antibiotics should be continued on an outpatient basis. The initial dose, either oral or parenteral, is administered prior to the discharge of the patient.

- Wounds greater than 8 to 12 hours old, especially of the hands and lower extremities
- Facial wounds can be primarily sutured up to 24 hours after injury and are not treated with antibiotics. After that period, the extent of the wound, level of contamination, and other factors influence the decision to administer an antibiotic. An exception is an intraoral injury caused by the victim's own teeth. Antibiotics are prescribed at the time of the initial repair regardless of the time following injury
- Crushing (compression) mechanism wounds with potential for devitalization of those requiring extensive revision
- Significantly contaminated wounds requiring extensive cleansing and debridement

- Violation of ear cartilage
- Involvement of joint spaces, tendon, or bone
- Complex, extensive paronychia and felons
- Mammalian bites, particularly human bites and cat bites (see Chapter 14)
- Extensive or contaminated wounds in patients with pre-existing valvular heart disease.
- Conditions of immunosuppression or impaired host defenses (example: diabetes)

The choice of systemic prophylactic antibiotics has to take into account that the most common infecting agent is *Staphylococcus aureus*. In addition, however, gram-negative organisms occur with significant frequency and need to be combated as well. Because of the broad activity against gram-positive and gram-negative organisms, including penicillinase-producing *Staphylococcus aureus*, first-generation cephalosporins are reasonable to use when prophylaxis might be advisable. Examples include Keflex (cephalexin) and Duricef (cefadroxil). Some authorities believe that coverage for gram-positive organisms alone is sufficient and they recommend using the less expensive dicloxacillin. There is no evidence that cephalosporins are superior to dicloxacillin in the setting of wound prophylaxis. For penicillin-allergic patients, erythromycin can be used. In most prophylaxis situations, 3 to 5 days of therapy should suffice. Ciprofloxacin is another potentially useful prophylactic agent. For bite wounds, refer to Chapter 14.

ANALGESIA

Pain following wounding can be trivial or significant. Simple lacerations are usually tolerated by the patient. Abrasions and partial-thickness (second-degree) burns can be almost unbearable. For most patients with uncomplicated lacerations, aspirin, acetaminophen, or other nonsteroidal anti-inflammatory drugs will relieve residual discomfort after repair. Occasionally, codeine is necessary. Burn victims require more powerful analgesics such as oxycodone. In addition to drugs, pain relief can be greatly enhanced by elevation of the injured part, proper immobilization, and cool compresses to the affected area.

The pain of lacerations and burns tends to subside significantly within 24 to 48 hours. A key follow-up instruction to the patient is to be concerned if pain increases or recurs. The most likely cause of this change in the pain pattern is wound infection. If this occurs, immediate physician notification is necessary.

INSTRUCTIONS TO THE PATIENT
Wound Area Protection

Patients need to be carefully instructed about how to care for their wound at home. The key principles of home care are protection, elevation, and cleanliness. Most patients will instinctively protect wounds from further trauma, but occasionally they need to be reminded that, although sutures are in place, undue pressure or other mechanical forces on the wound can cause disruption and possible infection. Proper counseling and admonition against premature use of the repaired hand or foot is especially necessary for patients who are anxious to return to work or sporting activities.

Elevation is particularly important in extremity wounds. The tendency of lower extremities and hands to develop edema from lymphatic stasis is well recognized. Elevation will help prevent these complications and possibly improve wound healing. Lower-extremity wounds have a higher rate of wound infection, a complication that can be abetted by edema and stasis. Crutches and slings are recommended adjuncts for home wound care.

Dressing Change and Follow-Up Intervals

The vast majority of uncomplicated wounds are trouble-free. For simple, uncomplicated lacerations, dressings can be kept over the wound for up to 7 days. It is not always necessary to have the patient return in 2 or 3 days, except for wounds in which there is a high risk of infection. Low-risk patients can be instructed to watch for the signs of infection or excessive soilage, and they can be depended upon to return should any doubt or problem arise. They can also be instructed in changing their own dressings when necessary.

The safest practice for patients with a high risk for infection or those patients judged to be possibly impaired or unreliable is to have them return for a follow-up visit 48 hours after wound repair. If the injured area is pain-free (except for very mild discomfort) and no exudate is soiling the bandage, the bandage can be left in place. If there is any doubt, then a dressing change is in order. Often a smaller, less bulky dressing can be applied at this time. The second dressing usually remains in place until the sutures are removed.

Wounds in critical areas like the hand have to be inspected within 48 hours regardless of cleanliness. If any infection develops, it has to be treated vigorously and early in order to prevent a serious complication. All dressings are removed and changed at this time for wounds in these areas. Wounds with a high risk of infection, such as animal bites, those caused by crushing mechanisms or those falling in the categories listed above that require the use of prophylactic antibiotics need to be seen within 48 to 72 hours. As a rule, if a wound is infection-free for 3 to 5 days after repair, it will remain so for the remainder of the healing period.

Wound Cleansing

Cleanliness is an important issue in wound aftercare. Repaired wounds of the scalp and face can be left open, provided that they are kept clean. In a controlled study of 200 head and neck incisions and traumatic lacerations, the investigators concluded that early washing (8 to 24 hours) after wound repair did not significantly alter wound healing or increase the potential for infection.[11] The results were identical for early-wash and no-wash groups. In the experimental group, Neosporin ointment was applied. No oral antibiotics were given.

Patients with sutured lacerations at all sites can be allowed to bathe once a day, provided that the wound is not immersed and soaked in water except for brief moments. Showers are preferable to tub baths. Gentle soaping and rinsing is immediately followed by patting the wound dry with a soft towel. Patients can usually begin to bathe 12 to 24 hours after wound repair. Application of an antibiotic ointment or reapplication of a dressing is recommended after each washing.

Signs of Wound Infection

Every patient has to be instructed in the signs of wound infection. Should any of these signs develop, the patient needs to return immediately for examination. The first sign of infection is usually excessive discomfort. The majority of minor wounds are only mildly uncomfortable. Copious drainage, particularly purulent-appearing material, usually indicates an established infection. If purulence is present, the patient often notices that the wound dressing becomes wet or soiled with the drainage. Redness that extends well beyond the wound margins (more than 5 mm) with accompanying swelling, induration, or tenderness does not appear in normally healing wounds. Admittedly, these two signs can be difficult to interpret, depending on the nature and size of the wounded area. Normal neovascularization and capillary dilatation do provide some erythema to the wound edge. The best course of action is to be cautious and have the wound re-examined if there is any doubt. Lymphangitic streaks, local nodal enlargement, and fever are all advanced signs of infection.

Written Instructions

Finally, patients should be given specific written instructions reinforcing and detailing these general principles as well as any other specifics for the given wound problem. Follow-up visits, dates, and times, have to be clearly written and understood by the patient and, whenever possible, by accompanying family members.

NOTE: Occasionally, a patient will discover that there is loss of function or of sensation after repair of a hand or forearm injury. It may be prudent to advise patients of this possibility in high-risk wounds. They can be reassured that tendons and nerves can still be successfully repaired up to 3 weeks after the initial injury.

ADVISING PATIENTS ABOUT WOUND HEALING

Patients are most concerned about the size and appearance of the scar that will result. Because traumatic injuries occur randomly on the body surface, the final outcome, to a certain extent, is predetermined. It is the duty of the person repairing the wound to advise the patient about the kind of scar he or she will end up with. Candidly discussing various aspects of wound healing such as the effects of drugs, associated diseases, body region, and skin tension will allow the patient to better accept and cope with the healing process (see Chapter 3).

The appearance of a wound can change during the healing process, which often gives rise to questions in the patient's mind. Patients need to understand that although stitches are removed within days of the injury and the wound appears to be sealed, it actually has very low tensile strength. Reopening or dehiscence can occur if it is exposed to undue trauma. Wounds are often temperature- and touch-sensitive for weeks. Early scars appear red and raised, but eventual blanching and contraction will eliminate those characteristics. People with dark skin have to be informed that scars do not regain lost pigmentation and will be much lighter than the surrounding skin.

Finally, patients have to be counseled that scars mature and change in configuration for several months as they take on their final appearance. More often than not, an initially unsightly scar will eventually become acceptable to the patient. However, a plastic surgeon can be consulted to perform necessary scar revision if the patient is unhappy about the appearance of the scar.

References

1. Brand D et al: Adequacy of anti-tetanus prophylaxis in six hospital emergency departments, N Engl J Med 309:636-640, 1983.
2. Burke J: The effective period of preventive antibiotic action in experimental incisions and dermal lesions, Surgery 50:161-168, 1981.
3. Cardany R et al: The crush injury: a high risk wound, J Am Coll Emerg Phys 5:965-970, 1976.
4. Cody CL et al: Nature of adverse reactions associated with DTP and DT immunizations in infants and children, Pediatrics 68:650-660, 1981.
5. Crikelair CT: Skin suture marks, Am J Surg 96:631-632, 1958.
6. Crossby K et al: Tetanus and diphtheria immunity in urban Minnesota adults, JAMA 242:2298-2300, 1979.
7. Diphtheria, tetanus, and pertussis: guidelines for prophylaxis and other preventive measures, Morbid Mortal Weekly Rep 30, no 32:392-396, 401-407, 420, 1981.
8. Diphtheria, tetanus, and pertussis: guidelines for vaccine prophylaxis and other preventive measures, Morbid Mortal Weekly Rep 34:405-414, 419-426, 1985.
9. Edlich R, Smith Q, and Edgerton M: Resistance of surgical wound to antimicrobial prophylaxis and its mechanisms of development, Am J Surg 126:583-591, 1973.
10. Furste W: Fifth international conference on tetanus, Ronneby, Sweden, 1978, J Trauma 20:101-105, 1980.
11. Goldberg HM, Rosenthal SAE, and Nemetz JC: Effect of washing closed head and neck wounds on wound healing and infection, Am J Surg 141:358-359, 1981.
12. Grossman JAI, Adams JP, and Kunec J: Prophylactic antibiotics in simple hand lacerations, JAMA 245:1055-1056, 1981.
13. Haughey RE, Lammers RL, and Wagner DK: Use of antibiotics in the initial management of soft tissue hand wounds, Ann Emerg Med 10:187-192, 1981.

14. Hutton P, Jones B, and Law D: Depot penicillin as prophylaxis in accidental wounds, Br J Surg 65:549-550, 1978.

15. Immunization Practices Advisory Committee, Centers for Disease Control: diphtheria, tetanus, and pertussis, Ann Int Med 95:723-728, 1981.

16. Jacobs RL, Lowe RS, and Lanier BQ: Adverse reactions to tetanus toxoid, JAMA 247:40-42, 1982.

17. Thirlby R and Blair A: The value of prophylactic antibiotics for simple lacerations, Surg Gynecol Obstet 156:212-216, 1983.

Index

A

Abrasions, 256-259
  deep
    cheek, 161
    closure in, 146
    forehead, 155-156
    lacerations in, 146
Absorbable sutures, 20, 76-77
  scalp lacerations and, 152
Absorbant gauze sponges, 278
Ace wrap, 85
Acetaminophen, 315
  burns and, 271-272
Achilles tendon, 51
Acid burns, 272-273
Adaptic, 276
  abrasions and, 258
  burns and, 268
  finger dressing of, 212
Adhesives, wound, 78
Adrenalin; *see* Norepinephrine
Adson forceps, 194
Aerobic bacteria in bite wound, 229
Aftercare; *see* Follow-up care
Age
  skin changes and, 146-147
  wound healing and, 20
Airway cannulas, 35
Airway injury, 266-267
Allergy, 32
Alpha hemolytic streptococci, 236; *see also* Streptococci
Ambu-masks, 35
Amoxicillin
  cat bites and, 234
  ear lacerations and, 168
  hand injuries and, 212
  septal hematoma and, 163
Amputated parts of hand, 207
Anabolic steroids, 21
Anaerobic bacteria in bite wounds, 229
Analgesia, 315
Anatomy of wound healing; *see* Wound healing
Ancef; *see* Cefazolin
Anesthesia
  forehead lacerations and, 154
  local
    excitatory central nervous system effects of, 30-31

Anesthesia—cont'd
  local—cont'd
    hand injuries and, 180
    nerve block; *see* Nerve block
    of nose, 162
    wound cleansing and, 60
Animal bites, 227-228
  infection and, 24
  risk factors and, 231
  wound management for, 232-233
Animals
  identification of, in rabies exposure, 236-239
  quarantining of, 239, 242
  rabies in, 240-241
Ankle dressings, 302-308
Anterior nasal pack, 163
Antibiotics
  for cat bites, 234
  for dog bites, 233-234
  for hand wounds, 211-212
  for human bites, 235
  intravenous, 92-93
  prophylactic, 314-315
    burns and, 273
    dog bites and, 233
Anticoagulants, 21
Antineoplastic agents, 21
Aponeurosis, 150
Arrival of patient, 1-4
Asphalt, abrasions and, 258
Aspirin, 315
  burns and, 271-272
  healing and, 21
Auricle, sensory innervation of, 41
Auricular block, 41-42
Avulsion injuries
  of fingertip, 203-204
  partial, 132-135
  scalp lacerations and, 152-153
  tissue loss and, 204

B

Bacillus subtilis, 236
Bacteria
  in bite wound, 228-229
  gram-negative
    human bite infections and, 228-229
    povidone-iodine and, 57
  gram-positive; *see* Gram-positive organisms

Bactericidal activity, 26
Bactrim, 163
Band-Aid, 278
Bandaging, wound; *see* Dressings
Barb, fishhook, 254-255
Basic principles and techniques, 96-121
    definition of terms in, 96-97
    knot tying and, 97-109; *see also* Knot-tying
        techniques
    wound closure and, 110-121; *see also*
        Closure
Basilar skull fracture, 165
Bicuspid, mandibular, 41
Bite wounds, 227-246
    aftercare and follow-up in, 236-242
    animal, 227-234, 236-244
        cat bites in, 234
        dog bites in, 233-234
        fish bites in, 236
        management of, 232-233
        microbiology of, 228-229
        rabies and, 236-244
        rat bites in, 236
        risk factors for, 230-232
    definition of, 96
    human, 24, 227-228, 234-235
    microbiology of, 24, 228-229
    post-exposure prophylaxis in, 242-244
Biting species, 232
Blades
    #10, 75
    #11, 75
        paronychia drainage and, 207-208
    #15, 75
        closing dog ear with, 142
Blister, burn, 268
Block, nerve; *see* Nerve block
Blunt injuries of hand, 197-201
Buccal mucosal lacerations, 171-172
Bulb-type syringe, 62
Bupivacaine, 32, 33
    perineum and, 173
Burn dressings, 268-271
    application of, 269-270
Burns, 260-274
    acid, 272-273
    assessment of, 261-265
    body location of, 262
    chemical, 272-273
    cleansing of, 267
    depth of, 262-263
    epidermal, 267
    estimation of pediatric, 265
    extent of, 263-265
    follow-up and home management of, 271-272
    full-thickness, 272
    hospital admission and, 266
    hospital versus non-hospital guidelines for,
        266-267

Burns—cont'd
    management of, 260-261
        hospital versus non-hospital, 266-267
        minor, 267-273
        partial-thickness, 267-272
        patient assessment and, 260-261
Butyl-2-cyanoacrylate monomer, 78

C

Cactus spines, 252
Cannulas, airway, 35
Carbocaine; *see* Mepivacaine
Carbon monoxide exposure, 260-261
Cardiovascular reactions to local anesthetics,
        30-31
Cartilage injury
    ear, 167
    nose, 163
Cat bites, 232, 234
Cefadroxil, 315
Cefazolin, 93
Ceftriaxone, 234
Cefuroxime
    cat bites and, 234
    human bites and, 235
Cellular necrosis, 116
Cephalexin, 315
Cephalosporins
    cat bites and, 234
    ear lacerations and, 168
    hand injuries and, 212
    human bites and, 235
Cheek lacerations, 159-161
    closure of uncomplicated, 161
    mucosal, 171-172
    through-and-through, 161
Chemical burns, 272-273
Child
    with burns, 265
    Demerol for fearful, 35
    with lacerations, 2
Chlorhexidine, 56, 57
    chemical burns and, 272
    frostbite and, 273
Chromic gut suture, 76, 172
Cipro; *see* Ciprofloxacin
Ciprofloxacin, 93
    bite wounds and, 234
    hand injuries and, 212
    prophylactic, 315
    puncture wounds and, 254
Circulation of hand, 193-194
Cleanliness of wounds, 315-316
Cleansing, wound; *see* Wound cleansing and
        irrigation
Clearon, 214-215
Closure, 80-95
    of aged skin, 146-147
    of beveled edge laceration, 128-129

Closure—cont'd
of cheek lacerations, 161
of circular or irregular defect, 139-141
with completely non-viable flap, 135, 137
consultation guidelines for, 93-94
continuous, 97
over-and-over suture in, 123-128
of corner, 131-132, 133
debridement and, 88-92
deep, 97
abrasions and, 146
reducing wound tension and, 116
dermal
definition of, 97
pull-out, 130-131
of dog-ear deformities, 142, 143
drains and, 92
exploration and, 84-85
of eyebrow lacerations, 159
of flaps with non-viable edges, 135, 136
galeal, 152
of geographic wounds, 135-138
hemostasis and, 85-87
interrupted, 97
intravenous antibiotics and, 92-93
laceration exploration and, 84-85
of laceration in abrasion, 146
of lid lacerations, 158
of lips, 168
of medium-deep lacerations, 130
of parallel lacerations, 142, 144
percutaneous; *see* Percutaneous suture
closure
primary, secondary, and tertiary, 82
principles of, 110-121
dead space and, 120
layer matching in, 110
sequence and style in, 120-121
wound-edge eversion in, 110-115
wound tension and, 116-120
of scalp, 151-153
sequence of, 99-102, 120-121
skin, 97
style of, 120-121
of thin-edge, thick-edge wound, 145
timing of, 81-84
two-layered, 120
of wound with completely non-viable flap,
135, 137
Cocaine, 34
Codeine, 315
burns and, 271-272
Colchicine, 21
Collagen synthesis, 17-18
Comfort and safety, 1
Complicated lacerations and wounds, 122-147
abrasions and, 146
aged skin and, 146-147

Complicated lacerations and wounds—cont'd
beveled edges in, 128-129
corners and uncomplicated flaps in, 131-132,
133
dog-ear deformities and, 142, 143
flap and, 132-135
geographic lacerations in, 135-138
of lips, 169
long, straight lacerations in, 123-128
medium-deep lacerations in, 129-130
parallel lacerations in, 142, 144
pull-out dermal closure for, 130-131
thin-edge, thick-edge wound in, 142-145
tissue loss and, 139-141
Compression forces, 12, 13-14
Compression injuries, 15
Compression wrap over scalp dressing, 153
Connective tissue, loose, 151
Consultation guidelines, 93-94
Continuous closure, 97
over-and-over suture in, 123-128
Corners and uncomplicated flaps, 131-132, 133
Corticosteroids
collagen deposition and, 11
healing and, 3, 21
Cotton pledgets, 175
Crushing injuries to hand, 197-201
Curi-Strip, 214-215
Curved iris scissors, 73
Curved needle, cutting or tapered, 79
Curved tissue scissors, 73
Cutaneous layer, 6, 7; *see also* Skin
Cuticle, 196
Cuticular needle, 79
Cutting curved needle, 79

D

Dead space, 120
Debridement, 64, 88-92, 267-268
Debris, excision of, 88-89
Deep abrasions
of cheek, 161
closure in, 146
Deep closure
abrasions and, 146
definition of, 97
reducing wound tension and, 116
Deep fascia, 8
Deep-structure exploration, 86
Deep suture, 117
Delayed primary closure, 83-84
Demerol; *see* Meperidine
Dermal closure
abrasion and, 146
definition of, 97
pull-out, 130-131
Dermalon; *see* Monofilament suture
Dermis, 5, 6, 7
excision of damaged, 89-90

Dermis—cont'd
    initiating or scoring of, 90
    injection beneath, 36-37
    trimming of wound edge of, 89-90
Devitalized tissue, 88
Dexon Plus suture; *see* Polyglycolic acid suture
Dexon suture; *see* Polyglycolic acid suture
Diabetes, 20
Diazepam, 32
Dicloxacillin, 84
    cat bites and, 234
    dog bites and, 233
    ear lacerations and, 168
    hand injuries and, 212
    rat bites and, 236
Digit
    digital nerves of, 43
    dressings for, 290-299, 300, 302
    tourniquet application to, 87
Digital nerves
    anesthesia deposited in dorsal, 45
    block of, 42-46
        initiation of, 44
    illustration of, 43
    injury to, 186-187
Diphenhydramine, 32
Diphtheria, tetanus, and pertussis
    immunization, 310
Diphtheria toxoid, 310
    immunization schedule for, 311
Diphtheroids, 236
Direct wound infiltration, 36-37
Discharge; *see* Patient discharge and follow-up
    care
Dissection scissors, 66
Distal interphalangeal joint, 188
Dog bites, 233-234
    infection rate in, 232
Dog-ear deformities, 142, 143
Drainage, infection and, 317
Drains, surgical, 92
Dreft soap, 267
Dressings, 27, 275-308
    ankle, 302-308
    basic, 278-281
    burn, 268-271
    changes of, 316
    correct taping in, 282
    ear, 286-290
    elbow, 302, 303-304
    face, 286
    finger, 290-299, 300, 302
    follow-up intervals for, 316
    foot, 302-308
    groin, 290, 295
    hand, 212, 290-296, 297-299, 300, 301,
        302
    heel, 302-308
    hip, 290, 295

Dressings—cont'd
    knee, 302, 303-304
    mastoid, 286-290
    moist environment and, 276, 277
    neck, 290, 291
    non-adherent, porous base of, 287
    partial immobilization and, 277-278
    principles of, 275-278
    protection of, 277
    scalp, 281-285
    shoulder, 290, 292-294
    thigh, 290, 295
    tidiness of, 276
    for trunk, 290, 294
    for upper thigh, 290, 295
Drugs, 315
    anesthetic solutions as, 33
    hand injuries and, 180
    nerve block and; *see* Nerve block
DTP; *see* Diphtheria, tetanus, and pertussis
    immunization
Duoderm dressings, 258
Duricef; *see* Cefadroxil

E

Ear lacerations, 163-168
    aftercare and, 168
    of auricle, 41
    of cartilage, 167
    circumferential anesthesia around, 41
    dressings for, 286-290
    non-cartilaginous, 166
    perichondral hematoma and, 168
    preparation for repair of, 165-166
    uncomplicated, 166
Eikenella corrodens, 229, 235
Elastic wrap, 281
Elbow dressings, 302, 303-304
Elevation of wounds, 315-316
Ellipsing of flap, 135, 137, 139
Elmer's Glue-All, 252
Endotracheal tube sizes, 35
Enterobacter, 228
Epidermis, 5, 6, 7
    burns of, 261, 262, 267
    initiating or scoring of, 90
Epilock, 258
Epinephrine
    allergy and, 32
    contraindications to, 30, 85
    pharmacology of, 30
    scalp wounds and, 151
    with topical anesthesia, 34
Epithelialization, 17, 277
Eponychium, 196
Erysipelothrix, 236
Erythromycin, 84
    bite wounds and, 234, 235
    ear lacerations and, 168

Erythromycin—cont'd
  hand injuries and, 212
  lip lacerations and, 171
  puncture wounds and, 253-254
  rat bites and, 236
Ethilon suture; *see* Monofilament suture
Examination, physical, 3
Excision
  of damaged dermis, 89-90
  full wound, 90-92
  simple debris, 88-89
Exploration of laceration or wound, 84-85
Extensor tendon of hand
  anatomy, 190
  function of, 187-191
    testing for, 189
External ear, 165
Extremity, 174-175
  hemostasis and, 85, 87
Eye trauma, 157
Eyebrow lacerations, 156-159
Eyelid injury, 84, 156-159
Eyewear, protective, 59

F
Facial nerve, 159, 160
Facial trauma
  dressings for, 286
  fentanyl sedation and, 35
Fainting, 31
Fascia
  anatomy of, 5-8
  healing and, 134
  superficial, 5, 6-7
    fatty, 134
    inserting needle in, 37
    pull-out dermal closure and, 130
Felon, 210-211
Fentanyl, 35-36
Fibroblasts, 7
Fibrous septa, 197
Field block, 38-39
Figure-of-eight dressings, 302
Figure-of-eight suture technique, 206
Fine-pore sponges, 61
Finger; *see* Digit
Fingernail, 196
Fingertip
  anesthesia and, 43
  injuries of, 195-204
    avulsion, 203
First-degree burns, 261, 262
Fish bites, 236
Fishhooks, 254-256, 257
Flap laceration closure, 132-135
  of completely non-viable flaps, 135, 137
  corners and, 131-132, 133
  ellipsing in, 135, 137, 139
  of forehead, 155-156

Flap laceration closure—cont'd
  non-viable edges and, 135, 136
Flexor digitorum profundus tendon, 192
  testing for function of, 192
Flexor digitorum sublimis tendon, 47
Flexor digitorum superficialis tendon, 192
  testing for function of, 193
Flexor function of hand, 191-193
Flexor tendon laceration, 204
Foam dressings, 258
Follow-up care, 309-319
  analgesia and, 315
  for bite wounds, 236-242
  for burns, 271-272
  dressing change and, 316
  hand dressings and, 212
  instructions for, 315-317
  prophylactic antibiotics and, 314-315
  suture removal and, 311-314
  tetanus prophylaxis and, 309-311
  wound healing advice and, 317-318
  wound stapling and, 222, 225
  wound taping and, 220
Foot, 176
  dressings for, 302-308
  plantar surface of, 51
  puncture wound of, 309
Forceps, 69-72
  grasping tissue with, 71
  holding, 72
Forehead
  lacerations of, 154-156
    complex, 155-156
  nerve block for, 39-40
Foreign bodies, 84, 247-252
  non-inert, 248
  removal technique for, 248-252
Foreign material in wound, 60
Fractures, skull, 165
Free-running intravenous line, 35
Frontalis muscle, 152
Frostbite, 273
Full-thickness burns, 262, 263, 272
Full-thickness tissue loss, 139
Full wound excision, 90-92
Furacin, 275

G
Galea aponeurotica, 150, 152
Gauze
  petrolatum-impregnated, 258, 271
    burns and, 268
  tube, for finger bandage, 300
  Xeroform, 83, 276
    finger dressings and, 212
Gauze sponges, 277, 278
Gauze wrappings, 277, 278
  for finger, 212, 300
Gelfoam, 85

Gentamicin, 93
  Pseudomonas resistance and, 271
Geographic wound or laceration closure,
    135-138
Germinal matrix, 196
Gingival lacerations, 171-172
Glass as foreign body, 247-248
Gloves, protective, 59
Gram-negative organisms
  human bite infections and, 228-229
  povidone-iodine and, 57
Gram-positive organisms
  chlorhexidine and, 57
  hexachlorophene and, 58
  human bite infections and, 228-229
  paronychia and, 207
  povidone-iodine and, 57
Granulocytes, 16-17
Groin dressings, 290, 295
Gut suture, chromic, 76, 172

H

Hair removal, 59-60, 151
Half-buried horizontal mattress suture, 131,
    145
Hand, 177-213
  aftercare for, 212
  amputated parts of, 207
  anatomy of, 180, 181
    extensor tendon, 190
  antibiotics and, 211-212
  circulation of, 193-194
  dorsal surface of, 180
    dressing for, 301
  dressings for, 212, 290-296, 297-299, 300,
      301, 302
    palmar, 301
  examination of, 182-193
    nerve testing in, 182-187
    tendon function and, 187-193
  extensor function of, 187-191
  felon and, 210-211
  flexor function of, 191-193
  function components of, 188-189
  injuries of
    antibiotics for, 211-212
    blunt, 197-201
    burn, 262
    crushing, 197-201
    exploration of, 194-195
    fingertip, 195-204
    injection, 211
    nerve, 205-207
    pressure, 211
    tendon, 204-205
    uncomplicated, 195
  joints of, 180
  motor function of, 182-183, 184
  paronychia of, 207-210

Hand—cont'd
  patient history and, 178-180
  radiography of, 194
  ring removal and, 178, 179
  sensory function of, 183-187
  sensory innervation of, 186
  tendon function of, 187-193
  terminology and, 180
  treatment of, 177-178
  vascularity of, 194
Hand tie, 97, 103-109
Hand washing, 58-61
  chlorhexidine and, 57
  povidone-iodine and, 57
HDCV; *see* Human diploid cell vaccine
Healing of wounds; *see* Wound healing
Heated paper clip for nail injury, 197
Heel dressings, 302-308
Hematoma of ear, perichondral, 168
Hemolytic streptococci, 236; *see also*
    Streptococci
Hemostasis, 85-87
  hemorrhage control and, 151
  hemostat-clamped vessels for, 103-109
  initial, 1
Hemostat, 66, 74, 75, 118
  function of, 75
  for hemostasis, 103-109
  mosquito, 74
  standard, 74
  two-handed tie and, 103-109
  wound exploration and, 85
Heparin well arrangement, 35
Hexachlorophene, 56, 58
High-pressure irrigation, 232-233
Hip dressings, 290, 295
Histo acryl, 78
Home management of burns, 271-272
Hooks, skin, 66, 69-72
  hand exploration and, 194
Horizontal mattress suture, 115
  elderly skin and, 147
  half-buried, 131
  parallel lacerations and, 142
  for scalp wounds, 153
Horseshoe paronychia, 209
Hospital admission of burn victims, 266-267
Human bites, 227-228, 234-235
  infection and, 24
Human diploid cell vaccine, 242-244
Hydrocolloid dressings, 258
Hydrofluoric acid, 272-273
Hydrogen peroxide, 56, 58
Hydron gel, 271
Hypertension, 3
Hypertrophic scar, 21, 22, 23
Hyphema, 156-157
Hypotension, 3
Hypothenar eminence of hand, 180

I

Ibuprofen, 271-272
Immunization schedules, 310-311
  rabies and, 244
Index finger, 180
Infection
  potential for, 24-28
  signs of, 317
  topical control of, 63-64
Infiltration and nerve block anesthesia; *see*
    Nerve block
Inflammatory phase of wound healing, 16-17
Infraorbital nerve block, 39, 40
  for upper lip, 168
Inhalation injury, 260, 266-267
Injection, buffering to reduce pain of, 34-35
Injection injuries of hand, 211
Injury; *see also* specific site or type of injury
  immediate response to, 16
  mechanism of, 12-15
Instrument tie of standard suture closure,
    99-102
Instruments and suture materials, 66-79; *see*
    also Sutures
  absorbable suture materials and, 76-77
  forceps and, 69-72
  hemostats and, 74, 75
  knife blades and, 75-76
  knife handles and, 75-76
  needle holders and, 67-69
  needle types and, 78, 79
  non-absorbable suture materials and, 77
  scissors and, 73-75
  skin hooks and, 69-72
  wound adhesives and, 78
Interphalangeal joint, 188
Interrupted closure, 97
Intramuscular sedation, 35
Intravenous antibiotic therapy, 92-93
Intravenous line, 35
Introitus, vaginal, 173-174
Intubation blades, 35
Iodine in povidone-iodine; *see* Povidone-iodine
Iris scissors, 66
  curved, 73
Irregular defect closure, 139-141
Irrigation; *see* Wound cleansing and irrigation
Ischemia, 20
Ivory flakes, 267

J

Jewelry removal, 2
Joints of hand, 180

K

Keflex; *see* Cephalexin
Kefzol; *see* Cefazolin
Kelly clamp in removal of rings, 179

Keloid, 21, 22, 23
Knee, 174
  dressings for, 302, 303-304
Knife blades, 66, 75-76
Knife handles, 66, 75-76
  #3 standard Bard/Parker style, 75
Knot-tying techniques, 97-109
  square knot in, 102
  standard percutaneous suture closure in,
    99-102
  surgeon's knot in, 97, 102
  two-handed tie of hemostat-clamped vessels
    in, 97, 103-109

L

Labial lacerations, 173-174
Lacerations, 96-121; *see also* Basic principles
    and techniques; Wounds; specific
    anatomic site
  in abrasions, 146, 256-259
  avulsion
    fingertip, 203-204
    partial, 132-135
    scalp and, 152-153
    tissue loss and, 204
  child arriving with, 2
  closure of, 80-95; *see also* Closure
  complicated, 122-147
    abrasions and, 146, 256-259
    aged skin and, 146-147
    beveled edges in, 128-129
    corners and uncomplicated flaps in,
      131-132, 133
    dog-ear deformities and, 142, 143
    flaps and; *see* Flap laceration closure
    geographic lacerations in, 135-138
    lips and, 169
    long, straight lacerations in, 123-128
    medium-deep, 129-130
    parallel lacerations in, 142, 144
    pull-out dermal closure for, 130-131
    thin-edge, thick-edge wound in, 142-145
    tissue loss and, 139-141
    exploration of, 84-85
  flap; *see* Flap laceration closure
  follow-up care of, 309-311
  infiltration and nerve block anesthesia of,
    29-54; *see also* Nerve block
  irregular in both configuration and depth,
    135-138
  long, straight, 123-128
  medium-deep, 129-130
  patient arrival and, 1-4
  patient discharge and, 309-311
Layer matching, 110
Leg, lower, 174-175
  hemostasis and, 85, 87
Leukocyte phagocytic activity, 26
Levator palpebrae muscle, 156

Lid laceration closure, 84, 156-159
   extramarginal, 158
   intramarginal, 158
Lidocaine, 32, 33
   buccal mucosa and, 40
   digital block and, 43
   perineum and, 173
   scalp wounds and, 151
Lip lacerations, 84, 168-171
   upper, 40
Lithium, 272
Little finger, 180
Local anesthetics
   excitatory central nervous system effects of,
      30-31
   hand injuries and, 180
Long, straight lacerations, 123-128
Loose connective tissue, 151
Lower extremity, 174-175
   hemostasis and, 85, 87
Lymphocytes, 17

M
Macrophages, 17
Mandibular bicuspid, 41
Marcaine; *see* Bupivacaine
Mastoid dressings, 286-290
Mastoid retractor, 85
Matrix of fingernail, 196
Mattress suture
   horizontal, 115
      elderly skin and, 147
      half-buried, 131
      parallel lacerations and, 142
      scalp wounds and, 153
   vertical, 112, 114, 130
Maxono; *see* Polyglyconate
Mechanism of injury, 12-15
Medial palpebral ligament laceration, 156
Median nerve, 47, 186
   block of, 46-47
      level and position of injection in, 48
   of hand, 182
   testing for function of, 182, 184
Medications, 315
   anesthetic solutions as, 33
   hand injuries and, 180
   nerve block; *see* Nerve block
Medium-deep lacerations, 129-130
Membrane dressings, 258
Mental nerve block, 39, 41, 168
Mental nerve foramen, 41
Meperidine, 35
Mepivacaine, 32, 33
   digital block and, 43
Metacarpophalangeal joint, 188
Metal as foreign body, 247
Methylparaben, 32
Metzenbaum dissection scissors, 73, 118

Microbiology of wound infection, 25; *see also*
      Bacteria; Gram-positive organisms
Middle finger, 180
Minor burns; *see* Burns
Monofilament suture, 77
   4-0
      lower leg laceration and, 174
      scalp lacerations and, 152
   5-0, 152
   6-0
      cheek and, 161
      forehead and, 154
   non-absorbable; *see* Non-absorbable
      monofilament suture
Mosquito hemostat, 74
   hand exploration and, 194
Motor function of hand, 182-183, 184
Mucosal injection site, 41
Mucosal wounds
   of cheek, 171-172
   of nose, 163
Multiple small flaps of forehead, 155-156
Myelin sheath, 30

N
Nail, 196
   removal of, 201-202
Nail-bed injury, 196, 202
   with subungual hematoma, 199
Nail plate, 196
Nail root, 196
   avulsion of, 200
Nasal pack, 163
Nasal structures, 162-163
Neck dressings, 290, 291
Needle holders, 66, 67-69
Needle-nose pliers, 254
Needles, 78, 79
   16- or 18-gauge, 255, 256
   30-gauge, 36
   configurations of, 78
   curved, 78, 79
   cuticular, 79
   fishhook removal with, 255, 256
   nerve block and, 36
   plastic, 79
   reverse cutting, 78
   tapered, 78, 79
Neosporin, 275, 278
   burns and, 268
   cheek lacerations and, 161
   facial lacerations and, 286
   forehead injuries and, 156
   genital area and, 174
   tar dissolution with, 258
Neovascularization, 17
Nerve block, 29-54
   allergy and, 32
   auricular, 41-42

Nerve block—cont'd
  buffering to reduce pain of, 34-35
  digital, 42-46
  direct wound infiltration in, 36-37
  field, 38-39
  finger, 42-46
  forehead, 39-40
  infraorbital, 40
  median, 46-47
  mental nerve, 41
  needles and, 36
  parallel margin infiltration in, 38-39
  pharmacology and, 30
  radial, 49
  sedation and, 35-36
  solutions for, 33
  supraorbital, 39-40
  supratrochlear, 39-40
  sural, 49-53
  syringes for, 36
  techniques of, 36-53
  tibial, 49-53
  toe, 42-46
  topical, 34
  toxicity of, 30-32
  ulnar, 47-49
Nerve function of hand, 182
  injuries and, 205-207
  testing for, 182-187
Nichi-Strip, 214-215
Non-absorbable monofilament suture
  4-0, extensor tendon and, 205
  5-0
    eyebrow laceration and, 159
    hand injuries and, 195
  6-0
    ear lacerations and, 166
    eyebrow laceration and, 159
    lid laceration and, 158
    nose lacerations and, 163
Non-absorbable suture materials, 77
Non-adherent base, 278
Non-viable edges of flap, closure of, 135, 136, 137
Nonsteroidal anti-inflammatory agents, 21
Norepinephrine, 157
Nose lacerations, 162-163
Novafil; see Polybutester
Nylon suture, 77
  extensor tendon and, 205
  labia majora and, 174

O

O-silk suture
  fishhook removal with, 254-255
O-silk suture
  ring removal with, 178, 179
Oral cavity, 161, 171-173

Over-and-over suture, 123-128
Oxycodone, 315

P

Packing, nasal, 163
Pain
  buffering of nerve block to reduce, 34-35
  relief of, 2; see also Pain medications
Pain medications, 315
  hand injuries and, 180
Palmar surface of hand, 180
  dressings on, 301
  nerves of, 42, 49
Palmaris longus tendon, 47
Palpebral ligament laceration, 156
Paper clip
  foreign body removal and, 248-250
  heated, nail injury and, 197
Papillary dermis, 7
Parallel lacerations, 142, 144
Parallel margin infiltration, 38-39
Paronychia, 207-210
Parotid gland, 159, 160
Partial avulsion lacerations, 132-135
Partial-thickness burns, 262, 263, 267-272
  superficial, 261
Partial-thickness tissue loss, 139
Pasteurella multocida, 228, 234
Patient arrival, 1-4
Patient discharge and follow-up care, 309-319
  analgesia and, 315
  instructions for, 315-317
  prophylactic antibiotics and, 314-315
  suture removal and, 311-314
  tetanus prophylaxis and, 309-311
  wound healing advice and, 317-318
PDS; see Polydioxanone
Penicillamine, 21
Penicillin
  cat bites and, 234
  cheek lacerations and, 161
  dog bites and, 233
  felon and, 210
  fish bites and, 236
  human bites and, 235
  lip lacerations and, 171
  Staphylococcus aureus resistance and, 210
Penis, lacerations of, 173
Percutaneous suture closure, 99-102
  definition of, 97
  removal of sutures and, 312
  scalp shearing lacerations and, 152
Perichondral hematoma of ear, 168
Pericranium, injury of, 151
Perineum, 173-174
Periosteum, injury of, 151
Petrolatum-impregnated gauze, 271
  burns and, 268
PGA suture; see Polyglycolic acid suture

Phagocytic activity, 26
Pharmadine, 275
Phenergan, 35
Phenol burns, 272
Phenylbutazone, 21
Physical examination, 3
Pinprick stimulus for hand, 183, 185
Plantar surface of foot, 51
Plastic needle, 79
Polaxamer 188, 56, 57-58
    eyelid and, 157-158
    polyglycolic acid suture coated with, 76
Polybutester, 77, 130
Polydioxanone, 76-77
Polyglycolic acid suture, 76
    nasal mucosa laceration and, 163
    through-and-through lip laceration and, 170
Polyoxyethylene sorbitan, 258
Polypropylene suture, 77
    extensor tendon and, 205
    labia majora and, 174
    pull-out dermal stitch and, 130
Polysporin ointment, 278
    dissolving tar with, 258
Posterior tibial nerve block, 53
Povidone-iodine, 55-57
    bite wounds and, 232
    chemical burns and, 272
    eyelid and, 157-158
    nose cleansing and, 162
Precise Ten Shot stapler, 221
Preoperative skin preparation, 57; *see also*
    Povidone-iodine
Pressure injection injuries of hand, 211
Primary closure, 81, 82
    delayed, 83-84
    foot lacerations and, 176
Primary intention healing, 81
Principles and techniques, 96-121
    definition of terms in, 96-97
    knot tying and, 97-109; *see also* Knot-tying
        techniques
    wound closure and, 110-121; *see also* Closure
Procaine, 32
Prolene suture; *see* Polypropylene suture
Promethazine, 35
Prophylactic antibiotics, 314-315
    burns and, 273
    for dog-bite wounds, 233
Prophylaxis
    antibiotic; *see* Prophylactic antibiotics
    rabies exposure and, 236-244
    tetanus, 273, 309-311
Protection of wounds, 315-316
Protective eyewear, 59
Protective gloves, 59
Proximal interphalangeal joint, 188
Pseudomonas aeruginosa, 252
Pull-out dermal closure, 130-131

Puncture wounds, 252-254
    of hand, 178-179
Push-through technique for removing fishhooks,
    256, 257

Q
Quarantining of wild animal, 239, 242

R
Rabies exposure and prophylaxis, 236-242
    current recommendations for, 242-244
    decision steps for, 237-238
    geographic location of bite and, 239, 240-241
    immune globulin and, 244
    severity of bite and, 239
    status of attacking animal and, 239-242
Rabies immune globulin, 242-244
Radial nerve, 182, 185-186
    block of, 49, 50
Radiographs
    forehead, 154
    foreign objects and, 60, 248
    hand, 194
Ragged-edge lacerations of forehead, 156
Rat bites, 236
Reflex One stapling device, 221
Reticular dermis, 7
Retractors, 85
Reverse cutting needle, 78
Rigid splinting, 277
Ring finger, 180
Ring removal, 178, 179
Road tar in abrasions, 258
Rule of nines for burns, 263, 264

S
Safety, 1
Saline
    high-pressure streams of, 62
    nose irrigation and, 162
Scalding burns, 261-262
Scalp lacerations, 84, 149-153
    anatomy and, 150
    anesthesia for, 151
    closure of, 151-153
    compression, with irregular margins, 152
    dressings for, 281-285
Scar, 317-318
    abnormal, 21-23
Scissors, 73-75
    iris, 66, 73
Scoring of dermis or epidermis, 90
Screening physical examination, 3
Scrotum, lacerations of, 173
Scrubbing of wound, 61-62
Second-degree burns, 261, 262, 263
Secondary closure, 81, 82
Secondary intention healing, 81
Sedation, 35-36; *see also* Medications

Sensory function of hand, 183-187
  testing for, 185
Sensory innervation
  of auricle, 41
  of hand, 186
Septa, fibrous, 197
Septal hematoma, 162
  over septal cartilage, 163
  technique for draining, 164
Shearing injuries, 12, 13-14
  fingertip and, 202-203
Shoulder dressings, 290, 292-294
Shur Clens; *see* Polaxamer 188
Silk suture
  fishhook removal with, 254-255
  ring removal with, 178, 179
Silvadene, 275, 278
Simple debris excision, 88-89
Skin
  aged, 146-147
  anatomy of, 5-8
    alterations in, 11
Skin cleansing; *see* Wound cleansing and
    irrigation
Skin closure, 97; *see also* Closure
Skin hooks, 66, 69-72
  hand exploration and, 194
Skin lacerations; *see* Lacerations
Skin layer, 6, 7
Skin tension lines, 8-10
  forehead and, 154
Skull fracture, 165
Sodium, chemical burns and, 272
Sodium bicarbonate buffer, 34
Sodium hydroxide, 272
Sphygmomanometer, 87
Splinter removal, 251
Splinting
  foot lacerations and, 176
  rigid, 277
Sponges
  fine-pore, 61
  gauze, 277, 278
Square knot, 102
Staphylococcus aureus
  cat bites and, 228
  dog bites and, 228
  non-animal bite wounds and, 25
  paronychia and, 207
  prophylactic antibiotics and, 315
  puncture wounds and, 252
Staphylococcus epidermidis, 25
  dog bites and, 228
  rat bites and, 236
Stapling, 81, 214, 220-226
  aftercare of, 222, 225
  devices for, 221
  indications for, 220-221
  removing staples and, 225

Stapling—cont'd
  scalp lacerations and, 152
  technique for, 221-225
Steri-Strips, 214-215
Sterile matrix of nail bed, 196
Steroids, anabolic, 21; *see also* Corticosteroids
Straight lacerations, 123-128
Stratum corneum, 7
Stratum germinativum, 7
Streptococci, 25; *see also Streptococcus
    pyogenes*
  cat bites and, 228
  rat bites and, 236
Streptococcus pyogenes
  felon and, 210
  paronychia and, 207
  puncture wounds and, 252
Subcutaneous layer, 6-7
Sublimaze, 35
Subungual hematoma, 197
Sulfuric acid, 272
Superficial fascia, 5, 6-7
  fatty, 134
  inserting needle in, 37
  pull-out dermal closure and, 130
Superficial partial-thickness burns, 261
Supraorbital nerve block, 39-40
Supratrochlear nerve block, 39-40
Sural nerve block, 49-53
Surgeon's knot, 97, 102
Surgical drains, 92
Suture scissors, 66, 73, 314
Suture-Strip, 214-215
Sutures, 76-78, 81; *see also* Instruments and
    suture materials
  absorbable, 20, 76-77
    scalp shearing lacerations and, 152
  chromic gut, 76, 172
  continuous over-and-over, 123-128
  deep, 117
  guidelines for, 149
  for human bites, 234-235
  instrument tie of standard percutaneous,
    99-102
  mattress
    horizontal; *see* Horizontal mattress suture
    vertical, 112, 114, 130
  monofilament; *see* Monofilament suture
  non-absorbable; *see* Non-absorbable
    monofilament suture
  polyglycolic acid, 76
    nasal mucosa laceration and, 163
    through-and-through lip laceration and,
      170
  polypropylene, 77
    extensor tendon and, 205
    labia majora and, 174
    pull-out dermal stitch and, 130
  removal of, 311-314

Sutures—cont'd
  silk
    fishhook removal with, 254-255
    ring removal with, 178, 179
  wound infection and, 26
Syncope, 30-31
Syringes
  35-cc, 63
  bulb-type, 62
  nerve block and, 36

T

TAC; *see* Tetracaine with epinephrine and
      cocaine
Tapered curved needle, 79
Taping, 81, 214-220, 226
  aftercare of, 220
  elderly skin and, 147
  indications for, 215
  technique for, 215-220
Tar in abrasions, 258
Tear duct injury, 156
TEC; *see* Tetracaine with epinephrine and
      cocaine
Techniques, basic, 96-121
  definition of terms in, 96-97
  knot tying and, 97-109; *see also* Knot-tying
      techniques
  wound closure and, 110-121; *see also* Closure
Teeth, trauma to, 171
Tegaderm, 258, 271
Telfa, 258, 276
Tendons of hand
  function of, 187-193
  lacerations of, 84, 204-205
Tension, reduction of wound, 116-120
Tension forces in injury, 12, 13-14
Tension lines of skin, 8-10
Tertiary closure, 82, 83-84
Tetanus immune globulin, 273, 311
Tetanus prophylaxis, 273, 309-311
  hand injury and, 180
Tetanus toxoid, 273, 310
  complications of, 311
  hand injuries and, 180
  immunization schedule for, 311
Tetracaine, 32, 34
  with epinephrine and cocaine, 34
Tetracycline, 235
Thenar eminence of hand, 180
Thick-edge wound, 142-145
Thigh dressings, 290, 295
Thin-edge wound, 142-145
Third-degree burns, 262, 263
Through-and-through lacerations
  of cheek, 161
  of lip, 169
Throw, 97
Thumb, 180, 188, 189
Tibial nerve block, 49-53

Tie
  of hemostat-clamped vessels, 103-109
  of standard percutaneous suture closure,
      99-102
TIG; *see* Tetanus immune globulin
Timing decisions for closure; *see* Closure
Tincture of benzoin, 281
Tissue adhesives, 78
Tissue debridement, 88-92
Tissue defects of forehead, 156
Tissue forceps, 66
Tissue grasping instrument, 70
Tissue handling, infection and, 26
Tissue loss in wounds, 139-141
  of finger, 203-204
Tissue scissors, 66
  curved, 73
Tissue undermining, 118
Toe block, 42-46
  midline dorsal needlestick in, 43, 44
Tongue lacerations, 172-173
Topical infection control, 63-64
Topical nerve block, 34
Tourniquet application, 87
  digital, 87
  large-extremity, 87
Triangle flap conversion to ellipse, 137, 139
Truncal dressings, 290, 294
Tube gauze finger bandage, 300
Two-handed tie of hemostat-clamped vessels, ˙
      103-109
Two-layered closure, 120
Two-point discrimination, 185, 187

U

Ulnar nerve, 49, 182, 186
  block of, 47-49, 48
  dorsal branch of, 49
  testing for function of, 182, 183
Umbilical tape
  fishhook removal with, 254-255
  ring removal with, 178, 179
Upper lip lacerations, 40
Upper thigh dressings, 290, 295
Uremia, 20

V

V-closure, 135, 136
Vaccine schedules, 310-311
  rabies and, 244
Vaginal introitus lacerations, 173-174
Valium, 32
Vascularity of hand, 194
Vaseline gauze, 258, 268, 271
Vasoconstrictors with local anesthetics, 26
Vasovagal syncope, 30-31
Venous access, 35
Vertical mattress suture, 112, 114
  medium-deep lacerations and, 130

Vessel formation, 17
Vigilon wound coverings, 271
Vital signs, 3
Vitamin A, 21
Vitamin C, 21
Volar digital nerves, blocked, 43
Volar surface
  of hand, 180
  of wrist, 191

W

Webster needle holder, 67
Wheatlander retractor, 85
Windshield injury, 155-156
Wound adhesives, 78
Wound care; *see also* Wound cleansing and
    irrigation
  delay in, 2
  hand washing and, 58
  of lacerations; *see* Lacerations
Wound cleansing and irrigation, 55-65
  anesthesia and, 60
  bite wounds and, 232-233
  burns and, 267
    chemical, 272
  follow-up care and, 316-317
  foreign material and, 250
  material for, 61
  periphery scrubbing in, 61-62
  povidone-iodine and, 57
  preparation for, 58-61
  solutions for, 55-58
    improper use of, 26
  techniques for, 61-64
Wound closure; *see* Closure
Wound dressings; *see* Dressings
Wound edges, 91
  eversion of, 110-115
Wound healing, 5-11, 21-23
  advising patient about, 317-318
  alterations in, 19-21
  categories of, 19
  components of, 16
  drugs and, 21
  fascia and, 5-8
  normal, 15-19
  skin and, 5-8
    alterations of, 11
  skin tension lines and, 8-10
Wound infection; *see* Infection
Wound irrigation; *see* Wound cleansing and
    irrigation
Wound stapling; *see* Stapling
Wound taping; *see* Taping
Wound tension, 116-120
  technique for reducing, 119

Wounds; *see also* Lacerations; specific anatomic
    site
  aftercare and cleanliness of, 315-316
  bandaging of; *see* Dressings
  bite; *see* Bite wounds
  characteristics of, 25-26
  closure of, 80-95; *see also* Closure
  complicated, 122-147; *see also* Complicated
      lacerations and wounds
  contraction of, 18-19
  elevation of, 315-316
  epithelial cell covering of, 277
  exploration of, 84-85
    hand and, 194-195
  fishhook, 254-256, 257
  foreign bodies and, 247-252
  full excision of, 90-92, 91
  hair removal and, 59-60
  immersion of, 60-61
  infection potential of, 24-28
  infiltration and nerve block anesthesia of,
      29-54; *see also* Nerve block
  injury mechanism and, 12-15
  instruments for, 66-79; *see also* Instruments
      and suture materials
  minor burns and, 260-274; *see also* Burns
  patient arrival and, 1-4
  prophylactic antibiotics for, 314-315
  protection of, 315-316
  puncture; *see* Puncture wounds
  soaking of, 60-61
  suture materials for, 66-79; *see also*
      Sutures
  thick-edge or thin-edge, 142-145
  with tissue loss, 139-141
  undermining of, 116
Wrist, 188
  anatomy of, 47, 49, 191
  dorsal-radial aspect of, 49
  volar surface of, 191
Written instructions, 317

X

Xeroform gauze, 83, 276
  finger and, 212
Xeroradiography; *see* Radiographs
Xylocaine; *see* Lidocaine

Y

Y-closure, 135, 136

Z

Zinc deficiency, 21
Zinc sulfate, 21
Zygomatic area, 159-161